M. S. Premila, PhD

Ayurvedic Herbs
A Clinical Guide
to the Healing Plants
of Traditional Indian Medicine

Pre-publication
REVIEWS,
COMMENTARIES,
EVALUATIONS . . .

"**M**.S. Premila has prepared a book that will be useful to all serious students of Ayurveda and herbalism. The text is rich in scientific references, important to modern practitioners of medicine. After providing an overview of the history of plant usage and research in Ayurveda, the author delves deeply into research supporting the use of herbs for each system of body. While doing so, she discusses the herbal treatment of many important diseases commonly seen in an Ayurvedic practice.

This book adds to the list of important textbooks that belong on the shelves of Ayurvedic and herbal practitioners. While Ayurveda has been practiced for thousands of years in India with great success, its emergence in the Western world requires a scientific basis for understanding the use of traditional medicine. This book is an important bridge between East and West as well as past and present and contributes in an important way to the future of Ayurveda.

May all who read this book gain deeper insight into the use of herbs for alleviating the suffering of humanity."

Dr. Marc Halpern
President, California College of Ayurveda;
Co-founder, National Ayurvedic Medical Association;
Co-founder, California Association of Ayurvedic Medicine

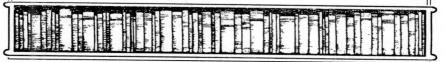

More pre-publication
REVIEWS, COMMENTARIES, EVALUATIONS . . .

"This is a wonderful work on Ayurvedic herbs. . . . Ayurvedic herbology—known as Dravyaguna in Sanskrit—is an integral part of the Ayurvedic approach to well-being. Traditional books written by great scholars have always given details regarding each herb based on the Ayurvedic principles of Rasa, Virya, Vipaka, and Prabhava. However, these books lack researched-based critical validation and efficacy on these herbs. The present work by Dr. Premila has very effectively filled the gap. . . . I am sure this will prove a great resource for all Ayurvedic physicians as well as Western herbalists. I feel no hesitation in recommending this book to all who are interested in using Ayurvedic herbs with more confidence in their practices."

Dr. S. Ajit, BAMS
Consultant Ayurvedic doctor;
Director, Planet Ayurveda

The Haworth Press, Inc.
New York • London • Oxford

Ayurvedic Herbs
A Clinical Guide
to the Healing Plants
of Traditional Indian Medicine

THE HAWORTH PRESS®
Titles of Related Interest

Concise Handbook of Psychoactive Herbs: Medicinal Herbs for Treating Psychological and Neurological Problems by Marcello Spinella

Herbal Medicine: Chaos in the Marketplace by Rowena K. Richter

Botanical Medicines: The Desk Reference for Major Herbal Supplements, Second Edition by Dennis J. McKenna, Kenneth Jones, and Kerry Hughes

Tyler's Tips: The Shopper's Guide for Herbal Remedies by George H. Constantine

Handbook of Psychotropic Herbs: A Scientific Analysis of Herbal Remedies for Psychiatric Conditions by Ethan B. Russo

Understanding Alternative Medicine: New Health Paths in America by Lawrence Tyler

Seasoning Savvy: How to Cook with Herbs, Spices, and Other Flavorings by Alice Arndt

Tyler's Honest Herbal: A Sensible Guide to the Use of Herbs and Related Remedies, Fourth Edition by Steven Foster and Varro E. Tyler

Tyler's Herbs of Choice: The Therapeutic Use of Phytomedicinals, Second Edition by James E. Robbers and Varro E. Tyler

Medicinal Herbs: A Compendium by Beatrice Gehrmann, Wolf-Gerald Koch, Claus O. Tschirch, and Helmut Brinkmann

Understanding Medicinal Plants: Their Chemistry and Therapeutic Action by Bryan Hanson

Anadenanthera: *Visionary Plant of Ancient South America* by Constantino Manuel Torres and David B. Repke

Ayurvedic Herbs
A Clinical Guide
to the Healing Plants
of Traditional Indian Medicine

M. S. Premila, PhD

The Haworth Press, Inc.
New York • London • Oxford

For more information on this book or to order, visit
http://www.haworthpress.com/store/product.asp?sku=5683

or call 1-800-HAWORTH (800-429-6784) in the United States and Canada
or (607) 722-5857 outside the United States and Canada

or contact orders@HaworthPress.com

Published by

The Haworth Press, Inc., 10 Alice Street, Binghamton, NY 13904-1580.

PUBLISHER'S NOTES
The development, preparation, and publication of this work has been undertaken with great care. However, the Publisher, author, employees, editors, and agents of The Haworth Press are not responsible for any errors contained herein or for consequences that may ensue from use of materials or information contained in this work. The Haworth Press is committed to the dissemination of ideas and information according to the highest standards of intellectual freedom and the free exchange of ideas. Statements made and opinions expressed in this publication do not necessarily reflect the views of the Publisher, Directors, management, or staff of The Haworth Press, Inc., or an endorsement by them.

This book has been published solely for educational purposes and is not intended to substitute for the medical advice of a treating physician. Medicine is an ever-changing science. As new research and clinical experience broaden our knowledge, changes in treatment may be required. While many potential treatment options are made herein, some or all of the options may not be applicable to a particular individual. Therefore, the author, editor, and publisher do not accept responsibility in the event of negative consequences incurred as a result of the information presented in this book. We do not claim that this information is necessarily accurate by the rigid scientific and regulatory standards applied for medical treatment. No warranty, expressed or implied, is furnished with respect to the material contained in this book. The reader is urged to consult with his/her personal physician with respect to the treatment of any medical condition.

Plant illustrations by M. S. Premila, © 2006.

Cover design by Marylouise E. Doyle.

Library of Congress Cataloging-in-Publication Data

Premila, M. S.
    Ayurvedic herbs : a clinical guide to the healing plants of traditional Indian medicine / M.S. Premila.
        p. cm.
    Includes bibliographical references and index.
    ISBN-13: 978-0-7890-1767-3 (hc. : alk. paper)
    ISBN-10: 0-7890-1767-9 (hc. : alk. paper)
    ISBN-13: 978-0-7890-1768-0 (pbk. : alk. paper)
    ISBN-10: 0-7890-1768-7 (pbk. : alk. paper)
    1. Herbs—Therapeutic use. 2. Medicine, Ayurvedic. 3. Materia medica, Vegetable. I. Title.
[DNLM: 1. Plants, Medicinal. 2. Phytotherapy. 3. Plant Preparations—therapeutic use. 4. Medicine, Ayurvedic. QV 770 J14
    P925a 2006]
    RM666.H33P737 2006
    615'.321—dc22
                                                                    2005034847

For my mother,
Lakshmi Sivaraman

And in memory of my father,
M. S. Sivaraman

ABOUT THE AUTHOR

M. S. Premila, PhD, retired as Chief Manager of Herbal Drugs at SPIC Pharmaceuticals Division, R&D Centre, in Maraimalai Nagar, India, with more than 30 years of experience in natural products. At SPIC, she was responsible for the development of scientifically validated herbal products based on Ayurveda. She previously worked as a Postdoctoral Fellow in the Pharmaceutical Institute of Tohuku University in Japan, was a Swiss National Science Foundation Fellow at the Institute of Organic Chemistry of the University of Zurich in Switzerland, and was a Research Scientist in Amrutanjan Ltd, Chennai. Dr. Premila has published several scientific papers and a book chapter on isoquinolines. She is a Fellow of the Society of Ethnobotanists and a member of the International Society for Ethnopharmacology, the Society for Medicinal Plant Research, and the Cucurbit Network.

© 2006 by The Haworth Press, Inc. All rights reserved.
doi:10.1300/5683_a

CONTENTS

Foreword

In the traditional medical system of India, the herbal drugs of Ayurvedic medicine form an important mainstay in therapy. Books of Ayurvedic medicine that date even from ancient times describe primarily historical aspects, the principles of Ayurveda, and the most common plants used for the prevention and therapy of diseases. The present text by Dr. M. S. Premila thus represents enormous progress, as it offers the first critical validation of traditional Ayurvedic medicine, which includes both clinically proven formulas and medicines that urgently require further research efforts. Each of the 12 chapters, dealing with the most prominent herbal drugs, enumerates the active chemical constituents, the relevant pharmacological and clinical data, and safety information, all extensively referenced. This first approach aims at what in Western terms is called evidence-based medicine. The documentation is a valuable guide for physicians and even Western-trained clinicians who are attentive to alternative and adjunctive therapies. It is a pleasure for me to recommend this book, without reservation, to all scientists in the field of phytomedicine. I wish the book much success and broad distribution beyond India.

H. Wagner, PhD
Professor Emeritus
Centre of Pharma Research
Institute of Pharmaceutical Biology
University of Munich
Munich, Germany

doi:10.1300/5683_b

Preface

Worldwide interest in Ayurveda is rapidly growing, especially in the United States, Europe, and Japan. Ayurveda, the major traditional system in India, is not just about herbs but is an entire system or a way of living aimed at achieving a state of total mental, physical, and spiritual well-being through lifestyle, diet, and drugs derived from herbs. Having worked on developing standardized and validated herbal products based on Ayurveda for around two decades, it never fails to amaze me how often Ayurvedic concepts and precepts receive scientific support. Therefore, when Professor Varro Tyler suggested a book on clinical data on Ayurvedic herbs, I was very happy to accede to his request. His suggestion was to put together the scattered information available on Western-style clinical trials on Ayurvedic herbs with descriptions, comments, and references, since there was a need for such a book owing to lack of information and limited access to these aspects.

This book attempts to bridge the knowledge gap and gather the scattered information on Ayurvedic herbs to see what scientific support there is for the traditional use of these plants. In doing so, I am aware of the fact that Ayurveda considers disease as an imbalance in *doshas,* or humors, and that healing is brought about by bringing back harmony to the "deranged" *doshas.* However, Ayurvedic herbs have also been classified according to their pharmacological action or indication. For many Ayurvedic disease entities and their symptoms described in Ayurveda, there are modern equivalent medicines; thus, there are a number of Western-style clinical studies conducted on single Ayurvedic herbs.

It has also long been my desire to be able to pull all the relevant information into a cohesive whole. The herbs have been dealt with according to body systems and indications in order to provide an easier overview.

Thus, after the two introductory chapters, which highlight the relevance of the background of Ayurveda, the herbs are covered in 12 chapters. Each chapter on herbs gives a short introduction of the Ayurvedic viewpoint, where relevant, after which the important plant monographs follow. Each plant monograph covers synonyms: names in Sanskrit, English, Hindi, and Tamil. The names are followed by a short introduction, a description of the plant and its distribution in India, traditional use, the part used as a drug, chemical constituents, pharmacology, clinical studies, and safety information.

Some herbs have names only in a particular language depending on the region where they grow predominantly. *Salacia* species, for example, have local names in Malayalam, the language used in Kerala, which are descriptive of the different species. Thus, *Salacia macrosperma,* with its sprawling habit, is called *anakoranti (ana:* "elephant"). *Salacia oblonga* and *S. reticulata* are called *ponkoranti (pon:* "gold") in reference to the yellow color of the root bark. *Salacia prinoides* is called *cherukoranti (cheru:* "small"). In cases where a plant occurrence is more regional, preference is given to the local name.

At this point, it should be mentioned that large variation exists in the way local names are spelled in English, and the spelling given by an author is often retained. This happens less often with botanical names.

The description of traditional use covers the major uses; similarly, the description of the plant covers details of what is important for its use.

The chemical constituents refer to active principles, where known, or to chemical classes or compounds that on the basis of current knowledge can be considered to contribute to the activity.

Some of the plants have more than one use. Thus, the same plant may occur in more than one chapter and in more than one section of a chapter. For example, ginger *(Zingiber officinale)* is used as an antiemetic and to treat malabsorption and finds place in two sections in Chapter 3, "Gastrointestinal agents." Ginger also finds place in Chapter 8, "Antirheumatic agents," for its anti-inflammatory effect. Turmeric *(Curcuma longa)* is a common ingredient of curry and is used for digestion (Chapter 3). In addition, it is used in the treatment of arthritis (Chapter 8), for asthma (Chapter 5, "Respiratory tract drugs") and oral cancer (Chapter 13, "*Rasayana* drugs").

Each portion on pharmacology deals only with studies that are relevant to the indication covered. Other known pharmacological studies for different uses not relevant to the particular indication are not cited. Only uses supported by clinical studies have been included. Thus, turmeric or curcumin is mentioned in discussions of the gastrointestinal tract, antirheumatic agents, asthma drugs, and anticancer drugs because some supporting clinical data are available. Similarly, *Commiphora mukul,* or *guggul*, finds a place in the discussions of hypolipidemic agents and antirheumatic agents, but not under agents used for thyroid stimulation even though experimental evidence is available.

In reporting clinical trials, the Ayurvedic indication and the modern medicine correlate as given by the authors have been included. For example, the condition known as *amlapitta* in Ayurveda is characterized by such symptoms as nausea, tiredness, sour vomiting, burning in the throat, thirst, vertigo, and hyperchlorhydria. *Amlapitta* has been variously described as acid dyspepsia, nonulcer dyspepsia, and gastritis syndrome. Some of the trials reported have certain basic data missing, such as the botanical name of the drug or the doses administered. As these trials correspond to traditional uses with supporting pharmacology, they could serve as indicators for further trials and have therefore been included. In some cases, specifications for the drug used should be urgently established so that it is possible to have reproducible results. This is especially true in the case of plants that have different eco- and chemotypes, for example, *Acorus calamus* and *Phyllanthus amarus.*

In addition, there have been problems in trying to group plants for a particular indication, as some of the trials are of an exploratory nature and cover several indications such as bronchial asthma, allergic rhinitis, or viral encephalitis. These have been grouped together under the same heading because, during the trial, the plant preparation would have been tried simultaneously for other indications as well, and presently, it would fragment information if grouped separately, since available information is scarce. Therefore, plants for peptic ulcer, nonulcer dyspepsia, and gastritis are grouped under antiulcer plants.

Safety information has been summarized under each monograph. Most of the plants have not been investigated adequately by modern standards of safety. Nonetheless, the herbs have been in use for a very long time and any toxicity should have become evident by now. In addition, Ayurveda prescribes the manner in which herbs are to be used or processed before use. For example, if *Commiphora mukul* resin is not processed using *triphala,* or an equivalent method, side effects are seen. In addition, the age of the resin influences its efficacy, as mentioned in the *Sushruta Samhita.*

In order to help locate the different plants and their indications for which information is available, an appendix has been added at the back of the book. This lists the names of plants, their indications, and chapter number. The chapter number in bold face is indicative of where introductory details of the plant are given.

Also included are color plates of watercolor paintings of 12 major Ayurvedic herbs, done by me.

I hope that this book will be of use not only to health care professionals but also to anyone interested in knowing more about Ayurvedic herbs.

M. S. Premila
Chennai
3.1.2005

Acknowledgments

First and foremost, I wish to thank my family and friends, who believed in me and gave constant encouragement, especially my mother, Mrs. Lakshmi Sivaraman.

I am grateful to Professor Varro Tyler for recommending this topic when I wrote to him with my own book suggestion. Unfortunately, he is not here to see the result. I am happy that I was able to meet him briefly in Chennai, during his very busy conference schedule in June 2001. Few of us at that time could have imagined that would be the last time we would see him.

Databases form the core of providing the numerous references that go into a book. Apart from numerous journals and my own personal literature collection, I have made extensive use of the *Medicinal and Aromatic Plants Abstracts (MAPA)* published by the National Institute of Science Communication and Information Resources NISCAIR (earlier known as Publications and Information Directorate), CSIR, New Delhi, and their earlier CD. Also very useful have been the Medline database provided by BioMedical Net (bmn) and PubMed of the National Medical Library, U.S.A. For access to some missing volumes of MAPA, I am grateful to Dr. P. K. Sehgal, CLRI, Chennai. Thanks are due also to Professor M. A. Iyengar for sending me a copy of his *Bibliography of Investigated Medicinal Plants (1950-1975)*. To obtain copies of original articles I received help from The Marketing Services Division of NISCAIR, which provides a unique service in hunting down the article and the source library and then providing photocopies. Help was also given by the National Medical Library, New Delhi, the Web site www.freemedicaljournals.com, Dr. Anju Chadha, Dr. Susan Raghavan, and Dr. M. Radhika.

I also wish to thank Mr. A. Kumaran for help in sorting the papers and Dr. Chitra Shastri for reading and commenting on the first three chapters. I thank Dr. P. Santhan for help in getting plant specimens to paint. I am also grateful to Dr. N. P. Damodaran for a specimen of *Commiphora mukul* from plants carefully nursed for over two decades in Coimbatore, Dr. P. R. Krishna Kumar for permission to pick specimens, and Dr. Padmamalini Sundararaghavan for getting the plant twigs for me.

Chapter 1

Drug Development and Evaluation in Ancient India

ORIGINS OF AYURVEDA

From time immemorial, plants have been used as medicines around the world and plant-based medicines have been the mainstay of traditional societies in dealing with health problems. The global search for alternative strategies for health care has been driven by a growing dissatisfaction with the inadequacy of modern medicines in certain disease areas, notably in chronic conditions such as arthritis and asthma, and with their distressing iatrogenic effects. This dissatisfaction is combined with the urge to adopt a more natural way of relating to the world and to return to nature. The search has led to worldwide interest in the scientific validation of the therapeutic efficacy of traditional plant-based medicines.

In India there arose some 3,000 years ago one of the most comprehensive and complete systems of medicine—Ayurveda, which in its holistic approach goes beyond the mere prescription of drugs. The aim of Ayurveda is twofold: to lead a healthy life full of vigor and, in the event of disease, to bring about healing. Disease is considered to be the absence of harmony, and Ayurveda involves taking measures to restore harmony and thereby health. This is achieved through a threefold plan of lifestyle, diet, and drugs in accordance with an individual's constitution and the season. Health is not merely the absence of disease but a state of total physical, mental, spiritual, and social well-being. In Ayurveda, drugs are one component of the therapeutic

doi:10.1300/5683_01

modality, and drugs of plant, mineral, and animal origin are used. However, herbs constitute approximately 70 percent of the Ayurvedic materia medica.

Ayurveda translates to "science or knowledge of life," with *Ayur* meaning "life" and *Veda* meaning "knowledge" or "science." Ayurveda is considered to be an auxiliary Veda *(upveda)* or sometimes as a fifth Veda, the first four being the *Rig Veda,* the *Yajur Veda,* the *Sama Veda,* and the *Atharva Veda.* The Vedas are a body of knowledge considered to be of nonhuman (divine) origin. Dismayed by the growing incidence of disease, the sages and other wise men in early times beseeched the divine creator for help in alleviating human suffering. In the tradition of the *Caraka Samhita,* the divine creator through various intermediaries transmitted the science of Ayurveda to Indra and from Indra to sages such as Bharadwaja, Atri, and others, who then taught Ayurveda to their disciples; however, in the tradition of the *Sushruta Samhita,* it is Dhanvantri who received the science from Indra.[1] A description of the first conclave on preventive health and therapeutic measures to treat disease appears in the first recorded text of Ayurveda, known as the *Caraka Samhita,* which is often dated to 700 BC. The next major texts were the *Sushruta Samhita,* which deals with surgery, and the *Astanga Hrdayam* of Vagbhata. The three physicians Caraka, Sushruta, and Vagbhata together form the so-called Greater Triad, or *Brihattrayi.*

Ayurvedic drugs were chosen by a combination of observation, experiment, intuition, and discussion among scholars. The intuitive element helped to select the most suitable plants, which were tried out on domestic animals such as cats, dogs, and cows. Their use was further refined by discussion among scholars, and disputes among scholars were resolved through regular meetings. The *Caraka Samhita* speaks of such meetings in the foothills of the Himalayas. Controversy was also resolved in each case by experimentation on human beings.[2]

What emerged from this long period of trial and experimentation on human beings is a large number of herbs of proven clinical utility. It is the results of this experimentation that are available today in the extremely terse written form known as *sutras.*

HISTORY OF DRUG EVALUATION

Medicinal plants and herbs are an important part of the Ayurvedic formulary. The use of more than 1,700 herbs has been described in Ayurveda. It is interesting at this point to review briefly the history of plant usage—drug collection, selection, and evaluation. Great attention was paid in ancient times to ensuring the quality, safety, and efficacy of the herbs used. The chemical contents of plants vary according to soil, location, season, time of day, time of year, manner of harvesting, and further processing. It is remarkable how these aspects were delineated several hundred years ago. In the *Kasyapa Samhita,* the steps to be followed before a plant can be used as medicine are enumerated: plants must be cultivated on suitable soil, in the proper season; they must be collected at the appropriate time, ensuring the absence of damage from heat, water, insects, stools, urine, and time; and they must be collected or grown in areas away from roadsides, cemeteries, and so on.[3]

In terms of the proper growing season, the *Caraka Samhita* mentions that leaves are to be collected in spring (March-April) and the rainy season (July-September).[4] Some scientific evidence corroborates this. *Adhatoda vasica* leaves are used for the treatment of coughs, colds, asthma, and bronchitis. In one study, the content of the major alkaloid and active principle and bronchodilator vasicine was analyzed throughout the year and plotted to yield a curve showing two major peaks in March-April and July-September corresponding to periods when the vasicine content was highest thereby showing good correlation with the guidelines of Caraka.[5]

The efficacy of herbs and their action was often a discussion point among scholars, with differing opinions resolved through observations on human beings. Unfortunately, the actual experimental procedures followed are no longer available to us. What have been written down are the final results of discussion and experimentation, consisting of the names of the plants to be used in various conditions and the treatment to be followed.

The tremendous regard for the safety of the drugs used and the manner in which they were to be processed led to any doubts being resolved by testing on domestic animals.[6] Processing was considered essential to reduce or remove toxicity and also to increase bioavailability. Many plants that are toxic or poisonous find use in Ayurveda after "purification," or *shodana*. The tubers of *Aconitum*, for example, are often used in Ayurveda although they contain the toxic alkaloid aconitine. This is possible because the drug is processed or detoxified before it is used. Boiling *Aconitum* tubers in water converts the toxic aconitine to aconine, which is less toxic.[7] *Commiphora mukul* gum resin is widely used in Ayurveda for the treatment of arthritis and is traditionally processed before use by boiling the resin in water or a decoction of *triphala*, or "three fruits" (a mixture of *Terminalia chebula, T. belerica,* and *Emblica officinalis*). During the development of *Commiphora mukul* as a hypolipidemic agent, it was found that the crude material produced minor side effects such as skin rashes, diarrhea, and irregular menstruation. After the material was purified in the traditional manner by boiling and skimming, it no longer caused skin rashes.[8]

PLANT USE IN AYURVEDA

A large number of plants are used in Ayurveda to maintain balance and harmony so that it is possible to enjoy good health. Plants were often combined to create synergy, reduce toxicity, and increase bioavailability. Multiplant preparations were and still are generally preferred, although a large number of single drugs were also used. However, very few studies have been carried out to provide scientific support to validate these combinations, not least because of the problems associated with devising a suitable methodology to do this.

Bioavailability

It has been possible to show an increase in bioavailability when either the traditional three-spice or pungent mixture known as *trikatu* (*tri:* "three"; *katu:* "pungent"), consisting of *Piper longum* (long pepper), *P. nigrum* (pepper), and *Zingiber officinale* (ginger), is added to formulations or the major alkaloid piperine of *P. longum* and *P. nigrum* is added.[9,10] This concept has also been used to reduce the required dosage of anti-TB drugs such as rifampicin or other drugs such as ciprofloxacin.[11] Controlled studies have also shown that in healthy volunteers the absorption of nutraceuticals such as β-carotene and curcumin can be increased severalfold—by 60 percent in the case of β-carotene through the addition of small quantities of piperine[12] and 2000 percent by addition of 20 mg piperine to 2 g curcumin.[13]

Synergy

A few clinical studies have shown the beneficial effects of combining drugs. Thus, combined therapy with *Semecarpus anacardium (bhallatak), Dalbergia lanceolaria (gourakh),* and *Commiphora mukul (guggul)* showed better results in osteoarthritis, frozen shoulder, and sciatica than the individual drugs alone.[14] Other examples include the addition of *Bacopa monnieri* to the combination of *Inula racemosa* and *Commiphora mukul* for the treatment of heart disease (see Chapter 6, "Cardiovascular drugs"), the combination of *Gymnema sylvestre* and *Eugenia jambolana* for diabetes (see Chapter 11, "Antidiabetic agents"), and the combination of *Zingiber officinale* and *Commiphora mukul* for arthritis (see Chapter 8, "Antirheumatic agents").

Any scientific study of Ayurvedic herbs would benefit greatly from a study of the ideas, concepts, and pronouncements given in early Ayurvedic texts regarding plant collection, processing, combination, selection, and use to see how these correlate with present-day scientific understanding. Even a brief look at the history of Ayurveda and drug development in ancient India and at some of the concepts used in drug formulation shows much can be learned and understood from the ancient texts. Such a venture could prove to be very rewarding.

NOTES

1. Sharma PV. Vedic medicine. In Sharma PV (ed.), *History of medicine in India* (p. 3). New Delhi: Indian National Science Academy, 1992.

2. Gaur DS, Gupta PL. A study of drug evaluation in ancient India. In Udupa KN (ed.), *Advances in research in Indian medicine* (pp. 357-385). Varanasi: Banaras Hindu University, 1970.

3. Vriddha Jivika, *Kasyapa samhita,* transl. and ed. Tewari PV, Kumar N, Sharma RD, Kumar A (p. 60, "Sutrasthana," chapter 26, verse 5). Varanasi: Chaukhambha Viswabharati, 2002.

4. *Caraka samhita,* 1st edn., transl. and ed. Sharma PV (vol. 2, pp. 539-540, "Kalpasthana," chapter 1, verse 10). Varanasi: Chaukhambha Orientalia, 1986.

5. Arambewela LSR, Ratnanayaka CK, Jayasekara JS, De Silva KTD. Vasicine contents and their seasonal variation in *Adhatoda vasica*. *Fitoterapia* 59:151-153 (1988).

6. Nitya Anand. Contribution of Ayurvedic medicine to medicinal chemistry. In Hansch C, Sammes PG, Taylor JB (eds.), *Comprehensive medicinal chemistry* (vol. 1, pp. 113-129). Oxford: Pergamon Press, 1990.

7. Hsu HY. A study of processing of some commonly used medicinal herbs. In Chang HM, Yeung HW, Tso WW, Koo A (eds.), *Advances in Chinese medicinal materials research* (p. 63). Singapore: World Scientific Publishing Co., 1985.

8. Satyavati GV. Gum *guggul:* The success story of an ancient insight leading to a modern discovery. *ICMR Bull* 17(1):1-6 (1987).

9. Atal CK, Zutshi U, Rao PG. Scientific evidence on the role of Ayurvedic herbals on the bioavailability of drugs. *J Ethnopharmacol* 4:229-232 (1981).

10. Johri RK, Zutshi U. An Ayurvedic formulation *"Trikatu"* and its constituents. *J Ethnopharmacol* 37:85-91 (1992).

11. Zutshi U, Bedi KL. Drug bioavailability enhancement—A new concept. In Handa SS, Kaul MK (eds.), *Supplement to cultivation and utilization of medicinal plants* (pp. 13-32). Jammu Tawi: Regional Research Laboratory, Council of Scientific and Industrial Research, 1996.

12. Dichek B. Enhancing the effect of nutraceuticals. *Scrip Magazine* May: 34-35 (1999).

13. Shoba G, Joy D, Joseph T, Majeed M, Rajendran R, Srinivas PSSR. Influence of piperine in the pharmakokinetics of curcumin in animals and human volunteers. *Planta Med* 64:353-356 (1998).

14. Majumdar A. Clinical studies of drugs *(bhallatak, gourakh* and *guggul)* in osteoarthritis and sciatica. *Rheumatism* 14:153-161 (1979).

Chapter 2

Scientific Investigation
of Indian Medicinal Plants

HISTORY OF RESEARCH

The scientific investigation of Indian medicinal plants, especially of those used in Ayurveda, started in the early part of the twentieth century with the extensive investigations of Dr. R. N. Chopra. His far-reaching work and documentation in the years 1930-1950 earned him the title "Father of Indian Pharmacology."[1-3] His work triggered major interest in the further exploration of the wealth of knowledge available in indigenous systems of medicine, mostly by chemical and pharmacological researchers, initially through individual effort in universities and then through team efforts in various institutions including the Indian Council of Medical Research[4,5] and the Indian Council for Research in Indian Medicine (now the Central Council for Research in Ayurveda and Siddha).[6] Broad-based screening of Indian medicinal plants was undertaken by the Central Drug Research Institute in Lucknow,[7-9] and specific research into individual plants and yoga therapy was carried out at the Faculty of Indian Medicine of the Institute of Medical Sciences at the Banaras Hindu University.[10] This list is not exhaustive.

The Ayurvedic literature on therapeutics and materia medica formed the basis for chemical, pharmacological, and clinical research. Important single-drug preparations and compound drugs comprising multiplant preparations were studied. The major efforts were

doi:10.1300/5683_02

expended in chemical and pharmacological studies, with an emphasis on what was possible based on the available materials and research facilities. Thus, for example, chemical work generally tended to use nonpolar solvents, probably because the methodology to deal with nonpolar compounds was better developed. Later, with the awareness that aqueous decoctions and infusions were the major mode of administration, researchers realized the need to look at polar compounds such as glycosides, tannins, and sugars. Working with such compounds was made easier by advances in separation science and the development of newer adsorbents such as Sephadex and new equipment based on countercurrent chromatography. A similar trend was seen in pharmacological and clinical work. Considering that in India paucity of funds has been a major constraint, the work that has been carried out is laudable.

Far less clinical work has been performed than pharmacological and chemical studies. A review of literature published between 1950 and 1975 shows that only 1.36 percent of the entries dealt with clinical trials, compared with 17.46 percent for pharmacological studies and 63.42 percent for chemical studies.[11,12]

Other problems include the fact that many of the clinical trials were of a preliminary or exploratory nature and were carried out on small numbers of patients. The methodology has often been far from satisfactory. In some cases, promising leads have not been followed up to confirm early results. Many of the results have been published in non-peer-reviewed journals that are difficult to access. Among the various problems faced in reporting clinical trials on herbs used in Ayurveda, one concerns relating Ayurvedic disease entities to modern parameters, or in other words the problem of Western-style clinical studies being applied to Ayurveda, which has its own concepts and basis. In addition, relatively few randomized, double-blind placebo-controlled trials have been carried out. Despite this, a tremendous amount of information has been generated that shows Ayurvedic herbs and concepts to have a very sound scientific basis. Any investigation of Ayurvedic drugs needs to look at the rationale behind their use, the mode of use, and the methods of drug collection and processing.

RESULTS OF SCIENTIFIC INVESTIGATION

As a result of scientific investigation into Ayurvedic herbs, a few trends or results can be seen.

1. There is better understanding of the specific role played by an herb.

It is now possible to understand the pharmacological profile of the drugs suited to certain disease areas so that a choice can be made with regard to the drug to be used. For example, Ayurvedic herbs for the liver are often used for the treatment of jaundice, which is a general term to describe inflammation of the liver and could result from the intake of alcohol or drugs or be of viral origin. Studies now enable better decisions to be made regarding whether a drug useful for jaundice has specific action against the Hepatitis B virus (say, by binding the Hepatitis B surface antigen), whether it is hepatoprotective or antihepatotoxic, whether it helps in liver cell regeneration, and whether it has anti-inflammatory activity or an antifibrotic effect.[13]

2. Modern methods confirm ancient concepts and use.

The gum resin of *Commiphora mukul,* or *guggul* in Sanskrit, which is widely used in arthritis, is also described as being a useful anti-obesity drug, and descriptions of its etiopathogenesis correspond remarkably well with modern ideas of how obesity arises. Research has now shown its effectiveness as a hypolipidemic agent with cholesterol-lowering properties.[14]

3. The elucidation of mechanisms of action explains use in different indications.

The gum resin of *Boswellia serrata* is traditionally used for a number of indications, including rheumatism, arthritis, asthma, gastrointestinal tract problems, and tumors. After the resin was shown to act to inhibit 5-lipoxygenase (and leukotriene synthesis), it was hypothesized that it would be useful in bronchial asthma, ulcerative colitis and Crohn's disease—that is, in conditions where leukotriene synthesis is considered responsible for initiation and perpetuation of the disease. This hypothesis has now been supported by clinical trials.[15]

4. Some crude drugs and their isolated components are COX-2 inhibitors.

COX-2 inhibitors are considered to be devoid of the usual side effects of nonsteroidal anti-inflammatory drugs (NSAIDs). Several crude drugs and their active principles have been shown to be COX-2 inhibitors, for example, turmeric, curcumin, holy basil (*Ocimum sanctum*), rosmarinic acid, and ursolic acid.[16-18]

5. Evidence supports the concept of anti-aging agents.

Two categories of drugs in Ayurveda, the *rasayana* and the *vayasthapana* drugs, are considered to be useful in reducing the effects of aging. Many of these drugs have powerful antioxidant properties.[19] For example, although turmeric is not a *rasayana* drug, curcuminoids from turmeric or *Curcuma longa* have a more powerful antioxidant effect than grape seed extract.[20] The ancient sage Chyavan is said to have rejuvenated himself using a concoction of herbs named after him: *Chyavanprash*. The major ingredient, *Emblica officinalis* or *amla,* is a potent antioxidant. *Amla* fruit, considered to be one of the richest sources of vitamin C, also contains other potent antioxidant compounds. The role of free radical scavengers in cancer, antiaging, diabetes, and so on is well recognized today.

6. The trend is toward use of enriched fractions.

A change is taking place in the way crude drugs are used. With the introduction of many standardized herbs, enriched fractions containing larger amounts of the active components are preferred, for example, Boswellic acids from *Boswellia serrata,* curcumin from *Curcuma longa,* and picroliv from *Picrorrhiza kurroa.*

NOTES

1. Chopra RN, Nayar SL, Chopra IC. *Glossary of Indian Medicinal Plants.* New Delhi: Council of Scientific and Industrial Research, 1956.

2. Chopra RN, Chopra IC, Verma BS. *Supplement to Glossary of Indian Medicinal Plants.* New Delhi: Publications and Information Directorate, Council of Scientific and Industrial Research, 1969.

3. Chopra RN, Chopra IC, Handa KL, Kapur LD. *Chopra's Indigenous Drugs of India,* 2nd edn. Calcutta: Academic Publishers, 1958.

4. Satyavati GV, Raina MK, Sharma M (eds.). *Medicinal Plants of India,* vol. 1. New Delhi: Indian Council of Medical Research, 1976. Satyavati GV, Gupta AK,

Tandon N (eds.). *Medicinal Plants of India*, vol. 2. New Delhi: Indian Council of Medical Research, 1987.

5. Gupta AK, Tandon N (eds.). *Reviews on Indian Medicinal Plants*, vols 1-3. New Delhi: Indian Council of Medical Research, 2004.

6. Sharma PC, Yelne MB, Dennis TJ (eds.). *Database on Medicinal Plants used in Ayurveda*, vols 1-5. New Delhi: Central Council for Research in Ayurveda and Siddha, 2000, 2001, 2001, 2002, 2002. Billore KV, Yelne MB, Dennis TJ, Chaudhari BG (eds.). *Database on Medicinal Plants used in Ayurveda*, vol. 6. New Delhi: Central Council for Research in Ayurveda and Siddha, 2004.

7. Rastogi RP, Dhawan BN. Research on medicinal plants at the Central Drug Research Institute, Lucknow (India). *Indian J Med Res* 76 (suppl.):27-45 (December 1982).

8. Rastogi RP, Dhawan BN, Dhar MM. Medicinal Plants. *Drugs and Pharmaceuticals, Industry Highlights* 11(2):1-26 (1988).

9. Dhawan BN (ed.). *Current Research on Medicinal Plants of India.* New Delhi: Indian National Science Academy, 1986.

10. Udupa KN, Chaturvedi GN, Tripathi SN (eds.). *Advances in Research in Indian Medicine*. Varanasi: Banaras Hindu University, 1970.

11. Vohora SB. Research on medicinal plants in India: A review on reviews. *Indian Drugs* 26:526-531 (1989).

12. Iyengar MA. *Bibliography of Investigated Indian Medicinal Plants (1950-1975)*, 1st edn. Manipal: College of Pharmacy, Manipal Medical College, 1976.

13. Premila MS. Emerging frontiers in the field of hepatoprotective herbal drugs. *Indian J Nat Prod* 11(Special Issue):3-12 (1995).

14. Satyavati GV. Gum *Guggul*: The success story of an ancient insight leading to a modern discovery. *ICMR Bull* 17(1):1-6 (1987).

15. Ammon HPT. Ayurveda—Arzneimittel aus indischer Kultur. *Z Phytother* 22:136-142 (2001).

16. Ramsewak RS, DeWitt DL, Nair MG. Cytotoxicity, antioxidant and anti-inflammatory activities of curcumins I-III from *Curcuma longa*. *Phytomedicine* 7:303-308 (2000).

17. Hong CH, Hur SK, Oh OJ, Kim SS, Nam KA, Lee SK. Evaluation of natural products on inhibition of inducible cyclooxygenase (COX-2) and nitric oxide synthase (iNOS) in cultured mouse macrophage cells. *J Ethnopharmacol* 83:153-159 (2002).

18. Kelm MA, Nair MG, Strasburg GM, DeWitt DL. Antioxidant and cyclooxygenase inhibitory phenolic compounds from *Ocimum sanctum* Linn. *Phytomedicine* 7:7-13 (2000).

19. Scartezzini P, Speroni E. Review on some plants of Indian traditional medicine with antioxidant activity. *J Ethnopharmacol* 71:23-43 (2000).

20. Majeed M, Badmaev V, Shivakumar U, Rajendran R. *Curcuminoids— Antioxidant phytonutrients* (p. 40). New Jersey: Nutriscience Publishers, 1995.

Chapter 3

Gastrointestinal Agents

In Ayurveda, the gastrointestinal system plays a very important role in both the maintenance of health and the cause of disease, not only diseases of the gastrointestinal tract but all disorders. A weak digestion, known as *mandagni,* is considered to be the main cause of all diseases, including gastrointestinal disorders.[1] Therefore, spices and herbs have been commonly added to food or taken as drugs to improve digestion, aid absorption, and promote elimination. The two most commonly used spices in Indian cooking are ginger and turmeric. Clinical trials covering such common, classical uses are rare. However, a clinical trial has been carried out to evaluate the efficacy of ginger in malabsorption syndrome or *grahni roga.*[2]

MALABSORPTION SYNDROME

Zingiber officinale *Roscoe* (*Family: Zingiberaceae*)

Sanskrit: Adraka (fresh), sunthi (dry)	Tamil: Inji (fresh), sukku (dry)
Hindi: Adrak (fresh), sunth (dry)	English: Ginger

Zingiber officinale, or ginger, is a slender perennial herb with rhizomes that is cultivated widely throughout India. The rhizomes are very commonly used in Ayurvedic medicine in both fresh and dry forms, though more usually in the dry form. In Sanskrit, ginger is

doi:10.1300/5683_03

13

known as a universal medicine, or *vishwa bhesaj* (*vishwa*: universal; *bhesaj:* medicine). It is also referred to as a great medicine, or *maha aushadi* (*maha:* great; *aushadi:* medicine). The drug consists of the roots or rhizomes of the plant. Traditionally, ginger is used in Ayurveda as a stomachic, to promote digestion, and for dyspepsia, flatulence, colic, vomiting, fever, coughs, colds, asthma, gout, and chronic rheumatism. It is also used externally to treat headache and toothache and to improve blood circulation.[3] The drug is approved in the *Indian Herbal Pharmacopoeia,* 2002, for its carminative, antiemetic, and anti-inflammatory properties.[4] The use of ginger as an antiemetic is discussed later in this chapter, and its use as an anti-inflammatory agent is covered in Chapter 8 "Antirheumatic agents."

The rhizome contains 1-2 percent of an essential oil that has a variable composition, depending upon the variety and the location of the plant, and 5-8 percent of an oleoresin. The oleoresin contains the non-volatile pungent principles, the gingerols—mainly [6]-gingerol, and also [8]-gingerol and [10]-gingerol—which vary in terms of the length of their side chain and are considered to be among the active principles. The corresponding dehydration products, the shogaols that arise from the gingerols on drying, are generally not found in the fresh plant.[3,4]

In Ayurveda, ginger is considered to be useful at every stage of digestion: digestion *(dipan)*, absorption *(pachan)*, and elimination *(grahi)*. Thus, it is regarded as having a role in the prevention of accumulation of toxic materials *(ama)* in the body. Ginger has been shown to increase salivary [5] and gastric secretion,[6] act as a cholagogue,[7] display spasmolytic activity in animals,[8] and increase peristalsis on oral administration.[9] In combination with two other pungent spices, pepper and long pepper, known as *trikatu,* ginger is commonly used in Ayurveda to increase bioavailability of other drugs by promoting their absorption or by preventing their metabolism during their first passage through the liver.[10]

An open trial was conducted on 111 patients with *grahni roga,* or malabsorption syndrome.[2] Inclusion criteria were chronic history of alternating diarrhea and constipation, loss of appetite, indigestion, history of loose motions, physical weakness, and loss of weight. Three grams of dried ginger powder was given thrice daily with warm water for 1 month. Patients were admitted as in-patients for treatment with ginger and were given a hospital diet. The duration of the disease in the patients ranged from 1 month to 7 years; 36 patients had the disease for 1 to 2 years and formed the largest group. Most patients were generally anemic and had more than four motions a day. A total of 26 patients had *Giardia* infections, and 27 patients had *Entamoeba histolytica* cysts. Treatment resulted in reduction of the number of motions to one to two per day, increase in hemoglobin levels, increase in body weight and general health, and elimination of cysts in giardiasis and amoebiasis in a majority of patients.[2] Thus the beneficial effect that ginger has on absorption has been revealed. However, considering the potential usefulness of the drug, further controlled studies are required.

Ginger has a low acute toxicity. In one study on mice, an alcoholic extract given at a dose of 2.5 g·kg^{-1} body weight (equivalent to 75 g fresh rhizome) for 7 days showed no mortality and no side effects except for mild diarrhea in two animals.[11] No side effects have been reported in clinical trials.[12] Experiments to test the mutagenic and antimutagenic potential of ginger and isolated constituents have shown variable results depending upon the components present and the bacterial strain used.[13] Based on the possible mutagenic potential, some authors warn against the use of ginger during pregnancy in doses larger than the amount taken in food (1-2 g per day)[13,14] Also, the use of ginger in conjunction with diabetic, cardiac, and anticoagulant therapy is not advocated, because synergistic effects may result from taking ginger in excessive amounts owing to the prolonged hypoglycemic activity of ginger in vivo, its positive inotropic action, and its inhibiting action on platelet aggregation).[13] In sensitive patients, ginger may cause gastric irritation.[13]

NOTES

1. Chaturvedi GN, Kumar S. Glimpses of Ayurvedic gastroenterology. Editorial. *J Res Edu Indian Med* 1(4):iii-iv (1982).

2. Nanda GC, Tekari NS, Kishore P. Clinical evaluation of *Sunthi (Zingiber officinale)* in the treatment of *Grahni Roga. J Res Ayur Siddha* XIV(1-2):34-44 (1993).

3. Kapoor LD. *Handbook of Ayurvedic medicinal plants* (pp. 341-342). Boca Raton, FL: CRC Press, 2001.

4. *Indian herbal pharmacopoeia* (rev. new edn., pp. 479-490). Mumbai: Indian Drug Manufacturers' Association, 2002.

5. Glätzel H. Therapie der Dyspepsie mit Gewürzextrakten. *Deutsche Apoth Ztg* 110:5-6 (1970).

6. Chang HM, But PPH. (eds.). *Pharmacology and applications of Chinese materia medica* (vol. 1, pp. 341-344). Singapore: World Scientific Publishing, 1986.

7. Yamahara J, Miki K, Chisaka T, Sawada T, Fujimura H, Tomimatsu T, Nakano K, Nohara T. Cholagogic effect of ginger and its active constituents. *J Ethnopharmacol* 13:217-225 (1985).

8. Suekawa M, Ishige A, Yuasa K, Sudo K, Aburada M, Hosoya E. Pharmacological actions of pungent constituents [6]-gingerol and [6]-shogaol. *J Pharmacobiodyn* 7:836-848 (1984).

9. Yamahara J, Huang QR, Li YH, Xu L, Fujimura H. Gastrointestinal motility enhancing effect of ginger and its active constituents. *Chem Pharm Bull* 38:430-431 (1990).

10. Johri RK, Zutshi U. An Ayurvedic formulation "trikatu" and its constituents. *J Ethnopharmacol* 37:85-91 (1992).

11. Mascolo N, Jain R, Jain RC, Capasso F. Ethnopharmacologic investigation of ginger *(Zingiber officinale)* L. *J Ethnopharmacol* 27:129-140 (1989).

12. Ernst E, Pittler MH. Efficacy of ginger for nausea and vomiting: A systematic review of randomized clinical trials. *Brit J Anaesthesia* 84:367-371 (2000).

13. Falch B, Reichling J, Saller R. Ingwer—Nicht nur ein Gewürz. Untersuchungen zur Wirkungen and Wirksamkeit. *Deutsche Apoth Ztg* 137:4267-4278 (1997).

14. Bone K. Ginger. *Brit J Phytother* 4(3):110-120 (1997).

DYSPEPSIA

The term *dyspepsia* is used to denote a feeling of fullness or pressing in the upper abdomen as a result of gas, leading to pain or discomfort. (See the section "Other antiulcer plants" below for *nonulcer dyspepsia.*) Reports of clinical trials use the term to denote the Ayurvedic condition known as *amlapitta*, which is associated with hyperacidity.

Curcuma longa *L. (Family: Zingiberaceae)*

Latin: Curcuma domestica Valeton	Hindi: Haldi
Sanskrit: Haridra	Tamil: Manjal
English: Turmeric	

Curcuma longa, or turmeric, is a slender perennial herb with fleshy roots. It is cultivated as an annual crop throughout the warmer parts of India. In India, turmeric is very commonly used as a spice and as an ingredient of curry, giving it a characteristic yellow color. Turmeric is also considered auspicious and is used in Hindu rituals. It is widely used by women as a cosmetic to protect the skin and prevent growth of body and facial hair.

Traditionally, it has been used as a stomachic and carminative, the powdered drug being given for flatulence and dyspepsia. It is mixed in milk and taken as an expectorant in household cough and cold remedies, and used externally either by itself or as a paste with *neem* *(Azadirachta indica)* leaves for its antiseptic and healing action. The dried rhizomes are listed in the *Indian Herbal Pharmacopoeia, 2002,* as an anti-inflammatory, stomachic, and tonic agent.[1]

The rhizome contains 3-5 percent yellow coloring chemicals known as curcuminoids (curcumin, curcumin I, or diferuloylmethane [50-60 percent]); monodemethoxycurcumin, or curcumin II, and bisdemethoxycurcumin, or curcumin III, as minor constituents; 2-7 percent of an essential oil with a high content of bisabolane derivatives; and the polysaccharides ukonan A, B, and C.[1,2]

Turmeric powder increases the mucin content of gastric juice in rabbits; it may thus exert a protective effect on the gastric mucosa in gastric disorders.[3] In isolated guinea pig ileum, the soluble sodium salt of curcumin—sodium curcuminate—exerts an antispasmodic effect against various spasmogens.[4] In addition, turmeric oil suppresses the growth of some intestinal, pathogenic, and toxigenic bacteria.[5] In vitro, curcumin at 0.05 percent concentration reduces intestinal gas formation by *Clostridium perfringens;* in vivo, curcumin at 0.1 percent concentration reduces intestinal gas formation on feeding rats along with chickpea flour—a known flatulent diet.[6] In studies from the 1950s,[7-9] the choleretic and cholagogic effects of the essential oil and sodium curcuminate administered intravenously were demonstrated. In more recent studies, curcuminoids and the essential oil stimulated bile secretion in isolated perfused rat liver . An increase both in the production of bile and in the bile concentration was seen.[10] In a rat bile fistula model, a choleretic effect was shown by a mixture of the three curcuminoids, by curcumin I, and also by curcumin III, which had earlier been considered to be inactive as a choleretic.[11,12] In cholestatis caused by cyclosporine, bisdemethoxycurcumin and the curcuminoid mixture caused a reduction in cholestatis, with the effect of bisdemethoxycurcumin being much greater than that of the mixture.[12] A potent cholagogic effect has also been reported for the essential oil.[13]

In a randomized, double-blind, study on 106 patients with acid dyspepsia, flatulent dyspepsia, or atonic dyspepsia patients were randomized to one of three groups—turmeric, placebo, or a multiplant preparation known as "Flatulence." Thus in 38 patients 500 mg turmeric powder was given four times a day for 1 week. At the end of 7 days the group of 38 patients on turmeric showed a statistically significant difference from the placebo group (38 patients); 30 patients were on "Flatulence," a multiplant preparation, for comparison and results comparable to turmeric were obtained.[14]

Another study examined 440 patients with dyspeptic symptoms of 17 weeks' duration. Of those, 36 percent had irritable bowel syndrome, 34 percent dyspepsia, 18 percent functional disturbances of the gall bladder, and 12 percent other digestive disturbances. In addition, 78 percent of patients presented a psychosomatic disease component symptoms worsening with mental stress. The trial preparation consisted of capsules containing 81 mg of 96 percent ethanolic *Curcuma longa* extract, which extracts the active components—the essential oil and the curcuminoids. Two capsules were given daily for 4 weeks. The results showed a definite reduction (67.8 percent) in dyspeptic symptoms, especially pain in the upper and lower abdomen, the feeling of pressure, the feeling of fullness, and abdominal bloating. Most patients could feel a difference after an average of 6 days of treatment. The good compliance was attributed to the dosage schedule of only two capsules per day. In addition, the global tolerance was evaluated by 95.3 percent of patients as either "excellent" or "very good."[15,16]

Turmeric is generally regarded as safe. In individuals not previously exposed to turmeric the possibility of allergic reactions has been reported,[1] although turmeric is itself considered to have an anti-allergic effect. The literature on the safety of turmeric and curcumin has been extensively reviewed, and they have been found to be safe even at high doses. However, turmeric can cause gastric irritation in susceptible individuals.[17] In a trial on patients with bronchial asthma who were given 12 g·day⁻¹ of turmeric powder, a few patients complained of dryness of the mouth and throat, which was assuaged by a reduction of the dose.[18]

NOTES

1. *Indian herbal pharmacopoeia* (rev. new edn., pp. 169-180). Mumbai: Indian Drug Manufacturers' Association, 2002.

2. Bisset NG, Wichtl M. *Herbal drugs and phytopharmaceuticals* (2nd edn., pp. 173-175). Stuttgart: Medpharm Scientific Publishers, 2001.

3. Mukerjee B, Zaidi SH, Singh GB. Spices and gastric function: Effects of *Curcuma longa* on the gastric secretion in rabbits. *J Sci Ind Res* 20C:25-28 (1961).

4. Rao TS, Basu N, Siddiqui HH. Antiinflammatory activity of curcumin analogues. *Indian J Med Res* 75:574-578 (1982).

5. Bhavani Shankar TN, Murthy VS. Effect of turmeric *(Curcuma longa)* fractions on the growth of some intestinal and pathogenic bacteria in vitro. *J Exp Biol* 17:1363-1366 (1979).

6. Bhavani Shankar TN, Murthy VS. Inhibitory effect of curcumin on intestinal gas formation by *Clostridium perfringens*. *Nutr Rep Int* 32:1285-1292 (1985).

7. Ramprasad C, Sirsi M. Studies on Indian medicinal plants: *Curcuma longa* Linn—Effect of curcumin & the essential oil of *Curcuma longa* on bile secretion. *J Sci Ind Res* 15C:262-265 (1956).

8. Ramprasad C, Sirsi MJ. Observations on the pharmacology of *Curcuma longa* Linn. Pharmacodynamic and toxicological studies of sodium curcuminate. *Indian J Physiol Pharmacol* 1:136-143 (1957).

9. Ramprasad C, Sirsi M. *Curcuma longa* and bile secretion—Quantitative changes in the bile constituents induced by sodium curcuminate. *J Sci Ind Res* 16C:108-110 (1957).

10. Fintelmann V, Wegner T. *Curcuma longa*—Eine unterschätzte Heilpflanze. *Deutsche Apoth Ztg* 141:3735-3743 (2001).

11. Siegers CP, Deters M, Strubelt O, Hänsel W. Choleretic properties of different curcuminoids in the rat bile fistula model. *Pharm Pharmacol Lett* 7:87-89 (1997).

12. Deters M, Siegers CP, Muhl P, Hänsel W. Choleretic effects of curcuminoids on an acute cyclosporin-induced cholestatis in the rat. *Planta Med* 65:610-613 (1999).

13. Ozaki Y, Liang OB. Cholagogic action of the essential oil of *Curcuma xanthorrhiza* Roxb. *Shoyakugaku Zasshi* 42:257-263 (1988).

14. Thamlikitkul V, Dechatiwongse T, Chantrakul C et al. Randomized double blind study of *Curcuma domestica* Val. for dyspepsia. *J Med Assoc Thai* 72:613-620 (1989).

15. Deitelhoff P, Petrowicz O, Müller B. Antidyspeptic properties of turmeric root extract (TRE). *Third International Conference on Phytomedicine. Phytomedicine* 7 (suppl. II):Abstract no. P-71, p. 92 (2000).

16. Kammerer E, Fintelmann V. *Curcuma* Wurzelsstock bei dyspeptische Beschwerden—Ergebnisse einer Anwendungsbeobachtung an 440 Patienten. *Naturmed* 16:18-24 (2001).

17. Chainani-Wu N. Safety and anti-inflammatory activity of curcumin: A component of turmeric *(Curcuma longa). J Altern Complement Med* 9:161-168 (2003).

18. *Selected medicinal plants of India: A monograph on identity, safety and clinical usage* (pp. 121-124). Bombay: Chemexcil, Basic Chemicals, Pharmaceuticals and Cosmetics Export Promotion Council, 1992.

ANTIULCER PLANTS

Peptic ulcers are a chronic disorder of the gut caused by a number of predisposing factors such as stress, genetic factors, acid pepsin secretion, and mucosal resistance. The bacterium *Helicobacter pylori* and the use of nonsteroidal anti-inflammatory drugs (NSAIDS) are considered major contributory factors.[1] Peptic ulcer has been equated with the disease entity known as *parinam shula* in Ayurveda. Hyperacidity, or *amlapitta,* is considered to form part of the same spectrum and is therefore often included as part of the same clinical trials. A number of plants have been used in Ayurveda for the management of the two conditions.[2]

Asparagus racemosus *Willd. (Family: Liliaceae)*

Sanskrit: Shatavari	Tamil: Ammaikodi
Hindi: Satavari	English: Asparagus

Asparagus racemosus, or *shatavari,* is a much-branched, extensive, spinous climbing shrub that is covered with a mass of small white flowers after the rains. It has numerous succulent tuberous roots that form the drug. It is found throughout the tropical and subtropical parts of India. *Shatavari* is best known for promoting milk production and for helping a pregnancy run to its full term. Its use in protecting the stomach against irritation is also well known. Despite the widespread use of *shatavari* as a nutritive tonic, only limited scientific information is available. It is mentioned in the ancient texts as being useful for peptic ulcers. A number of saponins have been isolated from the roots and of these shatavarin IV has been shown to have antioxytocic activity.[3]

Asparagus racemosus has been shown to exert a protective effect in experimentally induced abdominal sepsis in rats.[4]

Many minor studies have been conducted with few patients by different authors and it is deduced that there seems to be a beneficial effect of *shatavari* on ulcers. However, more major studies are needed with greater numbers of patients and dose-searching studies to better delineate both the quality of the drug and the dosage required.

In an exploratory study, *shatavari* was given in doses of four 0.5 g tablets of root powder six times a day in a number of conditions diagnosed by Ayurvedic and allopathic doctors to be *amlapitta* (hyperacidity), *parinam shool* (peptic ulcer), *pitaj shool* (acute or chronic gastritis) *vataj shool* (spastic colon), *kaphaj shool* (flatulence), *atisar* (diarrhea), *pravahika* (dysentry), *grahani* (amebic or ulcerative colitis), and was found to be more effective in acute diarrhea, dysentry and gastritis, and in some cases of gastric ulcer and hyperacidity.[5] Three grams of *shatavari* root powder was given four times a day to 32 patients with proven duodenal ulcer for an average of 6 weeks. Most of the patients were relieved of the distressing symptoms. It did not exhibit any antacid activity. This effect was attributed to *shatavari's* direct healing effect on ulcers by strengthening the mucosal resistance or by cytoprotection.[6] It has also been shown to help heal duodenal ulcers. Twenty-three patients with duodenal ulcer were treated with 25 mL of freshly expressed juice of *Asparagus racemosus* roots with 10 mL of honey 2-3 times a day for 45 days along with specific diet. Fourteen patients had complete relief, seven patients felt partial relief, and there were two dropouts.[7] Twenty patients with duodenal ulcer confirmed by Barium meal, X-ray, and gastric analysis were given 20 g per day of *shatavari* root powder in three divided doses with milk for 1 month. Of the 20 patients, 15 had hyperacidity, whereas the remaining 5 had normal levels of gastric acidity. There was significant reduction in total acids and free hydrochloric acid of gastric juice. The results were evaluated as "excellent" in 50 percent and "good" in 30 percent of duodenal ulcer cases although 15 percent showed poor response.[8] In eight healthy normal male volunteers, 2 g of *shatavari* was found to be equally effective in accelerating the gastric emptying as metoclopramide, a drug used in dyspepsia.[9]

A clinical trial was conducted on 109 patients with acid dyspepsia *(amlapitta)* in order to compare the efficacy of three different *shatavari* preparations—the single drug, *shatavari* in combination with other herbs, and a herbomineral preparation. All the three preparations were found equally effective; efficacy not being altered by addition of either herbs or minerals.[10]

In doses used clinically, no adverse reactions have been reported.[11] Using two species and dose levels of 50 mg·kg⁻¹ to 1 g·kg⁻¹ body weight, the acute (for 72 hours) and subacute toxicity (for 4 weeks) of the aqueous extract has been studied and found to be nontoxic. No organ toxicity was seen and there was improvement in phagocytic and killing capacity of monocytes and polymorphonuclear cells.[12]

Emblica officinalis *Gaertn. (Family: Euphorbiaceae)*

Latin: *Phyllanthus emblica* Linn.	Tamil: Nelli
Sanskrit: Amalaki	Hindi: Amla
English: Indian gooseberry, Emblic myrobalan	

Emblica officinalis (see Plate 1 in color gallery) is a medium-sized deciduous tree found both in the wild and cultivated throughout the tropical parts of India up to an elevation of 1,500 m. The yellowish green fruits are borne in bunches and are used widely in Indian cuisine to make preserves—jams, pickles, or wedges—sun-dried in order to ensure a supply throughout the year when the tree is not in fruit. The fruits of *amalaki* occupy a prominent place in Ayurveda, well known for its powerful antioxidant effect and for its high content of Vitamin C, several fold that of orange. The drug consists of the fresh and dried fruits. The fruits are listed in the *Indian Herbal Pharmacopoeia,* 2002, as antacid.[13]

The fruit contains Vitamin C, pectin, a number of polyphenolic compounds, gallic acid, ellagic acid, corilagin, alkaloids—phyllantidine and phyllantine.[14] Hydrolysable tannins punigluconin, pedunculagin, emblicanin A and B have been isolated from fresh pericarp of the fruit.[15] It has been suggested that there is no Vitamin C present in the fruit based on experiments.[15]

The ethyl acetate–soluble fraction of the methanolic extract of *amalaki* at 50 mg·kg[-1] body weight when tested on albino rats showed anti-ulcer and antisecretory activity. In addition, three compounds active at 10 mg·kg[-1] body weight were isolated that prevented stress ulcers in albino rats. The ethyl acetate and the three compounds showed H^+K^+ATPase activity.[16] Extracts of *amalaki* have been shown to have a healing effect on peptic ulcer in rats and humans. In a study published as abstract, patients with peptic ulcer who received 3 g of the drug twice a day after food for 15 days showed endoscopic improvement.[17]

In a pilot study, 20 patients with gastritis syndrome *(amlapitta)*, which is characterized by pain in the epigastric region, nausea, acid eructation, and burning sensation in the abdomen, were chosen for the study. Before the study, patients were kept as in-patients on a restricted diet for 5 days and gastric analysis was done on the sixth day, after which therapy was started. Patients were kept on a restricted bland diet of milk and *chapattis*—a kind of unleavened bread. Powdered *amalaki* was given to patients at dose of 3 g thrice a day for 7 days. On the eighth day gastric analysis was done to find out changes in the gastric acidity. Most patients showed relief in symptoms from the second day with relief in all patients within 2-5 days of taking the drug. The level of acidity also came back to normal levels in most of the cases. However, the drug was effective only in cases of hyperchlorhydria and not in cases with hypochlorhydria.[18]

An open comparative trial examined 38 patients with dyspepsia: 10 with ulcer and 28 without ulcer.[19] Patients were included in the trial if they had at least four of the following nine symptoms for a minimum of 2 weeks during the last 8 weeks prior to the entry into the study—belching, abdominal distension, feeling of fullness after meals, upper gastric burning, heartburn, regurgitation of bitter fluid, nausea, vomiting, and inability to finish normal meals. Parasitic infections were excluded by testing. In the ulcer dyspepsia group of 10 cases, patients were assigned to one of two treatment groups—five patients were given 3 g of *amalaki* powder three times a day for

4 weeks and five patients were given 30 ml gel antacid every 3 hour daily for 4 weeks. Endoscopically all five patients in the antacid group showed healing, whereas in the *amalaki* group four out of five patients showed evidence of complete healing.

In the nonulcer dyspepsia group with peak acid output between 16 and 40 mEq·h^{-1} patients were again divided into two groups: 15 on antacids and 13 on *amalaki*. *Amalaki* produced a significant improvement in dyspeptic symptoms and a decrease in acid output, both treatment modalities being comparable. Four patients on antacids complained of pain and weakness of lower limbs, whereas three patients on *amalaki* had vomiting and loose motions controlled in 2 days without stopping the drug. *Amalaki* is a known mild laxative. It has earlier been suggested[20] that *amalaki* strengthens the gastric and duodenal mucosa leading to rapid healing of the ulcers. Considering the high tannin content of *amalaki* this is likely to be the case, with the tannin forming a protective covering allowing the ulcer to heal underneath.

In another preliminary trial[20] 39 cases of duodenal ulcer and 21 cases of nonulcer dyspepsia were given 3 g of *amalaki rasayana* with water thrice daily for 10 days initially and subsequently twice daily. No other drug—antacid, tranquillizer, or anticholinergic drug was given during this period. *Amalaki rasayana* is a traditional Ayurvedic preparation obtained by adding a decoction of *amalaki* to the fruit powder and drying it. This process of adding the decoction and drying is repeated 21 times. Patients were selected after Barium meal, X-ray, and the history of their disease. Normal diet was advised with restrictions on sour, fried, and very spicy food, large quantities of rice and pulses. In cases of intolerable pain, a bland diet of milk and unleavened bread *(chapattis)* was advised. The duration of the complaint ranged from 6 weeks to 12 years. It was found that there was marked relief from pain within 2-10 days of treatment in 82 percent of the cases. There was also relief in other symptoms like pyrosis, flatulence, reduced appetite, constipation, vomiting, hemetemesis, and melena in a majority of cases.

Amalaki fruits are considered safe and have been used for a very long time in India, for their health benefits, in the form of food items like pickles, dried fruit powder mixed in yogurt, or just preserved in honey. In long-term trials a few patients complained of loose motions and nausea, which was controlled without stopping the drug, attributable to the known laxative effect of the *amalaki*.[19] The acute and sub-acute toxicity of *Emblica officinalis* has neither revealed any toxic effect nor was any toxic effect seen on liver and kidney, and it improved the phagocytic and killing capacity of monocytes and poly-morphonuclear cells.[21] No cellular toxicity was seen when added to fresh sheep erythrocytes.[22] The aqueous extract showed potent antimutagenic activity in vitro.[23]

Musa sapientum *L. var. paradisiaca (Family: Musaceae)*

Sanskrit: Kadali	Tamil: Vazhai
Hindi: Kela	English: Banana, plantain

Musa sapientum var. paradisiaca is cultivated throughout India for culinary use. The unripe fruits are commonly cooked and eaten as a vegetable in India. They are also considered to be useful for gastric disorders.[24]

Both raw and ripe banana skin and pulp contain 5-hydroxy-tryptamine, with maximum content in raw fruit pulp.[25] The pulp is rich in flavonoids, mostly leucoanthocyanidins especially leucodel-phinidin and leucocyanidin.[26] Leucocyanidin obtained from the pulp has been shown to exhibit a significant protective effect against aspirin-induced ulcers.[27]

Banana's antiulcerogenic effect in different small animal models has been summarized[28]—those using histamine in guinea pigs[25,29] and mice,[30] phenylbutazone-induced gastric ulcers in guinea pigs,[31,32] in restraint ulcers in rats,[33,34] aspirin-induced gastric ulcer in rats[35,36] and those using Thai *Musa* species.[37]

Banana powder presumably acts by strengthening the mucosal resistance against ulcerogens[28,38] and promotes healing by inducing cell proliferation[28] and increasing cellular mucus.[38] To obtain an active powder, drying of the pulp is best done below 40°C.[27] An active extract is obtained by extraction with water[27,35] or aqueous alcohol[35] at temperatures below 50°C, beyond which activity is lost. The aqueous extract is rich in leucocyanidin, which is an active compound.[27] Other components of green banana like pectin and phosphatidyl choline may protect the gastric mucosa by adding strength to the mucous phospholipid layer.[36] An ethanol extract increases eicosanoids accumulation in human gastric mucosa.[39] The anti-ulcerative activity of banana is influenced by the type of soil, season, maturity and species.[40]

An open clinical trial carried out on 24 peptic ulcer patients (2 gastric and 22 duodenal ulcer) with radiologically or endoscopically confirmed diagnosis. Banana powder at a dose level of 1 g four times a day was given half an hour before meals for 12 weeks. A total of 19 patients completed the treatment. Of the patients 84 percent showed symptomatic relief.[41] In a double-blind, multicentric study, there was complete healing in 70 percent patients as determined endoscopically compared to 40 percent in the placebo group. In the treatment group, 24 percent showed partial healing, whereas no partial healing was observed in the placebo group.[42]

Green bananas are commonly eaten as a vegetable in India and are considered to be safe without any adverse effects. There appear to be no specific studies on the toxicity of the fruit although some information is available on the leaf and stem alkali.[43]

NOTES

1. Andrew HS. Medical treatment of peptic ulcer disease. *J Am Med Assoc* 275:622-629 (1996).

2. Singh KP, Singh RH. Recent advances in the management of *amlapitta-parinama sula* (non-ulcer dyspepsia and peptic ulcer disease). *J Res Ayur Siddha* 6(2):132-147 (1985).

3. Sharma PC, Yelne MB, Dennis TJ (eds.). *Database on medicinal plants used in Ayurveda* (vol. I, pp. 418-430). New Delhi: Central Council for Research in Ayurveda and Siddha, 2000.

4. Dahanukar S, Thatte U, Pai N, More PB, Karandikar SM. Protective effects of *Asparagus racemosus* against induced abdominal sepsis. *Indian Drugs* 24:125-128 (1986).

5. Nanal BP, Sharma BN, Ranade SS, Nande CV. Clinical study of *shatavari (Asparagus racemosus)*. *J Res Indian Med* 9(3):23-29 (1974).

6. Singh KP, Singh RH. Clinical trial on *Satavari (Asparagus racemosus* Willd.) in duodenal ulcer disease. *J Res Ayur Siddha* 7(3-4):91-100 (1986).

7. Kishore P, Pandey PN, Pandey SN, Dash S. Treatment of duodenal ulcer with *Asparagus racemosus. J Res Ayur Siddha* 1:409-416 (1980).

8. Bharti , Maheshwari CM, Tewari SK. A clinical study of *parinamsula* and its treatment with *Satavari* (*Asparagus racemosus* Willd.). *Ancient Sci Life* 15:162-165 (1996).

9. Dalvi SS. Nadkarni PM, Gupta KC. Effect of *Asparagus racemosus* (*shatavari*) on gastric emptying time in normal healthy volunteers. *J Postgrad Med* 36:91-94 (1990).

10. Pande TN, Rajagopalan SS. Comparative study of three regimen containing *satavari* on *amlapitta* (acid dyspepsia with or without ulcer). *J Res Ayur Siddha* 15:23-24 (1994).

11. *Selected medicinal plants of India* (pp. 43-46). Bombay: Chemexcil. Basic Chemicals, Pharmaceuticals and Cosmetics Export Promotion Council of India, 1992.

12. Rege NN, Thatte UM, Dahanukar SA. Adaptogenic properties of six *rasayana* herbs used in Ayurvedic medicine. *Phytother Res* 13:275-291 (1999).

13. *Indian herbal pharmacopoeia* (rev. new edn., pp. 214-222). Mumbai: Indian Drug Manufacturers' Association, 2002.

14. Sharma PC, Yelne MB, Dennis TJ (eds.). *Database on medicinal plants used in Ayurveda* (vol. 3, pp. 11-56). New Delhi: Central Council for Research in Ayurveda and Siddha, 2001.

15. Ghosal S, Tripathi VK, Chauhan S. Active constituents of *Emblica officinalis:* Part I—The chemistry and antioxidative effects of two new hydrolysable tannins—Emblicanin A and B. *Indian J Chem* 35B:941-948 (1996).

16. Mathew SM, Rao SB, Nair GR, Nair CRS. Anti-ulcer activity of *amla* extract. *International seminar on recent trends in pharmaceutical sciences* (Abstract no A7). Ootacamund, 18-20 February, 1995.

17. Pakrashi A, Bandopadhyay S. Effect of *Phyllanthus emblica* extract on peptic ulcer. *Phytomedicine* 3 (suppl. 1):66 (1996).

18. Singh BN, Sharma PV. Effect of *amalaki* on *amlapitta. J Res Indian Med* 5:223-229 (1971).

19. Chawla YK, Dubey P, Singh R, Nundy S, Tandon BN. Treatment of dyspepsia with *amalaki* (*Emblica officinalis* Linn)—An Ayurvedic drug. *Indian J Med Res* 76 (suppl.):95-98 (1982).

20. Varma MD, Singh RH, Gupta JP, Udupa KN. *Amalaki rasayana* in the treatment of chronic peptic ulcer. *J Indian Med Yoga Homeo* 12(4):1-9 (1977).

21. Rege NN, Thatte UM, Dahanukar SA. Adaptogenic properties of six *rasayana* herbs used in Ayurvedic medicine. *Phytother Res* 13:275-291 (1999).

22. Ahmad I, Mehmood Z, Mohammad F. Screening of some Indian medicinal plants for their antimicrobial properties. *J Ethnopharmacol* 62:183-193 (1998).

23. Sharma N, Trikha P, Athar M, Raisuddin S. In vitro inhibition of carcinogen-induced mutagenicity by *Cassia occidentalis* and *Emblica officinalis. Drug Chem Toxicol* 23:477-484 (2000).

24. *The wealth of India, raw materials* (vol. VI, pp. 452-468). New Delhi: Publications and Information Directorate, CSIR, 1962.

25. Sinha SN, Sanyal AK, Sinha YK. Some observations on 5-hydroxy-tryptamine content of edible fruits and vegetables and its effect on gastric acidities. *Indian J Med Res* 49:681-687 (1961).

26. Simmonds NW. Anthocyanins in banana. *Nature* 173:402-403 (1954).

27. Lewis DA, Fields WN, Shaw GP. A natural flavonoid present in unripe plantain banana pulp (*Musa sapientum* L. var *paradisiaca*) protects the gastric mucosa from aspirin induced erosions. *J Ethnopharmacol* 65:283-288 (1999).

28. Goel RK, Gupta S, Shankar R, Sanyal AK. Anti–ulcerogenic effect of banana powder (*Musa sapientum* var. *paradisiaca*) and its effect on mucosal resistance. *J Ethnopharmacol* 18:33-44 (1986).

29. Sanyal AK, Das PK, Sinha S, Sinha YK. Banana and gastric secretion (letters to the editor). *J Pharm Pharmacol* 13:318-319 (1961).

30. Elliot RC, Heward GJF. The effect of a banana supplemented diet on gastric ulcers in mice. *Pharmacol Res Commun* 8:167-171 (1976).

31. Sanyal AK, Gupta KK, Chowdhury NK. Banana and experimental peptic ulcer (letters to the editor). *J Pharm Pharmacol* 15:283-284 (1963).

32. Sanyal AK, Gupta KK, Chowdhury NK. Studies in peptic ulceration part I—Role of banana in phenylbutazone induced ulcers. *Arch Int Pharmacodyn Ther* 149:393-400 (1964).

33. Sanyal AK, Banerjee CR, Das PK. Banana and restraint ulcers in albino rats (letters to the editor). *J Pharm Pharmacol* 15:775-776 (1963).

34. Sanyal AK, Banerjea CR, Das PK, Studies in peptic ulceration part II—Role of banana in restraint and prednisolone induced ulcer in albino rats. *Arch Int Pharmacodyn Ther* 155:244-248 (1965).

35. Best R, Lewis DA, Nasser N. The anti-ulcerogenic activity of the unripe plantain banana (*Musa* species). *Br J Pharmacol* 82:107-116 (1984).

36. Dunjic BS, Svensson I, Axelson J, Adlercreutz P, Ar'rajab A, Larsson K, Bengmark S. Green banana protection of gastric mucosa against aspirin induced injuries in rats. A multicomponent mechanism? *Scand J Gastroenterol* 28:894-898 (1993).

37. Pannangpetch P, Vuttivirojana A, Kularbkaew C, Tesana S, Kongyingyoes B, Kukongviriyapan V. The antiulcerative effect of Thai *Musa* species in rats. *Phytother Res* 15:407-410 (2001).

38. Mukhopadhyaya K, Bhattacharya D, Chakraborty A, Goel RK, Sanyal AK. Effect of banana powder (*Musa sapientum var. paradisiaca*) on gastric mucosal shedding. *J Ethnopharmacol* 21:11-19 (1987).

39. Goel RK, Tavares IA, Bennet A. Stimulation of gastric and colonic mucosal eicosanoid synthesis by plantain banana. *J Pharm Pharmacol* 41:747-750 (1989).

40. Goel RK, Chakrabarti A, Sanyal AK. The effect of biological variables on the anti-ulcerogenic effect of vegetable plantain banana. *Planta Med* 51:85-88 (1985).

41. Goel RK. Effect of vegetable banana on gastric secretion—An experimental and clinical study, PhD thesis. Varanasi, India: Banaras Hindu University, 1983.

42. Das PK, Dasgupta G, Mishra AK. Clinical studies on medicinal plants of India. In Dhawan BN (ed.), *Current research on medicinal plants of India* (pp. 72-86). New Delhi: Indian National Science Academy, 1986.

43. Satyavati GV, Gupta AK, Tandon N (eds.). *Medicinal plants of India* (vol. 2, pp. 299-303). New Delhi: Indian Council of Medical Research, 1987.

OTHER ANTIULCER PLANTS

The exploratory clinical evaluation of some other plants at Banaras Hindu University have been summarized.[1] Thus *Adhatoda vasica, Eclipta alba,* and *Glycyrrhiza glabra* have been tried out on small groups of patients.

Adhatoda vasica *Nees (Family: Acanthaceae)*

Latin: *Adhatoda zeylanica* Medicus, *Justicia adhatoda* Linn.	Hindi: Arusa
Sanskrit: Vasa	Tamil: Adhatodai
English: Malabar Nut Tree	

The leaves of *Adhatoda vasica* or *vasa* are widely used for the treatment of cough, cold, and asthma (see Chapter 5, "Respiratory tract drugs"). The plant is reputed in Ayurveda for use in bleeding disorders and hence it was tried out in cases of *"amlapitta,"* which was earlier explicated as nonulcer acid dyspepsia in modern parlance.[2] Thus 20 patients of hyperacidity and hyperchlorhydria were treated as in-patients and given *vasa* as a syrup—three teaspoons four times a day equivalent to 30 g per day of crude drug in four divided doses for 6 weeks. Symptoms were carefully recorded. There was clinical improvement and reduction in the free and total gastric acidity, with 85 percent responding "well" to treatment. The assessment was that 7 patients were cured and 10 improved, whereas 3 remained unchanged.[3]

Eclipta alba *(Linn.) Hassk (Family: Asteraceae)*

Latin: *Eclipta erecta* Linn, *Eclipta prostrata* Linn.	Hindi: Bhangra
Sanskrit: Bhringaraja, Kesharaja	Tamil: Karasalanganni
English: Trailing eclipta	

This plant is well known in Ayurveda for its hepatoprotective activity and has been covered in Chapter 4 "Hepatoprotective agents." *Eclipta alba* juice is used as a soaking agent in various Ayurvedic antiulcer preparations. A series of studies were conducted in Banaras Hindu University to evaluate the efficacy of the drug in nonulcer dyspepsia and duodenal ulcer.

In an exploratory study, 22 patients with nonulcer dyspepsia and 8 patients with duodenal ulcer were given *Eclipta alba* whole plant as a syrup in a dose of 20 ml·day^{-1} (from 20 g crude drug) in two divided doses for 6 weeks. Of dyspeptic patients 90 percent were cured and improvement was seen in 87 percent of ulcer patients.[4]

As a result of these findings, 60 patients were given 30 g of the whole-plant powder in three divided doses. Thus 35 cases of nonulcer dyspepsia received the drug for a period of 1 month and 25 patients with duodenal ulcer were administered the drug for a period of 3 months. Most of the patients showed marked symptomatic relief. Patients with nonulcer dyspepsia were relieved of epigastric pain, nausea, and throat burning, whereas patients with peptic ulcer were relieved of nocturnal pain, acid reflex and nausea. Both groups showed significant reduction in gastric acidity with 80 percent of patients with nonulcer dyspepsia showing good response. Radiological improvement was observed in 75 percent of patients who were followed up. It was assessed that excellent results were obtained with 48 percent of patients with duodenal ulcer.[5] However, considering the small number of patients, the large dosage of 30 g of drug used, and given the fact that *Eclipta alba* contains wedelolactone that is a potent 5-lipoxygenase inhibitor, further studies are needed to evaluate the usefulness of the drug.[6] Subsequently, in another study the same dosage of 30 g of whole-plant powder was given to 35 cases with duodenal ulcer for a period of 3-6 months and found to be effective in 60 percent of the cases.[7]

Glycyrrhiza glabra *Linn. (Family: Fabaceae)*

Sanskrit: Yashtimadhu	Tamil: Atimadhuram
Hindi: Mulethi	English: Liquorice, licorice

Rhizomes and roots of *Glycyrrhiza glabra* are commonly used in Ayurveda in cough remedies, skin preparations, and in combination with other plants for the treatment of ulcer. The drug is approved in the *Indian Herbal Pharmacopoeia, 2002,* for its anti-inflammatory activity and its antiulcer effect.[8] The major constituents[9,10] are the triterpenoid glycyrrhizin, which is the sweet-tasting calcium and potassium salt of glycyrrhizic acid and numerous flavonoids, of which liquiritin is the major constituent that on hydrolysis yields liquiritigenin and isoliquiritigenin.

In a study on 10 cases of nonulcer dyspepsia and 15 cases of peptic ulcer, 2 g of drug powder was given thrice daily for 1 month to the nonulcer dyspepsia group and 3 g thrice a day was given for 3 months to the peptic ulcer group. There was considerable symptomatic improvement and reduction in gastric acidity. In the nonulcer dyspepsia group, 30 percent showed excellent response and 30 percent showed good response. Most patients of peptic ulcer showed more than 50 percent radiological improvement, in addition to reduction in duodenal spasm and other symptomatic improvement.[11,12]

Extracts of *Glycyrrhiza glabra* were tested for antiulcerogenic activity against indomethacin-induced gastric ulcers in rats and their antisecretory and cytoprotective activity. The extract showed a dose-dependent antiulcerogenic activity associated with a reduced acid output and an increased mucin secretion, an increase in prostaglandin E_2 release and a decrease in leukotriene. It has been suggested that the cytoprotective effect may be due to the flavonoids present, which act as free radical scavengers.[13] The flavonoids glabridin and glabrene inhibited in vitro the growth of *Helicobacter pylori*.[14]

The use of *Glycyrrhiza glabra* can cause water retention, edema, and an increase in the blood pressure because of its corticosteroidal effect. This effect is due to deficiency or inhibition of 11-β-hydroxysteroid dehydrogenase,[15] an enzyme that catalyzes conversion of cortisol to cortisone, by a metabolite of glycyrrhetinic acid, 3-monoglcuronylglycyrrhetinic acid,[16] as a result of which cortisol levels increase in the kidney. In other parts of the world the use of deglycyrrhinated licorice (with glycyrrhizin removed) is preferred for the treatment of ulcers. Its use is not recommended for patients with high blood pressure, heart disease, and diabetes, problems with the kidney or liver, and for periods exceeding 4-6 weeks. Recommended average daily doses of crude root range from 5 to15 g corresponding to 200-800 mg of glycyrrhizin.[17] In Ayurveda licorice is generally combined with other plants in antiulcer preparations and therefore dosage is reduced to lower and hence safer levels.

This was also noted in the trial of Revers,[18] who noted that 20 percent of peptic ulcer patients treated with a paste containing 40 percent licorice suffered from edema, which disappeared on discontinuation of the drug.

NOTES

1. Singh KP, Singh RP. Recent advances in the management of *amlapitta-parinam sula* (non-ulcer dyspepsia and peptic ulcer disease). *J Res Ayur Siddha* 6:132-147 (1985).

2. Chaturvedi GN, Mohan K, Ariyawansa HAS. Clinical correlation of *amlapitta* and its treatment with indigenous drug *vasa (Adhatoda vasica* Nees). *Nagarjun* XXIV (8):170-174 (1981).

3. Chaturvedi GN, Rai NP, Dhani R, Tiwari SK. Clinical trial of *Adhatoda vasica* syrup *(vasa)* in patients of non-ulcer dyspepsia *(amlapitta). Ancient Sci Life* III (1):19-23 (1983).

4. Dhani R, Chaturvedi GN. Studies of effect of certain Ayurvedic drugs on gastric secretion *(Bhringaraja-Eclipta alba-Soota Shekara Rasa).* D.Ay. M. thesis, Varanasi: Department of Kayachikitsa, Institute of Medical Sciences, Banaras Hindu University, 1976.

5. Tiwari SK, Gupta JP, Chaturvedi GN. Comparative studies on gastroduodenal diseases *(amlapitta and parinama sula)* in Ayurveda and modern medicine with therapeutic evaluation of *Bhringaraja (Eclipta alba)* in peptic ulcer and non-ulcer dyspepsia. PhD thesis. Varanasi: Department of Kayachikitsa, Institute of Medical Sciences, Banaras Hindu University, 1979.

6. Wagner H, Fessler B. In-vitro-5-Lipoxygenasehemmung durch *Eclipta alba* Extrakte und das Coumestan–Derivat Wedelolacton. *Planta Med* 52:374-377 (1986).

7. Rai NP, Tripathi SN, Gupta P. A clinical study on peptic ulcer with special reference to population survey, human constitution studies and drug trial. PhD thesis. Varanasi: Department of Kayachikitsa, Institute of Medical Sciences, Banaras Hindu University, 1984.

8. *Indian herbal pharmacopoeia* (rev. new edn., pp. 243-253). Mumbai: Indian Drug Manufacturers' Association, 2002.

9. Pandey VN, Malhotra SC. Eds. *Phytochemical investigations of certain medicinal plants used in Ayurveda* (pp. 232-236). New Delhi: Central Council for Research in Ayurveda and Siddha, 1990.

10. Wagner H. *Pharmazeutische Biologie 2. Drogen und ihre Inhaltsstoffe* (4th edn., pp. 159, 249). Stuttgart: Gustav Fischer Verlag, 1988.

11. Prasad M, Gupta JP, Chaturvedi GN. Clinical and experimental studies on *Yastimadhu (Glycyrrhiza glabra)* in non-ulcer dyspepsia. MD (Ay) thesis. Varanasi: Department of Kayachikitsa, Institute of Medical Sciences, Banaras Hindu University, 1978.

12. Chaturvedi GN, Mahadeo Prasad, Agrawal AK, Gupta JP. Some clinical and experimental studies on whole roots of *Glycyrrhiza glabra* Linn. *(Yastimadhu)* in peptic ulcer. *Indian Med Gazz* 113:200-205 (1979).

13. Khayyal MT, el-Ghazaly MA, Kenawy SA, Seif-el-Nasr M, Mahran LG, Kafafi YA, Okpanyi SN. Anti-ulcerogenic effect of some gastrointestinally acting plant extracts and their combination. *Arzneimittelforsch* 51:545-553 (2001).

14. Fukai T, Marumo A, Kaitou K, Kanda T, Terada S, Nomura T. Anti-*Helicobacter pylori* flavonoids from licorice extract. *Life Sci* 71:1449-1463 (2002).

15. Stewart PM, Wallace AM, Valentino R, Burt D, Shackleton CHL, Edwards CRW. Mineral corticosteroid activity of liquorice: 11-beta-hydroxysteroid dehydrogenase deficiency comes of age. *Lancet* ii:821-823 (1987).

16. Kato H, Kanaoka M, Yano S, Kobayashi M. 3-Monoglucuronyl-glycyrrhetinic acid is a major metabolite that causes licorice-induced pseudoaldosteronism. *J Clin Endocrinol Metab* 80:1929-1930 (1995).

17. *WHO monographs on selected medicinal plants* (vol. 1, pp. 183-194). Geneva: World Health Organization, 1999.

18. Revers FE. Heeft succus liquiritae een genezender werking op demaagzweer? *Ned Tydschr Geneskd* 90:135-137 (1946).

INFLAMMATORY BOWEL DISEASE

Ulcerative colitis and Crohn's disease are two chronic inflammatory bowel diseases whose incidence is increasing in the West. Seen mostly in young adults,[1] it is the cause of much morbidity. It is believed that the increased formation of the inflammatory mediators known as leukotrienes plays an important role in causing and maintaining chronic inflammation. Therefore attempts have been made to find specific inhibitors of leukotriene synthesis. However, such products, on evaluation showed unsuitable attributes like poor bioavailability, susceptibility to oxidation, side effects and were toxic.[2] The gum resin of the tree *Boswellia serrata,* shown to be a specific inhibitor of leukotriene synthesis, is used in Ayurveda in a variety of inflammatory conditions.[3]

Boswellia serrata *Roxb. ex Coleb (Family: Burseraceae)*

Latin: *Boswellia glabra* Roxb.	Hindi: *Salai guggul*
Sanskrit: Sallaki	Tamil: Parangi sambrani
English: Indian Frankincense, Indian Olibanum	

Boswellia serrata or *salai guggul* (see Plate 2 in color gallery) is a medium-sized, deciduous tree that grows to a height of 17 m found throughout India in the dry hilly forests. The gum resin is found under the bark and is obtained by peeling the bark or by making an incision and allowing the gum to flow out, which is collected after 1 month.[4] The gum resin from the tree has been prescribed in Ayurveda for a variety of inflammatory conditions. It is used in rheumatism, skin diseases, asthma, diarrhea, and dysentery, etc.[5,6]

The gum resin contains essential oil, terpenoids, and gum. The active portion of the gum resin are the boswellic acids—β-boswellic acid, acetyl-β-boswellic acid, and especially what are now considered the main active principles 11-keto-β-boswellic acid and acetyl-11-keto-β-boswellic acid.[7]

In Ayurveda, *salai guggul* is considered to be a useful anti-inflammatory and antiarthritic drug. The gum resin shows a potent analgesic and sedative effect in small animals.[8] The alcoholic extract of *salai guggul* has a marked anti-inflammatory effect in rats and mice.[9] The alcoholic extract, as shown later by Ammon *et al.*, inhibits formation of leukotriene B4 (LTB4) and other 5-lipoxygenase products in isolated rat peritoneal neutrophils.[10] The boswellic acids more specifically acetyl-11-keto-β-boswellic acid (AKBA) was found to be the most active in inhibiting leukotriene synthesis.[7] They act by binding to a pentacyclic triterpene selective effector site, thereby inhibiting 5-lipoxygenase, and in turn inhibiting the synthesis of leukotrienes, while having no action on the synthesis of prostaglandins.[11] Apart from the inhibition of leukotriene synthesis, there is inhibition of leukocyte elastase, which causes damage in arthritis.[12] In an experimental model of inflammatory bowel disease in rats, *Boswellia* extract or AKBA was seen to cause significant reduction of inflammation associated with indomethacin administration.[13] In addition, boswellic acids have been shown to inhibit the complement system, which is another inflammatory mediator.[14]

Boswellic acids are selective and specific inhibitors of leukotriene synthesis. Therefore, they can be useful in a number of disease conditions in which increased leukotriene formation is considered to cause and perpetuate inflammation, for example polyarthritis and bronchial asthma, and inflammatory bowel diseases like Crohn's disease, chronic colitis, and ulcerative colitis. They have also been used to treat edema associated with certain brain tumors like astrocytoma and glioma.

These conditions have been clinically evaluated and are covered in the relevant chapter. Crohn's disease, ulcerative colitis, and chronic colitis are covered in this chapter. Asthma is covered in Chapter 5, arthritis is covered in Chapter 8 "Anti-rheumatic agents," and the brain tumor edema trials are covered in Chapter 13. Other disease conditions in which enhanced leukotriene synthesis plays a role are psoriasis, urticaria, allergic rhinitis, multiple sclerosis, lupus erthyromatosus, myocardial ischemia, and muscividosis. These have not yet been clinically evaluated.

Crohn's disease

In a randomized double blind trial,[15] 102 patients were treated with the *Boswellia* extract H15 or mesalazine for 8 weeks. A detailed history was recorded before start of the trial and clinical symptoms and laboratory parameters were noted. Patients also maintained a diary regarding their health, stool frequency and consistency, and occurrence of stomach pain based on which their status was evaluated using Crohn Disease Activity (CDA) index. Eighty-three patients completed the study, of which 44 patients received one 400 mg tablet containing a standardized *Boswellia serrata* extract three times a day. In the comparative group, 33 patients received thrice daily 1,500 mg mesalazine. Patients were followed up every 2 weeks by checking the diary entries and by determination of the CDA index.

The improvement in the CDA index was definitely better in the case of the *Boswellia serrata* extract, however, when computed statistically, was not significant. The side-effect profile of *Boswellia serrata* was better than mesalazine, with four infections in the case of *Boswellia serrata* as compared to eight with mesalazine. Considering that treatment with mesalazine is considered state-of-the-art treatment for Crohn's disease and that the *Boswellia* extract is as good as mesalazine, with a better side-effect profile, treatment with *Boswellia* extract H15 must be evaluated better than mesalazine based on the favorable benefit-risk advantage that it offers.

There are certain other substances in *Salai guggul* that enhance leukotriene synthesis and worsen the clinical picture. Therefore, the intake of *Salai guggul* extracts needs to be supervised by a doctor. In addition, there is in vitro evidence that there is a concentration-dependent inhibition or potentiation of 5-lipoxygenase.[16]

Ulcerative colitis

Ulcerative colitis is a nonspecific chronic inflammatory disease of the bowel, which can attack the entire colon from the rectum upwards. Usually, however, it is the lateral part of the intestines that is affected. With no cure, episodes of acute phase alternate with periods of remission. The disease is characterized by blood in the stools, pain, etc. It is treated with steroids in the acute phase and 5-aminosalicylic acid derivatives in the remission phase and also during the acute phase.[17]

In an open study, patients with ulcerative colitis grade II and III were treated with 350 mg *Boswellia serrata* extract thrice daily or 1 g sulfasalazine thrice daily for 6 weeks. There was marked reduction in loose motions, mucous in stool, blood in stool, and abdominal pain. Improvement was also seen in the inflammatory appearance of the intestinal mucosa—in crypts, abscess, and erosion of the mucosa. A total of 30 patients were examined in the *Boswellia* group. Results in both arms of the trial were comparable, with 82 percent remission in the resin group and 75 percent in the sulfasalazine group.[18]

Chronic colitis

Chronic colitis is a variant of ulcerative colitis characterized by vague lower abdominal pain, rectal bleeding with diarrhea, and tender palpable colon. In an open nonrandomized clinical trial, 30 patients with chronic colitis were included in the study. Twenty patients received 300 mg of a preparation from *Boswellia serrata* gum resin thrice daily for 6 weeks, and ten patients received 1 g of sulfasalazine thrice daily for 6 weeks and served as controls. Of the 20 patients on *Boswellia* 18 showed improvement, while in the control group six out of ten patients showed improvement. The remission rate was 14 out of 20 for *Boswellia* and it was four out of ten in the sulfasalazine group.[19]

The LD_{50} of an alcoholic extract was greater than 2 $g \cdot kg^{-1}$ body weight. No significant effect was seen on the cardiovascular, respiratory, and central nervous systems.[10] In a chronic study with controls on monkeys using the defatted alcoholic extract of *Boswellia serrata* at three dose levels, namely at two, five, and ten times the ED_{50} for 6 months, was found not to produce any biochemical, hematological, and histopathological toxicity.[20] In a small percentage of patients, gastrointestinal side effects like heart burn and hyperacidity are seen that increase with increasing dosage.[21] Also seen is skin irritation.[21]

In the clinical study on ulcerative colitis with a dose of 350 mg thrice daily for 6 weeks 6 patients out of 34 patients complained of heart burn and loss of appetite. In the bronchial asthma trial (see Chapter 5) with 300 mg thrice daily 2 out of 40 patients complained of epigastric pain, nausea and hyperacidity. In the glioblastoma trial (see Chapter 13, section "Cancer therapy," note 18) with increased dosages up to 1,200 mg thrice daily some patients complained of nausea and vomiting and two patients complained of skin irritation, which was reversible on stoppage. In the trial with children, no side effects were seen when they received a maximum dose of 126 $mg \cdot kg^{-1}$ bodyweight (see Chapter 13, section "Cancer therapy," note 20) and also in the trial of Streffer[21] (see also Chapter 13, section "Cancer therapy," note 19).

NOTES

1. Ditzel P, Hellwig B. Entzündliche Darmerkrankungen. Morbus Crohn and Colitis ulcerosa. *Deutsche Apoth Ztg* 136:2070-2071 (1996).

2. Safayhi H, Boden SE, Schweizer S, Ammon HPT. Concentration-dependent potentiating and inhibitory effects of *Boswellia* extracts on 5-lipoxygenase product

formation in stimulated PMNL. *Planta Med* 66:110-113 (2000) and references cited therein.

3. Ammon HPT. Ayurveda—Arzneimittel aus indischer Kultur. *Z Phytotherap* 22:136-142 (2001).

4. *The wealth of India, raw materials* (vol. 2, pp. 203-209). New Delhi: Publications and Information Directorate, CSIR, 1988.

5. Sharma PV. *Classical uses of medicinal plants* (pp. 361-362). Varanasi: Chaukhambha Visvabharati, 1996.

6. Chopra RN, Nayar SL, Chopra IC. *Glossary of Indian medicinal plants* (p. 39). New Delhi: Publications and Information Directorate, CSIR, 1986.

7. Safayhi H, Mack T, Sabieraj J, Anazodo M, Subramanian LR, Ammon HPT. Boswellic acids: Novel, specific, non-redox inhibitors of 5-lipoxygenase. *J Pharmacol Exp Ther* 261:1143-1146 (1992).

8. Menon MK, Kar A. Analgesic and psychopharmacological effects of the gum resin of *Boswellia serrata*. *Planta Med* 19:333-341 (1971).

9. Singh GB, Atal CK. Pharmacology of an extract of *salai guggal* ex—*Boswellia serrata*, a new non-steroidal anti-inflammatory agent. *Agents Actions* 18:407-412 (1986).

10. Ammon HPT, Mack T, Singh GB, Safayhi H. Inhibition of leukotriene B$_4$ formation in rat peritoneal neutrophils by an ethanolic extract of the gum resin exudate of *Boswellia serrata*. *Planta Med* 57:203-207 (1991).

11. Safayhi H, Sailer ER, Ammon HPT. Mechanism of 5-lipoxygenase inhibition by acetyl-11-keto-β-boswellic acid. *Mol Pharmacol* 47:1212-1216 (1995).

12. Safayhi H, Rall B, Sailer ER, Ammon HPT. Inhibition of boswellic acids of human leukocyte elastase. *J Pharmacol Exp Ther* 281:460-463 (1997).

13. Kriegelstein CF, Anthoni C, Rijcken EJ, Laukötter M, Spiegel HU, Boden SE, Schweizer S, Safayhi H, Senninger N, Schürmann G. Acetyl-11-keto-β-boswellic acid, a constituent of a herbal medicine from *Boswellia serrata* resin, attenuates experimental ileitis. *Intl J Colorectal Dis* 16:88-95 (2001).

14. Wagner H, Kraus U, Jordan E. Pflanzeninhaltsstoffe mit Wirkung auf das Komplementsystem. *Z Phytotherap* 8:148-149 (1987).

15. Gerhardt H, Seifert F, Buvari P, Vogelsang H, Repges R. Therapie des aktiven Morbus Crohn mit *Boswellia-serrata*—Extrakt H 15. *Z. Gastroenterol* 39:11-17 (2001). Reprinted in *Z Phytotherapie* 22:69-75 (2001).

16. Safayhi H, Boden SE, Schweizer S, Ammon HPT. Concentration-dependent potentiating and inhibitory effects of *Boswellia* extracts on 5-lipoxygenase product formation in stimulated PMNL. *Planta Med* 66:110-113 (2000).

17. Baumgärtner M. Ein bewährtes Therapieprinzip in der Behandlung der Colitis ulcerosa. *Deutsche Apoth Ztg* 137:2918-2921 (1997).

18. Gupta I, Parihar A, Malhotra P, Singh GB, Lüdtke R, Safayhi H, Ammon HPT. Effects of *Boswellia serrata* gum resin in patients with ulcerative colitis. *Eur J Med Res* 2:37-43 (1997).

19. Gupta I, Parihar A, Malhotra P, Gupta S, Lüdtke R, Safayhi H, Ammon HPT. Effects of gum resin of *Boswellia serrata* in patients with chronic colitis. *Planta Med* 67:391-395 (2001).

20. Gupta VN, Yadav DS, Jain MP, Atal CK. Chemistry and pharmacology of gum resin of *Boswellia serrata (Salai guggal)*. *Indian Drugs* 24:221-231 (1987).

21. Ammon HPT. Boswelliasäuren (Inhaltstoffe des Weihrauchs) zur Behandlung chronisch entzündlicher Erkrankungen. *Med Monatssch Pharmazeut* 26:309-315 (2003) and references cited therein.

ANTIEMETIC AGENTS

Nausea and vomiting can arise from indigestion, motion sickness, as a side effect of medicines used in cancer chemotherapy, in pregnancy in the form of morning sickness, anticipatory nausea, infections, certain internal endocrinological and neurological disorders, and after surgery.[1] In allopathic medicine, depending on the cause of nausea, different drugs are employed. Some of the drugs used to combat nausea are antihistaminic in nature and therefore cause drowsiness and loss of alertness. However, ginger has been shown to have wide-ranging antiemetic effects, without these side effects.

Zingiber officinale *Roscoe (Family: Zingiberaceae)*

Sanskrit: Adraka (fresh), Sunthi (dry)	Tamil: Inji (fresh), sukku (dry)
Hindi: Adrak (fresh), sunth (dry)	English: Ginger

Ginger is widely used in Ayurveda for its antiemetic effects. Fresh ginger is cut into small bits and taken along with honey, or fresh ginger juice is combined with lime and/or lemon juice in the form of syrup and taken to treat morning sickness. There is concern in Germany that ginger could cause problems in pregnancy not only because of the reported mutagenicity of ginger in certain test systems[2] but also because of the possibility of testosterone binding.[3] There are also reports that ginger has antimutagenic potential.[2]

Motion and sea sickness

The first reports of the use of ginger in motion sickness, caused by a motorized revolving chair, observed that 940 mg of powdered ginger root proved more effective than 100 mg Dramamine (dimenhydrinate) in reducing the gastrointestinal effects of motion sickness without the drowsiness caused by Dramamine. The study concluded that ginger was acting directly on the gastrointestinal tract increasing gastrointestinal motility and absorption of neutralizing toxins and acids, and not by its central action on the vomiting center.[4]

The use of powdered ginger as a prophylactic in seasickness has been studied in a double-blind randomized study with 80 cadets. One gram of ginger powder as a single dose was statistically better than placebo in reducing the incidence of vomiting and cold sweating 4 hours after ingestion.[5] In another trial with 1,741 volunteers, ginger powder when compared with seven other OTC and prescription antiemetic drugs proved equally effective as the tested drugs.[6]

Other studies[7-10] that investigated the effect of ginger on motion sickness have been divided in their opinion as to the effectiveness of the prophylactic use of ginger root in preventing nausea and vomiting. The varying results could arise from the variable quality or, as has been suggested,[11] because of the different focus in the trials—thus trials, which looked at the gastrointestinal effects reported better results as compared with trials that looked at the response of the central nervous system.[11] Positive results have been obtained using a standardized ginger root powder in two double-blind studies[12,13] one trial being conducted in children in the age group of four to eight years, who were susceptible to motion sickness when travelling in a bus, train, or on the merry-go-round. Doses were varied from 250 to 500 mg of ginger depending upon the age of the children and given half an hour before travel and repeated if necessary every 4 hours.[13]

Hyperemesis gravidarum

In a double-blind randomized crossover trial 250 mg powdered ginger four times a day for 4 days was compared against placebo given in a similar capsule also four times a day to 30 patients suffering from severe morning sickness admitted to the hospital. Nineteen patients evaluated both on subjective and objective parameters showed that ginger was significantly better than placebo in reducing or eliminating the symptoms of hyperemesis gravidarum.[14]

Postoperative nausea

In two randomized double-blind studies, 60 and 120 patients, respectively, received before the operation, a single dose of 10 mg metoclopramide, placebo, or 0.5 g[15] or 1 g[16] powdered ginger, incidence of nausea and vomiting was reduced to similar extents in metoclopramide and ginger and much less when compared to placebo.[15,16] Also, patients receiving ginger needed fewer postoperative antiemetics.[16] However, another double-blind clinical study concluded that ginger prepared according to the British pharmacopoeia was ineffective in reducing postoperative nausea and vomiting.[17]

Drug-induced nausea

Psoralens are taken before undergoing photophoresis. In 11 patients who regularly experienced nausea after ingestion of 8-methoxypsoralen (8-MOP), were treated with three 530 mg capsules of ginger powder taken prior to administration of 8-MOP experienced significantly reduced nausea.[18]

In a randomized double-blind placebo-controlled trial with leukemia patients who regularly took prochlorperazine when undergoing chemotherapy, the addition of ginger reduced both the time and the intensity of nausea when taking prochlorperazine alone, although there was no difference in the vomiting.[19]

Cisplatin, which is used in cancer chemotherapy, induces nausea, vomiting, and delay in gastric emptying. Experimentally acetone and alcoholic extracts of ginger has been shown to significantly reduce cisplatin-induced nausea in dogs.[20] In rats, ginger juice, acetone and 50 percent ethanolic extract have been shown to significantly reverse cisplatin-induced gastric emptying, with the reversal caused by the acetone extract being similar to odansetron that is usually used for this purpose.[21]

NOTES

1. Wöhrle M. Antiemetika: Mittel zur Behandlung des Erbrechens. *Deutsche Apoth Ztg* 138:1753-1756 (1998).

2. Ernst E, Pittler MH. Efficacy of ginger for nausea and vomiting: A systematic review of randomized clinical trials. *Brit J Anaesthesia* 84:367-371 (2000) and references cited therein.

3. Backon J. Ginger in preventing nausea and vomiting of pregnancy: A caveat due to the thromboxane synthetase activity and effect on testosterone binding. [Letter]. *Eur J Obstet Gynec Reprod Biol* 42:163-164 (1991).

4. Mowrey DB, Clayson DE. Motion sickness, ginger and psychophysics. *Lancet* i:655-657 (1982).

5. Grøntved A, Brask T, Kambskard J, Hentzer E. Ginger root against seasickness. A controlled trial on the open sea. *Acta Otolaryngol* 105(1-2):45-49 (1988).

6. Schmid R, Schick T, Steffen R, Tschopp A, Wilk T. Comparison of seven commonly used agents for prophylaxis of seasickness. *J Travel Med* 1:203-206 (1994).

7. Stewart JJ, Wood MJ, Wood CD, Mims ME. Effects of ginger on motion sickness susceptibility and gastric function. *Pharmacol* 42:111-120 (1991).

8. Wood CD, Manno JE, Wood MJ, Manno BR, Mims ME. Comparison of efficacy of ginger with various antimotion sickness drugs. *Clin Res Pract & Drug Reg Affairs* 6:129-136 (1988).

9. Stott JRR, Hubble MP, Spencer MB. A double blind comparative trial of powdered ginger root, hyosine hydrobromide, and cinnarizine in the prophylaxis of motion sickness induced by cross coupled stimulation. *Advis Group Aerosp Res Dev, Conf Proc* 372 (39):1-6 (1985).

10. Holtmann S, Clarke AH, Scherer H, Höhn M. The anti-motion sickness mechanism of ginger: A comparative study with placebo and dimenhydrinate. *Acta Otolaryngol* 108:168-174 (1989).

11. *WHO monographs on selected medicinal plants* (vol. 1, pp. 277-287) Geneva: World Health Organization, 1999 and references cited therein.

12. Riebenfeld D, Borzone L. Randomized double-blind study comparing ginger (Zintona®) and dimenhydrinate in motion sickness. *Healthnotes Rev Complemen Integrat Med* 6:98-101 (1999).

13. Careddu P. Motion sickness in children: Results of a double blind study comparing ginger (Zintona®) and dimenhydrinate. *Healthnotes Rev Complemen Integrat Med* 6:102-107 (1999).

14. Fischer-Rasmussen W, Kjaer SK, Dahl C, Asping U. Ginger treatment of hyperemesis gravidarum. *Eur J Obstet Gynecol Reprod Biol* 38:19-24 (1990).

15. Bone ME, Wilkinson DJ, Young JR, McNeil J, Charlton S. Ginger root—A new antiemetic. The effect of ginger root on postoperative nausea and vomiting after major gynaecological surgery. *Anaesth* 45:669-671 (1990).

16. Phillips S, Ruggier RC, Hutchinson SE. *Zingiber officinale* (Ginger)—An antiemetic for day-case surgery. *Anaesth* 48:715-717 (1993).

17. Arfeen Z, Owen H, Plummer JL, Ilsley AH, Sorby-Adams RAC, Doecke LJ. A double-blind randomized controlled trial of ginger for postoperative nausea and vomiting. *Anaesth Intensive Care* 23:449-452 (1995).

18. Meyer K, Schwartz J, Crater D, Keyes B. *Zingiber officinale* (ginger) used to prevent 8-MOP associated nausea. *Dermatol Nurs* 7:242-244 (1995).

19. Pace JC. Oral ingestion of encapsulated ginger and reported self-care actions for the relief of chemotherapy-associated nausea and vomiting. *Diss Abstr Internat* 47:3297-B (1987).

20. Sharma SS, Kochupillai V, Gupta SK, Seth SD, Gupta YK. Antiemetic efficacy of ginger *(Zingiber officinale)* against cisplatin-induced emesis in dogs. *J Ethnopharmacol* 57:93-96 (1997).

21. Sharma SS, Gupta YK. Reversal of cisplatin-induced delay in gastric emptying in rats by ginger *(Zingiber officinale). J Ethnopharmacol* 62:49-55 (1998).

LAXATIVES

In Ayurveda it is considered important to maintain a healthy colon for which a number of laxatives are used. In fact, it is considered necessary to have a clean colon before attempting to administer drugs in order for drugs to be effective and especially before attempting the so-called rejuvenation treatment that has its own rules and regulations to be complied with. Thus before the actual process of rejuvenation is started there is a lengthy cleansing process that is undertaken. The most commonly used laxatives are psyllium seed and husk, senna leaves and pods, castor oil and chebulic myrobalan either by itself or together with belleric myrobalan and emblic myrobalan as the three fruit combination of *Terminalia chebula, Terminalia belerica,* and *Emblica officinalis,* known as *triphala.*

Cassia angustifolia *Vahl (Family: Caesalpiniaceae)*

Sanskrit: Markand	Tamil: Nilavari
Hindi: Sonamukhi	English: Indian senna, Tinnevely senna

Cassia angustifolia is a small shrub, which is grown for its leaves and pods that have a cathartic action, the pods having a milder effect than the leaves. The use of *Cassia angustifolia,* indigenous to North Africa, was introduced, by Arabian physicians, into Europe and India.[1] Interaction of Ayurvedic physicians with Unani physicians in medieval times led to the introduction of the plant into the Ayurvedic materia medica. The British introduced the plant for cultivation sometime in the early nineteenth century. It is cultivated extensively in South India, especially in the Tinnevely (Tirunelveli) district of Tamil Nadu, with estimates of 6,000 tons of senna leaves and pods being produced and exported.[2] Both leaves and pods are approved in the US and German pharmacopoeia, and several other pharmacopoeias for their laxative action. Apart from its laxative action, it is considered useful in Ayurveda for skin problems.[3]

Senna's laxative action is due to the anthraquinone glycosides present, mainly sennoside A and B, which are converted by the normal intestinal bacteria into the active constituent rhein anthrone, which stimulates peristalsis and evacuation.[4]

Clinical studies with standardized senna have shown its utility in long-term therapy of habitually constipated patients,[5] although it is presently recommended only for short-term treatment of constipation. Standardized senna preparation has also been tried in the treatment of constipation immediately after delivery[6] with average success rate of over 93-96 percent as compared to 51-59 percent with placebo. Mild cramping was seen in those treated with senna as compared to 4 percent with placebo. In this trial there was no evidence of the commonly held view that senna causes diarrhea in breastfed babies when the mother takes senna as laxative.

In combination with psyllium, senna (6.5 g + 1.5 g·day^{-1}) provided better relief (63 percent) as regards stool frequency and weight when compared to psyllium (7.2 g·day^{-1}; 48 percent).[7] In terminal cancer patients being treated with opioids, senna was found to be as effective as lactulose with similar adverse effect profile but senna was preferred because it was more cost effective.[8] In children below 15 years of age who were constipated, lactulose was preferred over senna. Twenty-one children in a crossover trial received either lactulose or senna in the first week followed by a wash-out period with no treatment and the alternative treatment in the third week. Normal stools were significantly better with lactulose and the side effects reported by senna were greater.[9]

Senna preparations have been found useful in readying patients for colonoscopy either by exclusively[10] or in addition to the usual lavage.[11] One study did not find any advantage in using senna.[12]

Senna pods cause less griping because of lower sennosides content. Other drugs of *Cassia* species like the fruit pulp of *Cassia fistula* are also used as laxative. It is considered a safe drug because of its milder action. This is due to the fact that it contains lower concentration of sennoside A and B, rhein and, other anthraquinones.[13] Senna is preferred for short-term therapy; long-term use is to be avoided because of the possible mutagenic role of anthraquinones.

Plantago ovata **Forsk.** *(Family: Plantaginaceae)*

Sanskrit: Ashwagola	Tamil: Ishappukol, Iskolvirai
Hindi: Isapghul, Isabgol	English: Psyllium or Plantago

Plantago ovata is a stemless, hairy, annual herb found growing in northwest India and cultivated in certain regions of Gujarat, Punjab, and Uttar Pradesh.[14] Indigenous to the Mediterranean region, it is not found in the early texts of Ayurveda, but was later introduced into India. It was first reported in the Ayurvedic text *Vaidyamrita* written in the late eighteenth century by Vaidyaraja Moneswara for the treatment of fever due to diarrhea, and subsequently finds mention in numerous Ayurvedic texts for treatment of intestinal complaints.[15] The seeds are listed in the *Indian Herbal Pharmacopoeia*, 2002, as a bulk forming laxative and antidiarrhoeal agent.[16] The seed husk is also used as a laxative since it separates readily from the seed and is the part which contains the mucilage.

Plantago ovata seeds contain 20-30 percent of mucilage, which is found in the outer seed coat or husk and is composed of arabin-oxylans. In addition, the seed contains fixed oil, protein, and small amounts of aucubin—an iridoid glycoside.[17,18] When the seeds are put in water, the mucilage swells rapidly and takes up several times its volume, the bulk helping peristalsis and evacuation. An unfermented gel component of the seed husk provides lubrication and thereby promotes laxation in humans.[19] The seed husk also contains an active principle-exhibiting acetylcholine-like action.[20]

A number of clinical studies have confirmed the mild laxative action of psyllium husk in the treatment of chronic constipation, irritable bowel syndrome, and constipation due to diverticulitis. An early open clinical study showed that 13.5 g of psyllium husk improved stool frequency in a 4-week study with 65 patients with an average stool frequency of less than three hard motions per week to 74 percent having a motion every 1-2 days after 4 weeks of treatment.[21]

Another placebo-controlled randomized 8-week study evaluated the effect of psyllium on stool characteristics, colon transit, and anorectal function in chronic idiopathic constipation. After a run-in period of 4 weeks, 22 patients were assigned to one of two groups—11 patients received 5 g psyllium twice a day, and 11 patients received placebo for 8 weeks. Patients maintained a diary to record daily stool frequency, difficulty in defecation, and weekly stool weight. There was significant improvement in stool frequency and stool weight. In addition there was improvement in stool consistency and pain on defecation.[22]

Other studies have compared psyllium alone (7.2 g) and a combination of senna and psyllium (1.5 + 6.5 g).[23] Both laxatives improved stool frequency and consistency. Objectively assessed on the basis of stool frequency and weight, laxation was achieved by 63 percent of the combination group, whereas with psyllium alone it was 48 percent. Psyllium has also been compared with lactulose[24] and methylcellulose,[25] docusate sodium[26] and with placebo.[27] *Isabgol* husk was effective for the treatment of simple constipation and achieved better stool consistency and fewer side effects when compared to lactulose.[24] Psyllium was also found superior to docusate sodium in laxative efficacy.[26]

In a double-blind crossover study in 26 patients with Irritable Bowel Syndrome (IBS) the effect of ispaghula husk was studied against placebo for 6 weeks.[28] Fifty percent of patients receiving ispaghula reported improvement as against 23 percent of patients who were on placebo. Results were better in patients with spastic colitis, little effect being seen in patients with mucous diarrhea. Another study with ispaghula in IBS in combination with *Aegle marmelos* and *Bacopa monnieri* is found under *Aegle marmelos* later in this chapter.

The long-term safety and tolerability of ispaghula husk was also studied in 93 healthy subjects for 52 weeks, the study dosage being 10.5 g per day as long-term treatment of hypercholesterolemia. The majority of adverse effects were of minor nature and of short duration.[29] However, the seeds contain allergenic protein that can cause allergic reactions by inhalation to the worker during processing of the product and also to the user when spooning the husk into the glass for consumption.[18,30] In the carefully prepared seed husk these proteins are absent. Occasionally, abdominal pain has been reported due to distention and flatulence. In cases of intestinal obstruction the use of psyllium is to be avoided.[18]

Ricinus communis *Linn. (Family: Euphorbiaceae)*

Sanskrit: Eranda	Tamil: Ammanaku
Hindi: Erand	English: Castor

Ricinus communis seed oil or castor oil has been used in Ayurveda since the time of Caraka and Sushruta as laxative and for the treatment of rheumatism. The oil is used externally for aching joints. When taken internally for constipation it also helps relieve joint pain and soothe the nervous system (See also Chapter 8 "Anti-inflammatory agents). Therefore, it is often added to formulations to treat pain, nervous disorders, and menstrual irregularities.[31] It has been a very commonly used household remedy as a laxative with one or two drops being given even to month-old infants as a laxative till its use fell into disrepute. Castor oil is listed as a stimulant cathartic, lactagogue, and antirheumatic in the *Indian herbal pharmacopoeia.*[32]

Castor grows throughout India. Two varieties are known—one with green stem and the other with red stem. The seed contains the highly poisonous lectin, ricin. The oil is cold-pressed below 40°C to prevent the toxic ricin from being carried over to the oil. The seed contains 40-50 percent oil, which is composed up to 80 percent of triricinolein, which is hydrolyzed in the small intestine to glycerol and ricinoleic acid, which is the laxative agent.[33] Ricinoleic acid increases fluid secretion, releases nitric oxide, increases mucosal permeability and cytotoxicity and disrupts normal intestinal motility.[34]

The oil is generally used only for a short duration with doses of 10-30 ml being used for adults. There are a number of trials confirming the efficacy of castor oil when given in doses of 15-60 ml and this has been reviewed.[35]

In a double-blind randomized study, the effectiveness of 0.6 g castor oil in soft gelatin capsules in doses of 1.2, 2.4, and 3.6 g per day was compared with 150 mg senna extract equivalent to 25 mg sennosides also in soft gelatin capsules. There were four runs of 1-week duration each and one to two washout periods. The aim of the study was to reach at least five motions per week with the minimum dose possible both for castor oil and for senna. In 15 patients (50 percent) bowel function was normalized with two castor oil capsules (1.2 g) per day, 13 patients required two capsules twice a day (2.4 g) to get the desired effect whereas in two patients the maximum dosage of 3.6 g was needed. With the senna extract (two capsules) 28 patients achieved normalization of bowel function. However, there were no side effects observed with castor oil capsules, whereas seven patients had cramps in the lower abdomen with senna. The stools were always of a soft well-formed mass with castor oil leading to a preference for the castor oil preparation.[36]

In another study, 75 doctors took part where the trial medication was 1 g castor oil in soft gelatin capsules. A total of 168 patients were observed up to 14 days each. A single intake of three to five capsules once in the morning was recommended. By the end of the observation period, the medication was evaluated by the participating doctors as being "good" to "very good" in 97 percent of patients.[37]

The safety and usage of castor oil has been extensively reviewed.[35] With normal dosages no side effects are observed; however, in sensitive individuals stomach irritation may arise and larger doses can give rise to nausea, vomiting, cramps, and purgation. With dosages of 2-3 ml in more than 200 patients no side effects were seen.[35]

Terminalia chebula *Retz. (Family: Combretaceae)*

Latin: *Terminalia reticulata* Roth, *T myrobalanus* Koeng	Hindi: Harad, Harar
Sanskrit: Haritaki	Tamil: Kaddukai
English: Chebulic myrobalan	

Terminalia chebula is a medium-sized tree found growing throughout India in deciduous forests. The drug consists of the dried rind of mature fruits; the color varies from yellowish brown to brown to black depending upon the source. The drug is approved in the *Indian Herbal Pharmacopoeia*, 2002, as a laxative and astringent.[38] The name *haritaki* is derived from the Sanskrit word *hara* (to conquer). The fruits are traditionally considered to be useful for a number of conditions: laxative, stomachic, and tonic.[39] The fruits are best known for their laxative properties either alone or in combination known as *triphala* or three fruits—with the fruits of embelic myrobalan or *Emblica officinalis* and belleric myrobalan or *Terminalia belerica*. Depending upon the dosage, *haritaki* is used as a laxative or to control diarrhea.

The fruit flesh is a rich source of tannins (32-34 percent).[39] Major constituents include polyphenolics such as chebulinic acid, chebulagic acid, chebulic acid, gallic acid, and ellagic acid and anthraquinones. Some of the other minor constituents include other polyphenolics like corilagin and galloylglucose, sugars like glucose and sorbitol, flavonoids, triterpene glycosides, amino acids, and some other acids.[38]

Haritaki is very widely used in Ayurveda as a laxative and has been shown clinically to be useful in cases of simple constipation.[40] Experimentally, *haritaki* has been shown to significantly increase gastric emptying[41-43] comparable to metoclopramide.[41] The laxative principle has variously been suggested to be the oil from the fruit[44] and an anthraquinone glycoside similar to sennoside A.[45]

In a preliminary trial, 10 patients were admitted as in-patients and underwent hematological, biochemical, and radiological investigations to check for absence of pathology. Symptoms evaluated were frequency of stools, consistency, completeness of evacuation, and minor disturbances like flatulence, mild abdominal pain, and diminished appetite. Six grams of powder of dried ripe fruits of the big variety of *Terminalia chebula* known as *bari harar* was given at bedtime after meals for 7 days. A daily progress record of the patients was maintained noting changes in symptoms. There was gradual reduction in complaints starting from the day after the start of therapy. At the end of 7 days, incomplete evacuation and reduced frequency had improved in all patients with improvement in consistency, flatulence, and difficulty in evacuation. Total response to the treatment was evaluated as "excellent" in 20 percent and "good" in 80 percent of patients.[40]

Traditionally, the drug *haritaki* is considered to be safe and better than a mother since it does not have adverse effects.[40] In the clinical trial conducted no side effects were seen.[40] No toxicity was seen in acute and subacute studies.[46] Also studied was the effect on liver and renal function parameters and the phagocytic and killing capacity of monocytes and polymorphonuclear cells.[46] The tannin fraction from *Terminalia chebula* and individual fractions showed antimutagenic effect.[47]

NOTES

1. Chopra RN, Chopra IC, Handa KL, Kapur LD. *Chopra's indigenous drugs of India* (2nd edn., pp. 98-100). Calcutta: Academic Publishers, 1958.

2. Bornkessel B. Senna-Ernte im Sari, *Deutsche Apoth Ztg* 131:171-174 (1991).

3. Gogte VM. *Ayurvedic pharmacology and therapeutic uses of medicinal plants* (pp. 692-693). Trans. SPARC, Bharatiya Vidya Bhavan, Mumbai, 2000.

4. Lemli J. Metabolism of sennosides—An overview. *Pharmacology* 36 (suppl. 1): 126-128 (1988).

5. Glätzel H. [Results of long-term therapy of 1,059 habitually constipated patients using a standardized senna preparation]. *Z Allgemeinmed* 48:654-656 (1972).

6. Shelton MG. Standardized senna in the management of constipation in the puerperium: A clinical trial. *S Afr Med J* 57:78-80 (1980).

7. Marlett JA, Li BU, Patrow CJ, Bass P. Comparative laxation of psyllium with and without senna in an ambulatory constipated population. *Am J Gastroenterol* 82:333-337 (1987).

8. Agra Y, Sacristán A, González M, Ferrari M, Potugués A, Calvo MJ. Efficacy of senna versus lactulose in terminal cancer patients treated with opioids. *J Pain Symptom Manage* 15:1-7 (1998).

9. Perkin JM. Constipation in childhood: A controlled comparison between lactulose and standardized senna. *Curr Med Res Opin* 4:540-543 (1977).

10. Gould SR, Williams CB. Castor oil or senna preparation before colonoscopy for inactive chronic ulcerative colitis. *Gastrointest Endosc* 28:6-8 (1982).

11. Ziegenhagen DJ, Zehnter E, Tacke E, Kruis W. Addition of senna improves colonoscopy preparation with lavage: A prospective randomized trial. *Gastrointest Endosc* 37:547-549 (1991).

12. Labenz J, Hopmann G, Leverkus F, Börsch G. [Bowel cleaning prior to colonoscopy. A prospective, randomized, blind comparative study]. *Med Klin* 85:581-585 (1990).

13. Wagner H. *Pharmazeutische Biologie 2. Drogen und ihre Inhaltsstoffe* (4th edn., p. 253) Stuttgart: Gustav Fischer Verlag, 1988.

14. *The wealth of India, raw materials* (vol. VIII, pp. 148-153). New Delhi: Publications and Information Directorate, CSIR, 1969.

15. Dash B. *Herbal treatment for constipation* (pp. 63-74) New Delhi: B. Jain Publishers, 1988.

16. *Indian herbal pharmacopoeia* (rev. new edn., pp. 327-334). Mumbai: Indian Drug Manufacturers Association, 2002.

17. Bisset NG, Wichtl M. *Herbal drugs and phytopharmaceuticals* (2nd edn., pp. 382-383) Stuttgart: Medpharm Scientific Publishers, 2001,.

18. *WHO monographs on selected medicinal plants* (vol. 1, pp. 202-212). Geneva: World Health Organization, 1999.

19. Marlett JA, Kajs TM, Fischer MH. An unfermented gel component of psyllium seed husk promotes laxation as a lubricant in humans. *Am J Clin Nutr* 72:784-789 (2000).

20. Gilani AH, Aziz N, Khan MA, Khan S, Zaman V. Laxative effect of *ispaghula*: Physical or chemical effect? *Phytother Res* 12:S63-S65 (1998).

21. Borgia M, Sepe N, Brancato V, Costa G, Simone P, Borgia R, Lungli R. Treatment of chronic constipation by a bulk-forming laxative (Fibrolax). *J Int Med Res* 11:124-127 (1983).

22. Ashraf W, Park F, Lof J, Quigley EM. Effects of psyllium therapy on stool characteristics, colon transit and anorectal function in chronic idiopathic constipation. *Ailment Pharmacol Ther* 9:639-647 (1995).

23. Marlett JA, Ulysses B, Li K, Patrow CJ, Bass P. Comparatve laxation of psyllium with and without senna in an ambulatory constipated population. *Am J Gastroenterol* 82:333-337 (1987).

24. Dettmar PW, Sykes J. A multi-centre, general practice comparison of ispaghula husk with lactulose and other laxatives in the treatment of simple constipation. *Curr Med Res Opin* 14:227-233 (1998).

25. Hamilton JW, Wagner J, Burdick BB, Bass P. Clinical evaluation of methylcellulose as a bulk laxative. *Dig Diss Sci* 33:993-998 (1988).

26. McRorie JW, Daggy BP, Morel JG, Diersing PS, Miner PB, Robinson M. Psyllium is superior to docusate sodium for treatment of chronic constipation. *Ailment Pharmacol Ther* 12:491-497 (1998).

27. Tomás-Ridocci M, Añón R, Mínguez M, Zaragoza A, Ballester J, Benages A. [The efficacy of *Plantago ovata* as a regulator of intestinal transit. A double-blind study compared to placebo]. *Rev Esp Enferm Dig* 82:17-22 (1992).

28. Golechha AC, Chadda VS, Chadda S, Sharma SK, Mishra SN. Role of Isapghula husk in the management of irritable bowel syndrome. A randomized double-blind crossover study. *J Assoc Physicians India* 30:353-355 (1982).

29. Oliver SD. The long term safety and tolerability of *ispaghula* husk. *J R Soc Health* 120:107-111 (2000).

30. Arlian LG, Vyszenski-Moher D, Lawrence AT, Schrotel KR, Ritz HL. Antigenic and allergenic analysis of psyllium seed component. *J Allergy Clin Immunol* 89:866-876 (1992).

31. Dash B. *Herbal treatment for constipation* (1st edn., pp. 75-80). New Delhi: B Jain Publishers (P) Ltd, 1988.

32. *Indian herbal pharmacopoeia* (rev. new edn., pp. 365-375). Mumbai: Indian Drug Manufacturers' Association, 2002.

33. Diener H. Rizinus: Giftpflanze und Öllieferant. *PTA Heute* 9:253-256 (1995).

34. Gaginella TS, Capasso F, Mascolo N, Perilli S. Castor oil: New lessons from an ancient oil. *Phytother Res* 12:S128-S130 (1998).

35. Büechi S. Rizinusöl. *Z Phytother* 21:312-318 (2000).

36. Pawlik A, Drozdzik M, Wojcicki J, Samochowiec L. Evaluation of effectiveness of castor oil from castor plant (*Ricinus communis* L) as compared with senna extract from Alexandrian senna (*Cassia senna* L.) in patients with simple chronic constipation. *Herba Polonica* 40(1-2):64-67 (1994).

37. Böneke H. Niedrig dosiertes Rizinusöl als Laxans. *Therapiewoche* 45:1784-1790 (1995).

38. *Indian herbal pharmacopoeia* (rev. new edn., pp. 439-448). Mumbai: Indian Drug Manufacturers Association, 2002.

39. *The wealth of India, raw materials* (vol. X, pp. 171-177). New Delhi: Publications and Information Directorate, CSIR, 1976.

40. Tripathi VN, Tewari SK, Gupta JP, Chaturvedi GN. Clinical trial of *haritaki (Terminalia chebula)* in treatment of simple constipation. *Sachitra Ayurved* 35:733-740 (1983).

41. Tamhane MD, Thorat SP, Rege NN, Dahanukar SA. Effect of oral administration of *Terminalia chebula* on gastric emptying: an experimental study. *J Postgrad Med* 43:12-13 (1997).

42. Patel RP, Derasari HR, Parikh SH. Purgative activity of *Terminalia chebula*. *Indian J Pharm* 21(5):131 (1959).

43. Inamdar MC, Rao MRR, Siddiqui HH. Purgative activity of *triphala*. *Indian J Pharm* 24(4):87-88 (1962).

44. Miglani BD, Sen P, Sanyal RK. Purgative action of an oil obtained from *Terminalia chebula*. *Indian J Med Res* 59:281-283 (1971).

45. Gaind KN, Saini TS. Identification of purgative principle of *Terminalia chebula* Retz. *Indian J Pharm* 30(10):233-234 (1968).

46. Rege NN, Thatte UM, Dahanukar SA. Adaptogenic properties of six rasayana herbs used in Ayurvedic medicine. *Phytother Res* 13:275-291 (1999).

47. Kaur S, Grover IS, Singh M, Kaur S. Antimutagenicity of hydrolysable tannins from *Terminalia chebula* in *Salmonella typhimurium*. *Mutat Res* 419:169-179 (1998).

OTHER LAXATIVE PLANTS

Picrorhiza kurroa *Royle ex Benth (Family: Scrophulariaceae)*

Sanskrit: Katuka, Katurohini	Tamil: Katukarogini
Hindi: Kutki	

Picrorhiza kurroa is best known for its hepatoprotective action (see Chapter 4) because of the extensive scientific work carried out on this aspect, especially on the activity of picroliv, an iridoid glycoside mixture isolated from *Picrorhiza kurroa*. However, in traditional medicine, it is known as a bitter tonic and laxative in small doses, although acting as a cathartic in larger doses.[1]

Kutkin, the iridoid glycoside mixture obtained by alcoholic extraction of *P. kurroa* rhizomes, and its two constituent organic acids, cinnamic acid and vanillic acid showed significant choleretic and laxative effects in dogs[2] and rats.[3] Extraction with ethanol leads to enrichment of the laxative effect. The order of activity is picroside I (3.55), kutkoside, kutkin (3), defatted alcoholic extract (2.79), and alcoholic extract (2.31) when compared to crude drug powder.[2]

One gram of the rhizome powder caused moderate cathartic effect, with a single motion 10 hours after intake. With higher doses of 6 g, drastic purgation was seen.[2] The powder was better than decoction and cold infusion, probably because of the insolubility of the active constituents in water.

In a comparative study, it was found that *kutlki* was weight/weight 1.5 times more potent than senna and 7.26 times more potent than castor oil.[2] The safety and tolerability of *kutlki* is covered in Chapter 4 "Hepatoprotective agents."

NOTES

1. Nadkarni AK. *Dr. KM Nadkarni's Indian materia medica* (vol. 1, pp. 953-956). Bombay: Popular Prakashan, 1976.

2. Chaturvedi GN, Gupta JP, Tiwari SK, Rai NP, Mishra A, Kumar S, Singh KP. Research progress in Ayurvedic gastroenterology. *J Res Edu Indian Med* 1(4):7-15 (1982) and references cited therein.

3. Das PK, Tripathi RM, Agarwal VK, Sanyal AK. Pharmacology of kutkin and its two organic acid constituents—Cinnamic acid and vanillic acid. *Indian J Exp Biol* 14:456-458 (1976).

DIARRHEA

Diarrhea is very common in India, especially the ones due to bacterial and protozoal infections. Thus infections like amoebiasis and giardiasis caused by protozoa and bacterial infections caused by *Escherichia coli* and *Vibrio cholerae* are common. It is also a major cause of morbidity and mortality and a large number of plants have been used in Ayurveda for control of diarrhea and dysentery.

Aegle marmelos *Correa (Family: Rutaceae)*

Sanskrit: Bilva	Tamil: Vilvam
Hindi: Bel	English: Stone Apple, Bengal Quince, Bael

Aegle marmelos is a medium-sized tree and all parts including root, bark, leaves, fruits, and root bark are used as medicine. However, it is the fruit that is most commonly used. The ripe fruit is considered an excellent laxative, whereas the unripe or half-ripe fruit is used for the treatment of chronic diarrhea and dysentery. In India, *Aegle marmelos* was so commonly used by Western doctors during the British rule that it found its way into the British pharmacopoeia. It is official in the *Indian Herbal Pharmacopoeia,* 2002, as an antidiarrheal agent.[1]

The fruit contains large quantities of pectin, apart from alkaloids, sterols, and coumarins that have also been isolated. The methanolic[2] (3-15 mg·animal^{-1}) and 50 percent ethanolic[3] extract (100-200 mg·kg^{-1}) of the unripe fruit has been found to exhibit an antidiarrheal effect in small animals.

A few clinical studies have been reported with preparations of unripe fruit. The syrup made from the fruits *(Sharbat-e-Bael),* a *Unani* preparation, which also uses the fruits, was studied at a dose level of

25 ml thrice a day for seven days in a number of cases of acute diarrhea and dysentery.[4]

In an open trial, 5 g of unripe fruit powder was given thrice daily to 25 patients of chronic dysentery for 21 days. Fifty-two percent of the patients were completely cured, 44 percent showed improvement, and 4 percent remained unaffected.[5]

In a study, the effect of unripe fruit on intestinal parasites was tried out clinically and it was concluded that the drug was effective against *Giardia, Entamoeba histolytica,* and *Ascaris lumbricoides.*[6] Twelve grams of the unripe fruit pulp was given in cases of intestinal amoebiasis in three divided doses for 15 days with the response being "excellent" in 81 percent of the cases.[7] In a randomized double-blind comparative trial to test the efficacy of dried unripe fruit powder in cases of shigellosis (dysentery caused by *Shigella*) it was not found useful, since it did not cause clinical improvement or bacteriological cure as compared to ampicillin.[8]

In another randomized double-blind clinical trial for 6 weeks with 169 patients with irritable bowel syndrome (IBS), a combination of *Aegle marmelos* and *Bacopa monnieri* was evaluated against standard therapy (clidinium bromide, chlordiazepoxide, and isaphagulla) and placebo. The Ayurvedic combination that was tried out in 57 patients was effective in 64.9 percent, whereas the standard therapy in 60 patients was effective in 78.3 percent. There was a 32.7 percent improvement in the placebo group of 52 patients. The Ayurvedic combination was more useful in diarrhea, whereas the standard therapy was useful in the painful form of IBS. However, follow-up for 6 months showed similar rates of relapse for both treatment forms as compared to placebo.[9]

The fruit of *Aegle marmelos* is edible and widely consumed as fruit, despite the hard outer shell of some varieties, or as a fruit drink made with pulp and sugar syrup for its useful action on the stomach,[10] especially in Bengal.

Cyperus rotundus *Linn. (Family: Cyperaceae)*

| Sanskrit: Musta | Tamil: Korai |
| Hindi: Koreti-jar | English: Nut Grass |

Cyperus rotundus is a common weed with aromatic tubers found growing throughout India. The root tuber is commonly used for diarrhea, dysentery, dyspepsia, indigestion, and piles.[11] The tubers contain 0.5-0.9 percent of an essential oil containing sesquiterpenes, β-sitosterol, and a flavonol glycoside.[12] The acetone and alcoholic extracts have shown broad spectrum antibacterial activity.[13]

Twenty patients with chronic diarrhea of more than 3 weeks duration, or those in which there was early recurrence after an acute attack, were given 2 g of fine powder of *Cyperus rotundus* root tuber thrice daily along with 50 ml decoction made from 50 g tuber powder given daily for 15 days. The frequency of defecation was controlled by the fifth day of treatment. In addition it helped decrease fat malabsorption and improved lactose intolerance. Forty percent of patients were considered cured, whereas there was improvement in 30 percent.[14] Further work is required to confirm and expand the scope of use.

Cyperus rotundus is generally considered safe and often used to treat stomach complaints in children. In commonly used doses of 1-3 g twice daily no adverse reactions have been reported.[15]

Holarrhena antidysentrica *(Linn.) Wall. (Family: Apocyanaceae)*

Latin: *Holarrhena pubescens* (Buch.-Ham.) Wallich ex Don	
Sanskrit: Kutaja	Tamil: Veppalai
English: Conessi, Kurchee	Hindi: Kurchi

Holarrhena antidysentrica is a small tree found growing throughout India up to 1,200 m elevation. The stem bark is best known as a single drug for the treatment of diarrhea and dysentery, although other parts like the seeds and leaves are also used medicinally. The bark contains up to 4 percent alkaloids, of which conessine has been shown to exhibit potent amoebicidal activity. Other constituents include gum, resin, and triterpenes like lupeol and β-sitosterol.[16]

Early pharmacological work on the antiamoebic activity of *kutaja* bark has been summarized.[17] *Kutaja* decoction has also been studied in vitro for its activity against diarrhea producing strains of *Escherichia coli* and found to be effective.[18]

In an open trial, 40 patients of amoebiasis and/or giardiasis were treated with 4 g of *kutaja* bark powder in three divided daily doses for 15 days. Cysts were cleared in 70 percent of patients with intestinal amoebiasis (15), whereas all patients showed good clinical improvement. A few patients complained of burning sensation in the abdomen, feet, and head, which was reversible on stopping the drug.[19]

Holarrhena antidysentrica is generally considered safe in doses of 2-4 g twice a day.[20] However, in the clinical trial on amoebiasis, side effects were burning in the abdomen, feet, and head, which subsided on stopping the drug.[19] In a study to assess side effects in 11 patients, the drug produced subjective symptoms and lowering of blood pressure in three patients.[21] However, alcoholic extract of *Holarrhena antidysentrica* showed no cellular toxicity when tested against fresh sheep erythrocytes.[22]

In a country like India, where amoebiasis and diarrhea are widespread, *kutaja* bark powder or in the form of the preparation known as *kutajarista,* which is well tolerated, in which the drug is extracted by self-generated alcohol, deserves to be further studied.

Terminalia belerica *Roxb. (Family: Combretaceae)*

Sanskrit: Bibhitaka	Tamil: Tanri
Hindi: Bahera	English: Belleric Myrobalan

Terminalia belerica is a large deciduous tree found growing in forests throughout India. The fruit rind is extensively used in Ayurveda. It is a constituent of the three-fruit combination known as *triphala* that is very commonly used as a laxative and bowel tonic and, depending upon the dosage, also finds application in control of diarrhea.

Bahera is listed in the *Indian Herbal Pharmacopoeia,* 2002, as expectorant, hypolipidemic, and laxative. Depending upon the dose administered it also finds use in control of diarrhea. It is a rich source (~17 percent) of phenolic acids and tannins from which gallic acid, ellagic acid, ethyl gallate, galloyl glucose, and chebulagic acid have been isolated.[23]

In vitro, the alcoholic extract of the fruit also has shown amoebicidal and bactericidal activity against a wide range of bacteria and is considered promising in various forms of dysentery.[24] This extract was found to be better than chloramphenicol.

As a follow-up to the promising in vitro results, the drug was evaluated clinically and 25 patients were included in an exploratory study, which took place in five different clinics. Patients were given either 1-2 tablets containing 150 mg per tablet of methanolic extract of *Terminalia belerica* fruit pericarp or placebo thrice a day for 14 days. Doctors were allowed to stop treatment depending upon response and to vary the dose from 1 tablet thrice a day to 2 tablets thrice a day depending upon severity. There were 12 patients on drug and 10 on placebo. All patients on drug responded to therapy and required 12 tablets for recovery. No side effects were observed. Patients on the drug who were found positive for cysts and bacteria became negative, whereas those patients on placebo continued to be positive even after the seventh day.[25] Considering the results of this trial it needs to be extended to larger number of patients, especially since *Terminalia belerica* is such a common drug, which would prove useful if the results can be confirmed.

Terminalia belerica is generally regarded as safe in the recommended dosages of 0.75-1.5 gram of the fruit powder taken twice a day.[26] Alcoholic extract of *Terminalia belerica* showed no cellular toxicity when tested against fresh sheep erythrocytes.[22]

NOTES

1. *Indian herbal pharmacopoeia* (rev. new edn., pp. 40-48). Mumbai: Indian Drug Manufacturers' Association, 2002.

2. Shoba FG, Thomas M. Study of antidiarrhoeal activity of four medicinal plants in castor oil induced diarrhoea. *J Ethnopharmacol* 76:73-76 (2001).

3. Rao CVA, Aziz I, Rawat AKS, Mehrotra S, Pushpangadan P. Antiulcer and antidiarrhoeal activity of *Aegle marmelos* Correa. *Herb: The Natural Alternative* (Abstract no. D-09). Gandhinagar, Gujarat: National Convention on Current Trends in Herbal Drugs. Ann Conf Indian Soc of Pharmacognosy, January 17-18, 2003.

4. Beg MZ, Khan NH. Effect of *Aegle marmelos* Corr. Syrup *(Sharbat-e-Bael)* in acute diarrhoea and dysentery cases (Abstract no. 23). Beenapara: Proc First Sem on Ilmul Advia, April 23-25, 1993.

5. Singh AK, Kumar A, Sharma KK. *Shriphal* powder: Antidysentric action. *Sachitra Ayurved* 46:574-576 (1993).

6. Trivedi VP, Nesamany S, Sharma VK. A clinical study of effects of *bilwa majja churna* on intestinal parasites *(Udar Krimi)*. *J Res Indian Med Yoga Homeopath* 13 (2):28-35 (1978).

7. Chaturvedi GN, Gupta JP, Tiwari SK, Rai NP, Mishra A, Kumar S, Singh KP. Research progress in Ayurvedic gastroenterology. *J Res Edu Ind Med* 1(4):7-15 (1982).

8. Haider R, Khan AK, Aziz KM, Chowdhury A, Kabir I. Evaluation of indigenous plants in the treatment of acute shigellosis. *Trop Geogr Med* 43:266-270 (1991).

9. Yadav AK, Jain AK, Tripathi SN, Gupta JP. Irritable bowel syndrome: Therapeutic evaluation of indigenous drugs. *Indian J Med Res* 90:496-503 (1989).

10. Nadkarni AK. *Dr. KM Nadkarni's Indian materia medica* (vol. 1, pp. 45-49). Bombay: Popular Prakashan, 1976.

11. Moos SN. *Single drug remedies* (pp. 55-56). Kottayam, India: Vaidyasarathy Press (P) Ltd, 1976.

12. *The wealth of India, raw materials* (first suppl. series, vol. 2, pp. 333-334). New Delhi: National Institute of Science Communication, CSIR, 2001.

13. Puratchikody A, Jaswanth A, Nagalakshmi A, Anagumeenal PK, Ruckmani K. Antibacterial activity of *Cyperus rotundus*. *Indian J Pharm Sci* 63:326-327 (2001).

14. Chaturvedi GN, Gupta JP, Tiwari SK, Rai NP, Mishra A, Kumar S, Singh KP. Research progress in Ayurvedic gastroenterology. *J Res Edu Ind Med* 1(4):7-15 (1982).

15. *Selected medicinal plants of India. A monograph on identity, safety and clinical usage* (pp. 128-130). Bombay: Chemexcil. Basic Chemicals, Pharmaceuticals and Cosmetics Export Promotion Council of India, 1992.

16. Chaturvedi GN, Singh KP, Gupta JP. Phytochemistry and pharmacology of *Holarrhena antidysentrica* Wall *(kutaja)*. *Nagarjun* 24(4):77-84 (1980).

17. Satyavati GV, Gupta AK, Tandon N. *Medicinal plants of India* (vol. 2, pp. 41-48). New Delhi: Indian Council of Medical Research, 1987.

18. Daswani PG, Birdi TJ, Antarkar DS, Antia ANH. Investigation of the antidiarrhoeal activity of *Holarrhena antidysentrica*. *Indian J Pharm Sci* 64(2):164-167 (2002).

19. Singh KP. Clinical studies on amoebiasis and giardiasis evaluating the efficacy of *kutaja (Holarrhena antidysentrica)* in *Entamoeba histolytica* cyst passers. *Ancient Sci Life* V:228-231 (1986).

20. *Selected medicinal plants of India. A monograph on identity, safety and clinical usage* (pp. 182-184). Bombay: Chemexcil. Basic Chemicals, Pharmaceuticals and Cosmetics Export Promotion Council of India, 1992.

21. Chaturvedi GN, Singh KP. Side effects of a traditional indigenous drug— *Kutaja (Holarrhena antidysentrica)* (letters to the editor). *Indian J Physiol Pharmacol* 27:255-256 (1983).

22. Ahmad I, Mehmood Z, Mohammad F. Screening of some Indian medicinal plants for their antimicrobial properties. *J Ethnopharmacol* 62:183-193 (1998).

23. *Indian herbal pharmacopoeia* (rev. new edn., pp. 429-438). Mumbai: Indian Drug Manufacturers' Association, 2002.

24. Bhutani KK, Kumar V, Kaur R, Sarin AN. Potential antidysentric candidates from Indian plants: A selective screening approach. *Indian Drugs* 24:508-513 (1987).

25. Patwardhan B, Bhutani KK, Patki PS, Dange SV, Gore DV, Borole DI, Shirolkar RB, Paranjpe PV. Clinical evaluation of *Terminalia belerica* in diarrhoea. *Ancient Sci Life* X(2):94-97 (1990).

26. *Selected medicinal plants of India. A monograph on identity, safety and clinical usage* (pp. 312-314). Bombay: Chemexcil. Basic Chemicals, Pharmaceuticals and Cosmetics Export Promotion Council of India, 1992.

Chapter 4

Hepatoprotective Agents

The liver is the largest solid organ in the body, and it carries out a number of important functions, including metabolism, detoxification, etc. The liver can be damaged by various factors: environmental toxins, such as chemicals; by ingestion of certain drugs, excessive alcohol, other hepatotoxins; and by virus. Thus, the liver is susceptible to a number of disorders because of this multifunctionality and constant exposure to toxins. Liver disorders such as hepatitis, hepatosis, and cirrhosis are a major cause of morbidity. Therefore, agents that can protect the liver from damage and help alleviate an already damaged liver would play an important role in health care, especially since no satisfactory remedy exists in modern allopathic medicine.

PLANT USE IN AYURVEDA

The importance of a healthy liver was realized long ago in India. Plants have been used for centuries in the Indian system of medicine, Ayurveda, for the treatment of liver disorders. In the classical recipes, several plants were combined in a preparation to be used as a remedy. The first recorded medical treatise on Ayurveda—the *Caraka Samhita*—dated to 700 BC describes the use of several multiplant preparations for the treatment of jaundice and other liver disorders.[1]

Plant combinations are still the most popular form of plant remedy today: be it the classical formulae based on traditional Ayurvedic texts or the newer proprietary formulations based on Ayurvedic concepts. It is in only in the past few years that a few single-plant

doi:10.1300/5683_04

remedies have been introduced in the market. However, single plants have always been commonly used as home remedies—the most popular ones being those based on *Phyllanthus amarus, Andrographis paniculata, Eclipta alba,* and *Picrorhiza kurroa.*

NOTE

1. *Caraka samhita,* ed. and trans. Sharma PV (vol. II, pp. 261-262, "Chikitsasthanam," chapter XV, verse 132-140) Varanasi: Chaukhambha Orientalia, 1983.

SCIENTIFIC STUDIES

There are approximately 40 hepatoprotective multiplant proprietary products available in the Indian market derived from some 93 plants belonging to 44 families.[1] Of these plants many have been studied individually to determine their chemical composition and to find out their pharmacological action. However, only a few of these plants have been tried out clinically. Most of the trials have been open trials using few patients. In early trials on viral hepatitis, viral markers were not examined. Double-blind placebo-controlled trials have been carried out with only four plants—*Berberis aristata, Phyllanthus amarus, Picrorhiza kurroa,* and *Tinospora cordifolia.*

A large number of experimental studies have been carried out on individual plants to test for hepatoprotective activity. A survey of literature published between 1986 and 1993 has reviewed the data on 43 plants used in India and elsewhere, of these 24, which included four combinations, showed hepatoprotective activity.[2] Emerging trends in the field of hepatoprotective plant drugs have been reviewed and several other reviews have been published, apart from a monograph that covers work on Ayurvedic plant drugs for liver diseases.[3-7]

Hepatoprotective plants that are interesting because of a combination of factors such as wide usage, traditional use, experimental, and clinical studies are *Andrographis paniculata, Boerhaavia diffusa, Eclipta alba, Picorhiza kurroa, Phyllanthus amarus,* and *Tinospora cordifolia.*

Andrographis paniculata *(Burm. f.) Wall. ex Nees* *(Family: Acanthaceae)*

Sanskrit: Bhunimba, Kirata	Tamil: Nilavembu
Hindi: Kalmegh	English: The Creat

Andrographis paniculata (see Plate 3 in color gallery) is a small herb found in the tropical and subtropical parts of India. The plant is included in the multiplant preparations mentioned in the *Caraka Samhita*.[8] It has been traditionally used for the following conditions: for sluggish liver; as an antidote to poisons; in cases of colic, dysentery, dyspepsia, fever; and in general debility.[9] The drug comprises the dried aerial parts of the plant: mostly leaves and stem. It has an intensely bitter taste, which is usually masked by the addition of aromatics. It is also one of the most widely used plants in Ayurvedic formulations for liver disorders, being found in 26 of 40 multiplant preparations.[10] *Andrographis paniculata* or *kalmegh,* the Hindi and Bengali name by which it is commonly known, has the official status in the *Indian Herbal Pharmacopoeia,*1998, as being a bitter tonic, febrifuge, and a hepatoprotective agent.[11]

Numerous chemical constituents have been isolated in *kalmegh,* such as diterpene lactones and flavonoids.[9,11] Andrographolide, a diterpene lactone, which is present up to 1 percent in the plant, has been shown to be the major active hepatoprotective constituent of *Andrographis paniculata.*[9,11,12] However, the extract from *Andrographis paniculata* is more active than andrographolide suggesting that there are other minor constituents that contribute to the hepatoprotective activity.[13]

The aqueous or alcohol extract of *Andrographis paniculata* has been shown to have hepatoprotective effects in a number of experimental models of liver damage—alcohol, carbon tetrachloride, and benzene hexachloride.[14-17] The aqueous extract prevented necrosis when given to rats for 3 days before the administration of carbon tetrachloride, whereas control rats showed massive necrosis of liver parenchyma cells. Increase in alanine aminotransferase ALT, aspartate aminotransferase AST, serum bilirubin, and free fatty acids was prevented.[15]

In another experiment, such pretreatment resulted in an increase of biliary flow and liver weight, while hexabarbitone sleeping time was reduced, suggesting the induction of microsomal enzymes.[18] The extract also decreased carbon tetrachloride-induced hepatic microsomal lipid peroxidation and inhibited hepatic microsomal enzymes in rats.[13,19]

Andrographolide, a diterpene lactone, which is the major constituent in the plant has shown hepatoprotective activity against carbon tetrachloride, galactosamine, and paracetamol- and ethanol-induced hepatotoxicity, apart from showing choleretic activity.[12,20-24]

In an open trial, patients of acute viral hepatitis were given 60 ml of a decoction of *Andrographis paniculata* extract equivalent to 40 g of crude drug in three divided doses, for an average period of 24 days. Patients were assessed both for clinical and biochemical parameters. There was considerable symptomatic relief and statistically significant decrease in serum bilirubin, ALT, AST, and serum alkaline phosphatase, and an increase in protein synthesis as shown by an increase in serum globulin.[25]

The drug has been used for centuries in India as a household remedy, as it is generally considered safe for use. No adverse effects are reported when administered standard doses; however, large oral doses have been reported to cause gastric discomfort, vomiting, and loss of appetite.[11] It is an official status as a drug in the *Indian Herbal Pharmacopoeia,* 1998.[11] When given orally, in animals, the minimum lethal dose for andrographolide, neoandrographolide, and deoxydidehydroandrographolide is greater than 20 $g \cdot kg^{-1}$.[26] A survey that reviewed the safety and efficacy of *Andrographis paniculata* in upper respiratory disorders reported the drug to be safe and the adverse events being mild and infrequent with few spontaneous reports of adverse events.[27]

Thus, although there is some evidence for its hepatoprotective activity from experimental studies and a preliminary clinical trial, further clinical work is needed for this much-used medicinal plant to delineate the range of therapeutic efficacy.

Eclipta alba *(Linn.) Hassk (Family: Asteraceae)*

Latin: *Eclipta erecta* Linn., *Eclipta prostrata* Linn.	Hindi: Bhangra
Sanskrit: Bhringaraja, Kesharaja	Tamil: Karasalanganni
English: Trailing eclipta	

Eclipta alba is a small creeping prostate or sometimes erect plant with white flower heads, it is found throughout India in the moist and wet areas up to an elevation of 2,000 m.[28] In Ayurveda, it is considered one of the best plants for the treatment of jaundice. Traditionally the whole plant or its leaves are used. It is also used as a single drug preferably in the fresh state.[29] It is one of the most widely used plants in Ayurvedic formulations for the liver with 16 out of 40 preparations in the market containing this plant as one of the ingredients.[30] It has an official status as a hepatoprotective agent in the *Indian Herbal Pharmacopoeia,* volume 1 published in 1998.[28]

Chemically the major constituents are the coumestans—wedelolactone (1.6 percent) and norwedelolactone or demethylwedelolactone, which were recognized as the main active constituents in 1986, 30 years after their first isolation.[28,31] Other constituents include polyacetylenes, thiophene derivatives, flavonoids, steroids, and triterpenoids.[28]

Several preparations of the plant, such as powdered aerial parts, fresh leaf juice, aqueous extracts, and alcoholic extracts have been tested for hepatoprotective activity in small animals using a variety of experimental models—carbon tetrachloride, alcohol, acetaminophen, and D-galactosamine.[32-35] The plant extract and the coumestans wedelolactone and demethylwedelolactone exhibited antihepatotoxic activity in in vitro assays employing carbon tetrachloride, galactosamine, and phalloidin-induced cytotoxicity in primary cultured rat hepatocytes. In vivo also ethyl acetate fraction protected mice from phalloidin toxicity, no mortality being seen in the group being pretreated with the drug, although the control group showed 70 percent mortality. In addition, ethyl acetate fraction, wedelolactone, and demethylwedeloactone showed significant stimulatory effect on liver cell regeneration.[31] Wedelolactone has also been shown to be one of the most potent 5-lipoxygenase inhibitors isolated from plants.[36] In vivo *Eclipta alba* has been shown to possess anti-inflammatory activity against carrageenin-induced rat paw edema. It also inhibits the enzyme phospholipase A2 thereby preventing the release of inflammatory prostaglandins by arachidonic acid.[32] This combination of anti-inflammatory and hepatoprotective activity makes *Eclipta alba* useful for the treatment of inflammatory liver diseases.

Eclipta alba extract has also been shown to have significant antioxidant activity. It is a potent inhibitor of lipid peroxidation and scavenges hydroxy radicals in vitro.[37] Extracts of *Eclipta alba* have shown in vitro inactivation of hepatitis B surface antigen (HBsAg) when incubated with HBsAg positive sera isolated from patients.[38] However, no further work on this property of *Eclipta alba* has been published.

Clinically, *Eclipta alba* plant powder at a dose level of 50 mg·kg^{-1} body weight in three divided doses was tried in two open preliminary trials: in 50 children with jaundice and in 20 adults with infective hepatitis.[39,40] The treatment period varied from 3 to 7 weeks. Clinical response and liver function tests, such as serum bilirubin, alkaline phosphatase, and ALT, were monitored. Testing was continued till patients showed complete biochemical recovery and were followed up for 2-3 months thereafter.

Clinical recovery was observed to be faster than biochemical normalization. Children showed a faster response to the drug when compared to adults; biochemical recovery being seen in 2-3 weeks of therapy. Acute viral hepatitis is for most part a self-limiting disease; however, in countries such as India it can be associated with high morbidity and mortality. Thus, any treatment that can hasten recovery deserves further study.

The aerial parts of *Eclipta alba* are commonly cooked and eaten as a vegetable in South India in order to protect the liver. The alcoholic extract of fresh *Eclipta alba*'s aerial parts did not show any sign of toxicity. When given orally and intraperitoneally in mice, the minimum lethal dose was greater than 2 g·kg^{-1}.[34] In the clinical trials no side effects were seen or reported.[39,40] In a chronic study in mice there was no weight loss, no behavioral changes, and no mortality. In addition, the histopathology of kidney, spleen, and liver of mice showed no significant difference from controls. In tissue culture studies in *vero* cells, no cytotoxicity and cytotonicity was observed when innoculated with *Eclipta alba* extracts.[41]

Picrorhiza kurroa *Royle ex Benth* *(Family: Scrophulariaceae)*

Sanskrit: Katuka, Katurohini   Tamil: Katukarogini

Hindi: Kutki

Picrorhiza kurroa is a perennial woody herb with grayish brown cylindrical irregularly curved roots 5-10 cm long, found in the North-western Himalayas at an elevation of 2,700-4,500 m. The drug consists of dried rhizome and roots and is widely used in Ayurveda for the treatment of epidemic jaundice.[42] It is commonly mixed in compound preparations for the liver. The rhizomes have official status as a bitter tonic and for their hepatoprotective action in the *Indian Herbal Pharmacopoeia,* volume I, published in 1998.[43]

Major chemical constituents of *Picrorhiza kurroa* are iridoid glycosides, picroside I, and kutkoside. Other minor constituents include some iridoid glycosides, such as picroside III, veronicoside, and minecoside, phenol and cucurbitacin glycosides.[43]

The alcoholic extracts of roots of *Picrorhiza kurroa* were found to be hepatoprotective in number of experimental models. *Picrorhiza kurroa* prevented damage caused to the liver by intraperitoneal administration of carbon tetrachloride, reversing the increase in transaminase levels in rabbits.[44] It also showed protection against carbon tetrachloride, paracetamol, and aflatoxin damage in rats, at a dose level of 20 mg·kg^{-1} once a day for 7 days, preventing significant rise of transaminase levels in all three models and restoring Na$^+$ K$^+$ATPase levels to normal in hepatic injury caused by paracetamol and aflatoxin.[45] In rats, pretreatment with *Picrorhiza kurroa* ethanolic extract prevented elevation of serum enzymes and glutathione-S-transferase activity by D-galactosamine and carbon tetrachloride, which is attributed to the overall antioxidant effect of the extract.[46-48] Among the six plant extracts tested, *Picrorhiza kurroa* was one of the two extracts with the most potent antioxidant activity.[49] Alcoholic extract of *Picrorhiza kurroa* has been shown to have a choleretic effect in dogs.[50]

Kutkin, the iridoid glycoside mixture from the alcoholic extract of *Picrorhiza kurroa*, has been shown to be the hepatoprotective agent, whereas kutkin-free extracts are not active.[51] Subsequently picroliv, which is a standardized fraction consisting of 55-60 percent of a mixture of two iridoid glycosides picroside 1 and kutkoside I in the ratio 1:1.5, has been studied extensively in a variety of in vivo and ex vivo experimental models: carbon tetrachloride, thioacetamide, alcohol, paracetamol, and galactosamine.[52-58]

In addition, picroliv stimulates nucleic acid and protein synthesis in the liver.[59] In partially hepatectomized rats, rate of recovery in several biochemical markers in regenerating liver was faster.[60] This was also observed in rats pretreated with picroliv before hepatectomy as compared with control rats.[61]

Picroliv showed a dose-dependent choleretic effect in conscious rats and anaesthetized guinea pigs.[62] It also possessed anticholestatic effect against paracetamol-, ethinylestradiol-, carbon tetrachloride-, and thioacetamide-induced cholestatis.[62-64]

In an open clinical study, 20 patients with acute hepatocellular jaundice were given 1 g of *Picrorhiza kurroa* root powder thrice daily for a mean period of 26 days. There was significant improvement in serum bilirubin and transaminase levels. It was also tried out in a small group of six chronic patients for an average of 27 days: one patient was considered cured and improvement was seen in the other five patients.[65] In a double-blind, randomized, placebo-controlled trial, patients with acute viral hepatitis of less than 10 days duration were given 375 mg *Picrorhiza kurroa* powder three times daily for 2 weeks. These patients showed marked clinical improvement in anorexia, malaise, nausea, vomiting, liver size, and tenderness. There was also significant reduction in serum bilirubin and transaminase levels. Bilirubin levels took an average of 75.9 days to fall to 2.5 mg·dl^{-1} with placebo, while *Picrorhiza kurroa*-treated patients took only 27.4 days to reach the same level. Thus, the drug is found to be useful in therapy of early viral hepatitis.[66]

Picrorhiza kurroa is widely used in India for several indications. In clinical trials on patients with viral hepatitis, no side effects have been noticed using a dosage of 375 mg thrice daily for 14 days.[66] It is considered to have a laxative effect at larger dose levels.[42] It has been reported to have a mild laxative effect at 1 g and drastic purgation at 6 g. Clinical trials have been reported with dose levels of 1g three times a day with no untoward effects.[67] See also Chapter 3 "Gastrointestinal agents." In a long-term clinical trial using up to 1 g of root powder for a period of 1 year in patients of bronchial asthma, no side effects were observed, although one patient complained of mild gastric irritation during the last 2 months of the trial. In rats and mice, the alcoholic extract did not affect the weight of spleen, thymus, and adrenals and caused no gastric mucosal damage.[42]

Tinospora cordifolia *(Willd.) Miers ex Hook f. & Thoms.* *(Family: Menispermaceae)*

Latin: *Tinospora glabra* (N.Brum.) Merr.	Hindi: Giloe
Sanskrit: Guduchi, Amrita	Tamil: Sindal

Tinospora cordifolia Miers (see Plate 4 in color gallery) is a woody climber found on trees and shrubs throughout the tropical and subtropical parts of India. It grows readily in different soils, the stem attaining a thickness of 6 cm diameter. Usually, however, the diameter is approximately 1 cm.[68] As a drug, the plant growing on neem (*Azadirachta indica*) trees is considered to be valuable and therefore prized. *Tinospora cordifolia*'s mature stem powder, the aqueous extract, the starch obtained from the stem by repeated washing of crushed stem with water are used in Ayurveda for debility, hepatitis, dyspepsia, jaundice, and other liver disorders.[69] It is an official drug in the *Indian Herbal Pharmacopoeia*, 1990, for its analgesic and antipyretic activity.[70]

Several classes of compounds have been isolated among them clerodane furanoditerpenes, alkaloids such as jatrorhizine, palmitine, berberine and tembeterine, steroids, flavonoids, lignans, and a few other compounds.[70] Anticomplement and immunostimulating activity has been ascribed to TC-1 (a clerodane furano diterpene glycoside), syringin, cordiol, cordioside, and cordifolioside A and B.[71]

In acute liver damage caused by carbon tetrachloride, pretreatment for 4 weeks with *Tinospora cordifolia* aqueous extract, prepared by decocting the stems at a dose of 100 mg·kg^{-1} body weight, was found to aggravate acute damage. However, it was effective in preventing fibrotic changes in the liver, and it enhanced parenchymal tissue regeneration in albino rats.[72] In a chronic liver disease model using Kupffer cells, *Tinospora cordifolia* was found to cause significant improvement in Kupffer cell functioning thereby preventing fibrous tissue deposition and tending toward normalization.[73] This suggests that the antifibrotic effect is mediated by activation of Kupffer cells.[73] An aqueous suspension of alcoholic extract of the stem of *Tinospora cordifolia* was shown to protect against liver damage caused by administration of carbon tetrachloride in mice, rats, and rabbits.[74] The aqueous extract of *Tinospora cordifolia* also showed significant anti-inflammatory activity in acute and chronic inflammation in rats.[75]

Immune suppression is caused by the development of cholestasis in rats and suggests the need for an immunomodulator such as *Tinospora cordifolia* in the treatment of obstructive jaundice. Thus, treatment with the aqueous extract (100 mg·kg^{-1}) of *Tinospora cordifolia* given orally twice daily for 7 days, 4 weeks after the development of cholestasis, resulted in the improvement of cellular immune function as evidenced by normalization of phagocytic activity of macrophages and polymorphonuclear cells, and the intracellular killing capacity of macrophages. Cholestatic rats were also more susceptible to infection; however, when receiving *Tinospora cordifolia* they better resisted infection caused by *Escherichia coli* with 16.67 percent mortality in the treated group as compared to 77.78 percent in the untreated group.[76]

This finding was used in a clinical study where 30 patients undergoing surgery for malignant obstructive jaundice were administered *Tinospora cordifolia* in addition to the conventional treatment of Vitamin K, antibiotics, and biliary drainage.[77] Thus, only those patients who additionally received 16 mg·kg·day^{-1} of *Tinospora cordifolia* aqueous extract for 3 weeks, after institution of biliary drainage, showed normalization of phagocytic and killing capacity of neutrophils, although in both groups hepatic function was comparable. None of the patients receiving *Tinospora cordifolia* treatment showed septicemia as compared to 50 percent of the patients who were on conventional treatment alone, although 92.4 percent of the *Tinospora cordifolia*–treated group survived, in contrast to 40 percent postoperative survival in the conventional treatment group.

Tinospora cordifolia is considered safe at the usual dose levels of 3-6 g.[78] In acute toxicity studies, the stem extract had almost no toxicity; rabbits and albino rats could be administered up to 1.6 g·kg^{-1} without untoward effects.[79] In another study on mice and rats, the aqueous extract of stem in a dose range of 50 mg to 1 g·kg^{-1} was found safe in acute (72 hours) and subacute (4 weeks) studies with no damage to liver and kidney.[80] The extract was also evaluated on organ function in healthy volunteers for 15 days.[80]

NOTES

1. Sharma A, Singh RT, Sehgal V, Handa SS. Antihepatotoxic activity of some plants used in herbal formulations. *Fitoterapia* LXII:131-138 (1991).

2. Doreswamy R, Sharma D. Plant drugs for liver disorders management. *Indian Drugs* 32:139-154 (1995).

3. Premila MS. Emerging frontiers in the area of hepatoprotective herbal drugs. *Indian J Nat Prod* 11 (special issue):3-12 (1995).

4. De S, Ravishankar B, Bhavsar GC. Plants with hepatoprotective activity— A review, *Indian Drugs* 30:355-363 (1993).

5. Bhatt AD, Bhatt NS. Indigenous drugs and liver disease. *Indian J Gastroenterol* 15(2):63-67 (1996).

6. Tyagi MG, Tripathi CD, Bapna JS. Current status of hepatoprotective plant products in India. *Acta Clinica Scientia* 1(2):79-86 (1991).

7. Chaturvedi GN, Singh G. *Clinical studies on* Kamala *(jaundice) and* Yakrt Rogas *(liver disorders) with Ayurvedic drugs.* New Delhi: Central Council for Research in Ayurveda and Siddha, 1988.

8. *Caraka samhita,* ed. and trans. Sharma PV (vol. II, p. 261, "Chikitsasthanam," chapter XV, verse 132-133). Varanasi: Chaukhambha Orientalia, 1983.

9. *The wealth of India, raw materials* (vol. I, pp. 264-266). New Delhi: Publications and Information Directorate, CSIR, 1985 and references cited therein.

10. Sharma A, Singh RT, Sehgal V, Handa SS. Antihepatotoxic activity of some plants used in herbal formulations, *Fitoterapia* LXII:131-138 (1991).

11. *Indian herbal pharmacopoeia* (vol. I, pp. 18-29). Mumbai: Indian Drug Manufacturers' Association and Jammu-Tawi: Regional Research Laboratory, 1998.

12. Handa SS, Sharma A. Hepatoprotective activity of andrographolide from *Andrographis paniculata* against carbon tetrachloride. *Indian J Med Res* [B] 92:276-283 (1990).

13. Choudhury BR, Haque SJ, Poddar MK. *In vivo* and *in vitro* effects of *kalmegh (Andrographis paniculata)* extract and andrographolide on hepatic microsomal drug metabolizing enzymes. *Planta Med* 53:135-140 (1987).

14. Choudhury BR, Poddar, MK. Effect of *kalmegh* extract on rat liver and serum enzymes. *Meth Find Exptl Clin Pharmacol* 5:727-730 (1983).

15. Shahid A. Protective effect of *Andrographia paniculata* Nees on experimental liver damage. *Hamdard Medicus* XXX (4):63-69 (1987).

16. Trivedi V, Rawal VM. Effect of aqueous extract of *Andrographis paniculata*. *Indian J Pharmacol* 30:318-322 (1998).

17. Rana AC, Avadhoot Y. Hepatoprotective effects of *Andrographis paniculata* against carbon tetrachloride-induced liver damage. *Arch Pharmacol Res* 14(1):93-95 (1991).

18. Chaudhri SK. Influence of *Andrographis paniculata (kalmegh)* on bile flow and hexabarbitone sleeping in experimental animals. *Indian J Exp Biol* 16:830-832 (1978).

19. Choudhury BR, Poddar MK. Andrographolide and *kalmegh (Andrographis paniculata)* extract: *In vivo* and *in vitro* effect on hepatic lipid peroxidation. *Meth Find Exptl Clin Pharmacol* 6:481-484 (1984).

20. Handa SS, Sharma A. Hepatoprotective activity of andrographolide against galactosamine and paracetamol intoxication in rats. *Indian J Med Res* [B] 92:284-292 (1990).

21. Saraswat B, Visen PKS, Patnaik GK, Dhawan BN. Effect of andrographolide against galactosamine-induced toxicity, *Fitoterapia* 66:415-420 (1995).

22. Choudhury BR, Poddar MK. Andrographolide and *kalmegh (Andrographis paniculata)* extract: Effect on rat liver and serum transaminases. *IRCS Med Sci* 12:466-467 (1984).

23. Shukla B, Visen PKS, Patnaik GK, Dhawan BN. Choleretic effect of andrographolide in rats and guinea pigs. *Planta Med* 58:146-149 (1992).

24. Tripathi GS, Tripathi YB. Choleretic effect of andrographolide obtained from *Andrographis paniculata* in rats. *Phytotherap Res* 5:176-178 (1991).

25. Chaturvedi GN, Tomar GS, Tiwari S.K, Singh, K.P. Clinical studies on *kalmegh (Andrographis paniculata* Nees) in infective hepatitis. *Ancient Sci Life* 2:208-215 (1983).

26. Deng WL, Nie RJ, Liu JY. Comparison of pharmacological effect of four andrographolides. *Chin Pharm Bull* 17:195-198 (1982).

27. Coon JT, Ernst E. *Andrographis paniculata* in the treatment of upper respiratory tract infections: A systematic review of safety and efficacy. *Planta Med* 70:293-298 (2004).

28. *Indian herbal pharmacopoeia* (vol. 1, pp. 81-88). Mumbai: Indian Drug Manufacturers' Association and Jammu Tawi: Regional Research Laboratory, 1998.

29. Lakshmipathi A. *One hundred useful drugs* (3rd edn., vol. III, section I, pp. 23-24). A Text Book of Ayurveda. Madras: Arogya Ashramam Samithi, 1973.

30. Sharma A, Singh RT, Sehgal V, Handa SS. Antihepatotoxic activity of some plants used in herbal formulations. *Fitoterapia* LXII:131-138 (1991).

31. Wagner H, Geyer B, Kiso Y, Hikino H, Rao GS. Coumestans as the main active principles of the liver drugs *Eclipta alba* and *Wedelia calendulaceae*. *Planta Med* 52:370-374 (1986).

32. Chandra T, Sadique J, Somasundaram S. Effect of *Eclipta alba* on inflammation and liver injury. *Fitoterapia* LVIII:23-32 (1987).

33. Ma-Ma K, Nyunt N, Tin KM. The protective effect of *Eclipta alba* on inflammation and liver injury. *Toxicol Appl Pharmacol* 45:723-728 (1978).

34. Singh B, Saxena AK, Chandan BK, Agarwal SG, Bhatia MS, Anand KK. Hepatoprotective effect of ethanolic extract of *Eclipta alba* on experimental liver damage in rats and mice. *Phytother Res* 7:154-158 (1993).

35. Lin SC, Yao CJ, Lin CC, Lin YH. Hepatoprotective activity of Taiwan folk medicine: *Eclipta prostrata* Linn. against various hepatotoxins induced acute hepatotoxicity. *Phytother Res* 10:483-490 (1996).

36. Wagner H, Fessler B. *In vitro* 5- Lipoxygenasehemmung durch *Eclipta alba* Extrakte and das Coumestan-Derivat Wedelolacton. *Planta Med* 52:374-377 (1986).

37. Joy KL, Kuttan R. Anti-oxidant activity of selected plant extracts. *Amala Res Bull* 15:68-71 (1995).

38. Thyagarajan SP, Thiruneelakantan K, Subramanian S, Sundaravelu T. *In vitro* inactivation of HBsAg by *Eclipta alba* Haask and *Phyllanthus niruri* Linn. *Indian J Med Res* 76 (suppl.):124-130 (1982).

39. Dixit SP, Achar MP. Study of *bhringaraja (Eclipta alba)* therapy in jaundice in children. *J Sci Res Pl & Med* 2(4):96-100 (1981).

40. Dixit SP, Achar MP. *Bhringaraja (Eclipta alba* Linn) in the treatment of infective hepatitis. *Curr Med Pract* 23:237-242 (1979).

41. Jayaram S, Thygarajan SP, Panchanandam M, Subramanian S. Anti-hepatitis-B properties of *Phyllanthus niruri* Linn and *Eclipta alba* Hassk: *In vitro* and *in vivo* safety studies. *Biomed* 7(2):9-16 (1987).

42. *Selected medicinal plants of India. A monograph of identity, safety and clinical usage* (pp. 238-240). Bombay: Chemexcil. Basic Chemicals, Pharmaceuticals and Cosmetics Export Promotion Council, 1992.

43. *Indian herbal pharmacopoeia* (vol. I, pp.106-113). Mumbai: Indian Drug Manufacturers' Association and Jammu Tawi: Regional Research Laboratory, 1998.

44. Pandey VN, Chaturvedi GN. Effect of alcoholic extract of *kutaki (Picrorhiza kurroa)* on experimentally induced abnormalities in the liver of rabbits. *J Res Indian Med* 3:25-35 (1968).

45. Mogre K, Vora KK, Sheth UK. Effect of *Picrorhiza kurroa* and *Eclipta alba* on $Na^+K^+ATPase$ in hepatic injury by hepatotoxic agents. *Indian J Pharmacol* 13:253-259 (1981).

46. Anandan R, Devaki T. Hepatoprotective effect of *Picrorhiza kurroa* on tissue defence system in D-galactosamine-induced hepatitis in rats. *Fitoterapia* 70:54-57 (1999).

47. Anandan R, Rekha RD, Devaki T. Protective effect of *Picrorhiza kurroa* on mitochondrial glutathione antioxidant system in D-galactosamine hepatitis in rats. *Curr Sci* 76:1543-1545 (1999).

48. Joy KL, Kuttan R. Protective effect of Lycovin and *Picrorhiza kurroa* extract against acute as well as chronic hepatotoxicity induced by CCl_4 in rats. *Amala Res Bull* 16:67-72 (1996).

49. Joy KL, Kuttan R. Anti-oxidant activity of selected plant extracts. *Amala Res Bull* 15:68-71 (1995).

50. Pandey VN, Chaturvedi GN. Effect of indigenous drug *kutaki (Picrorhiza kurroa)* on bile after producing biliary fistula in dogs. *J Res Indian Med* 5:11-24 (1971).

51. Ansari RA, Aswal BS, Chander R, Dhawan BN, Garg NK, Kapoor NK, Kulshreshta DK, Mehdi H, Mehrotra BN, Patnaik GK, Sharma SK. Hepatoprotective action of kutkin—the iridoid glycoside mixture of *Picrorhiza kurroa. Indian J Med Res* 87:401-404 (1988).

52. Ansari RA, Tripathi SC, Patnaik GK, Dhawan BN. Antihepatotoxic properties of picroliv: An active fraction from rhizomes of *Picrorhiza kurrooa. J Ethnopharmacol* 34:61-68 (1991).

53. Dwivedi Y, Rastogi R, Chander R, Sharma SK, Kapoor, NK, Garg NK, Dhawan BN. Hepatoprotective action of picroliv against carbon tetrachloride-induced liver damage *Indian J Med Res* 92B:195-200 (1990).

54. Dwivedi Y, Rastogi R, Sharma SK, Garg NK, Dhawan BN. Picroliv affords protection against thioacetamide-induced hepatic damage in rats. *Planta Med* 57:25-28 (1991).

55. Visen PKS, Shukla B, Patnaik GK, Chander R, Singh V, Kapoor NK, Dhawan BN. Hepatoprotective activity of picroliv isolated from *Picrorhiza kurroa* against thioacetamide toxicity on rat hepatocytes. *Phytother Res* 5:224-227 (1991).

56. Rastogi R, Saksena S, Garg NK, Kapoor NK, Agarwal DP, Dhawan BN. Picroliv protects against alcohol induced chronic hepatotoxicity in rats. *Planta Med* 62:283-285 (1996).

57. Dwivedi Y, Rastogi R, Garg NK, Dhawan BN. Prevention of paracetamol-induced hepatic damage in rats by picroliv, the standardized active fraction from *Picrorhiza kurroa. Phytother Res* 5:115-119 (1991).

58. Visen, PKS, Shukla B, Patnaik GK, Dhawan BN. Prevention of galactosamine-induced hepatic damage by picroliv: Study on bile flow and isolated hepatocytes *(ex vivo). Planta Med* 59:37-41 (1993).

59. Singh V, Kapoor NK, Dhawan BN. Effect of picroliv on protein and nucleic acid synthesis. *Indian J Exp Biol* 30:68-69 (1992).

60. Saksena S, Rastogi R, Garg NK, Dhawan BN. Effect of picroliv on regeneration of liver after partial hepatectomy in rats. *Phytother Res* 9:518-521 (1995).

61. Srivastava S, Srivastava AK, Patnaik GK, Dhawan BN. Effect of picroliv on liver regeneration. *Fitoterapia* 67:252-256 (1995).

62. Shukla B, Visen PKS, Patnaik GK, Dhawan BN. Choleretic effect of picroliv the hepatoprotective principle of *Picrorhiza kurroa. Planta Med* 57:29-33 (1991).

63. Saraswat B, Visen PKS, Patnaik GK, Dhawan BN. Anticholestatic effect of picroliv, active hepatoprotective principle of *Picrorhiza kurroa* against carbon tetrachloride induced cholestatis. *Indian J Exp Biol* 31:316-318 (1993).

64. Shukla B, Visen PKS, Patnaik GK, Dhawan BN. Reversal of thioacetamide induced cholestatis by picroliv in rodents. *Phytother Res* 6:53-55 (1992).

65. Chaturvedi GN, Singh G. *Clinical studies on Kamala (jaundice) and Yakrt Rogas (liver disorders) with Ayurvedic drugs.* (pp. 80-91, 131-132). New Delhi: Central Council for Research in Ayurveda and Siddha, 1988.

66. Vaidya AB, Antarkar DS, Doshi JC, Bhatt AD, Ramesh V, Vora PV, Perissond D, Baxi AJ, Kale PM. *Picrorhiza kurroa (Kutaki)* Royle ex Benth as a hepatoprotective agent—experimental and clinical studies. J Postgrad Med 42:105-108 (1996).

67. Chaturvedi GN, Gupta JP, Tiwari SK, Rai NP, Mishra A, Kumar S, Singh KP. Research progress in Ayurvedic gastroenterology. *J Res Edu Indian Med* 1(4):7-15 (1982) and references cited therein.

68. Srivastava VK, Singh BM, Gupta R. Variability in total bitters in *Tinospora cordifolia* (Willd) Miers populations. *Indian J Pl Genet Resources* 8(1) special issue (2):49-56 (1995).

69. Khory RN, Katrak NN. *Materia medica of India and their therapeutics* (3rd reprint edn., pp. 30-31) New Delhi: Neeraj Publishing House, 1985.

70. *Indian herbal pharmacopoeia* (vol. I, pp. 156-164). Mumbai: Indian Drug Manufacturers' Association and Jammu Tawi: Regional Research Laboratory, 1990.

71. Kapil A, Sharma J. Immunopotentiating compounds from *Tinospora cordifolia. J Ethnopharmacol* 58:89-95 (1997).

72. Rege N, Dahanukar S, Karandikar SM. Hepatoprotective effects of *Tinospora cordifolia* against carbon tetrachloride induced liver damage. *Indian Drugs* 21:544-555 (1984).

73. Nagarkatti DS, Rege NN, Desai NK, Dahanukar SA. Modulation of Kuppfer cell activity by *Tinospora cordifolia* in liver damage. *J Postgrad Med* 40(2):65-67 (1994).

74. Singh B, Sharma ML, Gupta DK, Atal CK, Arya RK. Protective effect of *Tinospora cordifolia* Miers on carbon tetrachloride induced hepatotoxicity. *Indian J Pharmacol* 16:139-142 (1984).

75. Pendse VK, Mahawar MM, Khanna NK, Somani KC, Gautam SK. Anti-inflammatory and related activity of water extract of *Tinospora cordifolia* (Tc-We) "Neem Giloe." *Indian Drugs* 19(10):14-21 (1981).

76. Rege NN, Nazareth HM, Bapat RD, Dahanukar SA. Modulation of immunosuppresion in obstructive jaundice by *Tinospora cordifolia. Indian J Med Res* 90:478-483 (1989).

77. Rege, N, Bapat RD, Koti R, Desai NK, Dahanukar S. Immunotherapy with *Tinospora cordifolia:* A new lead in the management of obstructive jaundice. *Indian J Gastroenterol* 12:5-8 (1993).

78. Gupta AK, co-ordinator, *Quality standards of Indian medicinal plants* (vol. 1, p. 218). New Delhi: Indian Council of Medical Research, 2003.

79. Ikram M, Khattak SG, Gilani SN. Antipyretic studies on some indigenous Pakistani medicinal plants II. *J Ethnopharmacol* 19:185-192 (1987).

80. Rege NN, Thatte UM, Dahanukar SA. Adaptogenic properties of six *rasayana* herbs used in Ayurvedic medicine. *Phytotherap Res* 13:275-291 (1999).

VIRAL HEPATITIS

Viral hepatitis is a major cause of mortality and morbidity especially in the developing world. Several types of virus have been identified—A, B, C, D, E, and G. Hepatitis A and E, which spread through infected food and water, are usually self-remitting. However, hepatitis B and C, which are transmitted parenterally through infected blood products, through sexual contact, or vertical transmission from mother to child, can become chronic.

Hepatitis B is the most common viral disease in the world with over 300 million chronic carriers. Although a major proportion of patients who contract hepatitis B clear the virus from the blood, a definite proportion of patients go on to become chronic carriers. These carriers serve as a reservoir for further transmission of the disease and they are themselves at a risk of developing liver cirrhosis and/or hepatocellular carcinoma.

Thus, there has been a great deal of interest in testing Indian medicinal plants for their activity against hepatitis B. Of these, the best studied is the plant known as *Phyllanthus amarus* or *bhumyamalaki* in Sanskrit. Earlier literature identifies *bhumyamalaki* as *Phyllanthus niruri* or *Phyllanthus fraternus* and is often reported in literature under this name. However, the plant has now been confirmed to be *Phyllanthus amarus*, with *Phyllanthus niruri* being an American species not found in India.[1]

Phyllanthus amarus *Schum & Thon.*
(Family: Euphorbiaceae)

Sanskrit: Bhumlyamalaki, tamalaki	Tamil: Keelanelli
Hindi: Bhuiavala	

Phyllanthus amarus (see Plate 5 in color gallery) is a small herb found throughout the hotter parts of India, especially after the rains. Traditionally, all parts of the plant are used medicinally—leaves, tender aerial parts, and roots. The plant known as *bhumyamalaki* or *tamalaki* in Sanskrit has been known for centuries in the treatment of jaundice. Interestingly the use of the plant tamalaki is first mentioned in multiplant preparations for jaundice in *Caraka Samhita*.[2] It is a commonly used, popular household remedy for the treatment of jaundice. In South India, a bolus of the whole plant is administered with buttermilk. It is traditionally used for jaundice, dyspepsia, colic, and as an appetite stimulant and a diuretic.[3] It has been studied extensively, following the discovery that it can bind the hepatitis B virus surface antigen (HBsAg).[4] The aerial parts of *Phyllanthus amarus* have official status in the *Indian Herbal Pharmacopoeia*, volume II, 1999, for antiviral activity.[5]

Phyllanthus amarus contains lignans, several tannins, flavonoids, sterols, and alkaloids. The lignans phyllanthin and hypophyllanthin have been shown to be hepatoprotective against carbon tetrachloride-induced hepatotoxicity in primary cultured hepatocytes.[6]

The plant has been shown to have an in vitro antiviral activity against hepatitis B.[4,7] The plant extracts have been shown to inhibit HBs-Anti HBs reaction and inhibit HBV DNA polymerase activity. In cell culture it downregulates HBV mRNA transcription and replication and inhibits enhancer I activity.[8,9] In woodchucks it has been shown to clear those infected with Woodchuck Hepatitis Virus (WHV) and prolong the mean survival time.[10] The hepatoprotective activity of *Phyllanthus amarus* on carbon tetrachloride and alcohol-induced damage has also been shown.[11,12]

In a double-blind, placebo-controlled trial, 59 percent of chronic hepatitis B patients became HBsAg negative after ingesting 200 mg powder of aerial parts of *Phyllanthus amarus* three times a day for 1 month, while seroconversion in the placebo group was 4 percent.[13] In another open trial with 28 chronic HBV carriers, clearance rate of 20 percent was seen in patients who were HBeAg negative, that is those who did not show active replication of the virus.[14] However, in Thailand, a double-blind, placebo-controlled trial using Thai *Phyllanthus amarus* failed to clear HBsAg from asymptomatic carriers.[15]

Similarly, seroconversion was not seen in a trial conducted in New Zealand using material from Madras (now Chennai), standardized using geraniin—a hydrolysable tannin— as a marker for standardization.[16]

Despite the fact that there have been negative clinical trials, *Phyllanthus amarus* must be considered a plant of potential use for viral hepatitis B. However, further work is required on choice of plant material, method of processing, dosage to be used, and period of treatment, especially because of the presence of ecotypes of *Phyllanthus amarus.*

In acute viral hepatitis, A, B, non-A, and non-B, 4 week-treatment with *Phyllanthus amarus* was compared with Essentiale (as essential phospholipid from soybean oil) and another control group of patients who were treated with vitamins. In acute viral hepatitis B, patients on *Phyllanthus amarus* had significantly faster recovery. *Phyllanthus amarus* also seemed to accelerate the clearance of HBsAg in 86.9 percent of patients of convalescing from acute viral hepatitis B cases in 3 months time, as against 48 percent in the Essentiale-treated group, and 50 percent in controls on vitamins.[17]

In an early open trial, in 160 children in the age group of 1-12 years, *Phyllanthus fraternus (Phyllanthus amarus)* was found useful in infective hepatitis at a dose level of $50 \text{ mg} \cdot \text{kg}^{-1}$ in three divided daily doses for 6 weeks. A total of 101 children who completed the trial were considered cured, although there were 59 dropouts. Clinical response was marked after 2 weeks and no side effects were seen.[18]

Phyllanthus amarus has been commonly and widely used in India for a very long time. In dosages commonly used (3-6 g of plant powder twice daily) no adverse reactions have been reported.[19] A 90-day study with mice did not show any mortality or weight loss.[20]

NOTES

1. Sivarajan VV, Balachandran I. *Ayurvedic drugs and their plant sources* (pp. 466-469). New Delhi: Oxford and IBH Publishing Co Pvt Ltd, 1994.

2. *Caraka samhita,* ed. and trans. Sharma PV (vol. II, p. 110, "Chikitsastanam," chapter VI, verse 118-121). Varanasi: Chaukhambha Orientalia, 1983.

3. *The wealth of India, raw materials* (vol. VIII, pp. 34-35). New Delhi: Publications and Information Directorate, CSIR, 1969.

4. Thyagarajan SP, Thiruneelakantan K, Subramanian S, Sundaravelu T. *In vitro* inactivation of HBsAg by *Eclipta alba* Haask and *Phyllanthus niruri* Linn. *Indian J Med Res* 76 (suppl.):124-130 (1982).

5. *Indian herbal pharmacopoeia* (vol. II, pp. 85-92). Mumbai: Indian Drug Manufacturers' Association and Jammu Tawi: Regional Research Laboratory, 1999.

6. Syamsundar KV, Singh B, Thakur RS, Husain A, Kiso Y, Hikino H. Antihepatotoxic principles of *Phyllanthus niruri* herb. *J Ethnopharmacol* 14:41-44 (1985).

7. Mehrotra R, Rawat S, Kulshreshtha DK, Goyal P, Patnaik GK, Dhawan BN. *In vitro* effect of *Phyllanthus amarus* on hepatitis B virus. *Indian J Med Res* 93:71-73 (1991).

8. Lee C-D, Ott M, Thyagarajan SP, Shafritz DA, Burk RD, Gupta S. *Phyllanthus amarus* down-regulates hepatitis B virus mRNA transcription and replication. *Eur J Clin Invest* 26:1069-1076 (1996).

9. Ott M, Thyagarajan SP, Gupta S. *Phyllanthus amarus* suppresses hepatitis B virus by interrupting interactions between HBV enhancer I and cellular transcription factors. *Eur J Clin Invest* 27:908-915 (1997).

10. Blumberg BS, Millman I, Venkateswaran PS, Thyagarajan SP. Hepatitis B virus and hepatocellular carcinoma—Treatment of HBV carriers with *Phyllanthus amarus*. *Cancer Detect Prevent* 14:195-201 (1989).

11. Rao YS. Experimental production of liver damage and its protection with *Phyllanthus niruri* and *Capparis spinosa* (both ingredients of Liv 52) in white albino rats. *Probe* 24:117-119 (1985).

12. Umarani D, Devaki T, Govindaraju P, Shanmugasundaram KR. Ethanol induced metabolic alterations and the effect of *Phyllanthus niruri* in their reversal. *Ancient Sci Life* IV:174-180 (1985).

13. Thyagarajan SP, Subramanian S, Thirunalasundari T, Venkateswaran PS, Blumberg BS. Effect of *Phyllanthus amarus* on chronic carriers of hepatitis B virus. *The Lancet* (Oct. 1) 2:764-766 (1988).

14. Thyagarajan SP, Jayaram S, Valliammai T, Madanagopalan N, Pal VG, Jayaraman K. *Phyllanthus amarus* and hepatitis B. *The Lancet* (Oct. 13) 336:949-950 (1990).

15. Leelarasamee A, Trakulsomboon S, Maunwongyathi P, Somanabandhu A, Pidetcha P, Matrakool B, Lebnak T, Ridthimat W, Chandanayingyong D. Failure of *Phyllanthus amarus* to eradicate hepatitis B surface antigen from symptomless carriers. *The Lancet* (June 30) 335:1600-1601 (1990).

16. Milne A, Hopkirk N, Lucas CR, Waldon J, Foo Y. Failure of New Zealand hepatitis B carriers to respond to *Phyllanthus amarus*. *N Z Med J* 107:243 (1994).

17. Jayaram S, Thyagarajan SP, Sumathi S, Manjula S, Malathi S, Madanagopalan N. Efficacy of *Phyllanthus amarus* treatment in acute viral hepatitis A, B, non A non B: An open clinical trial. *Indian J Virol* 13:59-64 (1997).

18. Dixit SP, Achar MP. Bhumyamalaki (*Phyllanthus niruri* Linn) and jaundice in children. *J National Integ Med Assn* 25:269-272 (1983).

19. *Selected medicinal plants of India. A monograph of identity, safety and clinical usage* (pp. 235-237). Bombay: Chemexcil. Basic Chemicals, Pharmaceuticals and Cosmetics Export Promotion Council, 1992.

20. Jayaram S, Thygarajan SP, Panchanandam M, Subramanian S. Anti-hepatitis-B properties of *Phyllanthus niruri* Linn and *Eclipta alba* Hassk: *In vitro* and *in vivo* safety studies. *Biomed* 7(2):9-16 (1987).

OTHER ANTIVIRAL PLANTS

Although a few other Indian plants were found active when tested for activity against hepatitis B, including picroliv from *Picrorhiza kurroa* that was found to bind HBsAg,[1] only *Picrorhiza kurroa* was tested clinically in a double-blind clinical trial on chronic carriers of hepatitis B and found to be inactive.[2] However, this should be considered only a preliminary result and further work is needed on this. In the trial, patients were divided into four groups and randomly allocated to receive 500 mg of *Phyllanthus amarus, Picrorhiza kurroa,* a 1:1 mixture of *Phyllanthus amarus* and *Picrorhiza kurroa,* or a placebo given thrice daily for 3 months. There was a 25-percent clearance in the *Phyllanthus amarus*–treated group, 11.1-percent clearance in the combination group, whereas there was no conversion in the *Picrorhiza kurroa* and placebo groups.

Other single plants that have undergone clinical evaluation are *Berberis aristata* DC. (Family: Berberidaceae) and *Luffa echinata* Roxb. (Family: Cucurbitaceae). In patients of acute viral hepatitis, *Berberis aristata* treatment led to rapid clinical and biochemical improvement.[3] In a comparative study of 42 uncomplicated cases of acute viral hepatitis, the effect of Ayurvedic drugs such as *Picrorhiza kurroa* root powder and *Berberis aristata* bark powder at a dose level of 2 g in four divided doses was studied against a placebo. Early clinical and biochemical improvement was seen in drug-treated cases as compared with the placebo group. A better response was seen in *Picrorhiza kurroa*–treated patients as compared to those treated with *Berberis aristata,* whereas clinical improvement was poor in patients on placebo.[4]

In six patients of viral hepatitis, single administration of drops of aqueous extract of *Luffa echinata* dried fruits into the nostrils lead to intense rhinorrhea and to a significant reduction of serum bilirubin and ALT levels within 2-7 days, and was accompanied by substantial relief in clinical symptoms. The nasal secretions contained total bilirubin ranging from 1.6 to 5.5 mg percent; however, the authors[5] feel that the possibility that there is nasal absorption of the drug and consequent action on the liver cannot be ruled out.

NOTES

1. Mehrotra R, Rawat S, Kulshreshtha DK, Patnaik GK, Dhawan BN. *In vitro* studies on the effect of certain natural products against hepatitis B virus. *Indian J Med Res* 92B:133-138 (1990).

2. Jayaram S. Studies on prevention and control of hepatitis B virus infection. PhD thesis, University of Madras, 1992 quoted in Thygarajan SP, Jayaram S. Natural history of *Phyllanthus amarus* in the treatment of hepatitis B. *Indian J Med Microbiol* 10:64-80 (1992).

3. Das Adhikary BM, Debnath PK. Preliminary report on *daruharidra (Berberis aristata)* on clinical jaundice. *Indian J Pharmacol* 13:61 (1981).

4. Singh DS, Gupta SS, Ansari SA, Singh RH. A comparative study of Ayurvedic drugs *Picrorrhiza kurroa (kutaki)* and *Berberis aristata (daruharidra)* in acute viral hepatitis at Varanasi. *J Res Edu Indian Med* X (4):1-4 (1991).

5. Vaidya AB, Bhatia CK, Mehta JM, Sheth UK. Therapeutic potential of *Luffa echinata* (Roxb.) in viral hepatitis. *Indian J Pharmacol* 8:245-246 (1976).

ASCITES

Boerhaavia diffusa L. (family Nyctaginaceae) has been tried out clinically in cases of ascites due to early liver and peritoneal conditions and has been found to be very beneficial with the drug producing marked diuresis leading in some cases to disappearance of ascites.[1] Experimentally the plant has been shown to have hepatoprotective, diuretic, and anti-inflammatory activity.[2-5] A study of the diuretic and anti-inflammatory activity of different parts of the plant showed that the water-soluble portion of the alcoholic extract of the root and leaf were more active than the whole-plant extract.[5] It has also been shown that the aqueous extract of the root was more active than the root powder, and it was most active when collected in the month of May.[6] The plant has official status as a hepatoprotective and diuretic in the *Indian Herbal Pharmacopoeia,* volume I, 1998[7] It is a commonly used plant for jaundice, and further studies need to be carried out.

NOTES

1. Chopra RN, Chopra IC, Handa KL, Kapur LD. *Chopra's indigenous drugs of India* (pp. 297-300). Calcutta: Academic Publishers, 1994.

2. Chandan BK, Sharma AK, Anand KK. *Boerhaavia diffusa:* A study of its hepatoprotective activity. *J Ethnopharmacol* 31:299-307 (1991).

3. Chakroborti KK, Handa SS. Antihepatotoxic activity of *Boerhaavia diffusa. Indian Drugs* 27:161-166 (1989).

4. Singh RH, Udupa KN. Studies on the indigenous drug *punarnava (Boerhaavia diffusa).* Part III. Experimental and pharmacological studies. *J Res Indian Med* 7(3):17-27 (1972).

5. Mudgal V. Comparative studies on the anti-inflammatory and diuretic action of different parts of the plant *Boerhaavia diffusa (punarnava). J Res Indian Med* 9(2):57-59 (1974).

6. Rawat AKS, Mehrotra S, Tripathi SC, Shome U. Hepatoprotective activity of *Boerhaavia diffusa* L. roots-a popular Indian ethnomedicine. *J Ethnopharmacol* 56:61-66 (1997).

7. *Indian herbal pharmacopoeia* (vol. I, pp. 38-46). Mumbai: Indian Drug Manufacturers' Association and Jammu Tawi: Regional Research Laboratory, 1998.

CHRONIC CHOLECYSTITIS

Single plants do not appear to have been tried out in chronic cholecystitis. However, the alkaloid berberine from *Berberis vulgaris,* either as a sulfate or hydrochloride, was shown to be effective in alleviating the clinical symptoms in chronic cholecystitis patients by reducing the bilirubin levels and increasing the gall bladder bile volume.[1] Isolated compounds cannot be considered to be plant drugs, but may point the way to activity in the crude drug or its extract.

Thus, despite the long history of clinical use of plants in Ayurveda for the treatment of liver diseases, few controlled clinical trials have been carried out. Many of the plants have been studied experimentally for hepatoprotective activity, some for choleretic and anticholestatic activity, and a few of them for liver cell regeneration and antiviral activity against the hepatitis B virus. Chemical work to identify active constituents has also been carried out. The result of the scientific studies so far has been the setting off of a differentiation in the pharmacological profile and therefore a change in the way we view these plants. For these plants to acquire a wider usage, further work is required in the universally acceptable standards of their quality, efficacy, and safety.

NOTE

1. Handa SS, Sharma A, Chakraborti KK. Natural products and plants as liver protecting drugs. *Fitoterapia LVII:*307-351 (1986).

Chapter 5

Respiratory Tract Drugs

In modern medicine, respiratory tract drugs include antiallergic drugs, antiasthmatic drugs, and antitussives.[1] In Ayurveda, respiratory problems are considered to arise from poor digestion[2] and therefore the herbs prescribed in Ayurveda for treatment of respiratory disorders not only improve digestion but also have other useful effects like antiallergic activity and immunostimulant activity. For example, *Piper longum* is a carminative agent that improves digestion, and has antianaphylactic and immunostimulant effects. A large number of herbs have been used to stimulate digestion, reduce the cough reflex, liquefy phlegm, and aid in the removal of phlegm through expectoration. Some of the conditions associated with respiratory tract problems have been classified as *kasa* (cough), *swasa* (dyspnea), and *kasa swasa (bronchial asthma)*. The most popular home remedies for these conditions include spices, such as ginger, turmeric, black, and long pepper, and common plants, such as *Adhatoda vasica, Solanum xanthocarpum, Solanum trilobatum,* etc.

NOTES

1. McGuire JL (ed.), *Pharmaceuticals, classes, therapeutic agents, areas of application* (vol. 2, p. 837). Weinheim: Wiley-VCH, 2000.
2. Frawley D. *Ayurvedic healing. A comprehensive guide* (p. 160). Delhi: Motilal Banarasidass Publishers Pvt Ltd, 1992.

doi:10.1300/5683_05

PLANTS FOR BRONCHIAL ASTHMA

Bronchial asthma is a chronic allergic condition caused by the sensitivity of the body, especially the respiratory organs, to external allergens, which are often harmless agents such as dust, pollen, temperature, etc. As a result of this hyperreactivity of the bronchial tissues, there is a production of excess phlegm, swelling, and partial blockage of the bronchial passage resulting in wheezing and breathlessness. The Ayurvedic concept and the pathogenesis of the disease are considered to be similar to that in Allopathy and these have been discussed.[1] The Ayurvedic term for bronchial asthma, *tamaka swasa* or less correctly *kasa swasa,* consists of the names of its two major symptoms—cough *(kasa)* and breathlessness *(swasa).* A number of plants recommended by Caraka are still in use today. There are 33 major herbs that have been listed[1] and 22 plants that have been tried out clinically and reviewed.[2]

Adhatoda vasica *Nees (Family: Acanthaceae)*

Latin: *Adhatoda zeylanica* Medicus, *Justicia adhatoda* Linn.	Hindi: Arusa
Sanskrit: Vasa	Tamil: Adhatodai
English: Malabar Nut Tree	

Adhatoda vasica is an evergreen perennial shrub found all over India up to an elevation of 600 m.[3] The name of the plant is derived from the Tamil *(adu:* goat, *thodathu:* will not touch) because the fetid smell of the leaves keeps goats away. Therefore, it is often used for fencing in villages, as it is safe from grazing animals, and also because it is then readily available for use. Medicinally the use of the plant—leaves, roots, and flowers— has been known for over 2,000 years. The *Caraka Samhita* recommends its use for cough. The leaf of *Adhatoda vasica* is traditionally used in Ayurveda for the treatment of cold, cough, bronchitis, and asthma. It is considered an expectorant, and aids in the liquefying and removal of phlegm.[3,4] Not only is it used as a hemostatic agent in bleeding disorders, it also helps in the healing of wounds, in peptic ulcer (see Chapter 3), and in pyorrhea and bleeding gums (see Chapter 14).[5] The leaf of *Adhatoda vasica* has the official status in the *Indian Herbal Pharmacopoeia, 2002*, as a bronchodilator and an expectorant.[6]

Among the constituents of *Adhatoda vasica* are an essential oil containing limonene, flavonoids, resin, and several alkaloids of which the major alkaloid is vasicine (~1 percent),[3] which has been shown to possess brochodilatory activity.[7] Vasicinone, a minor alkaloid, has been shown in vitro to be a potent vasodilator.[8] In vivo vasicinone was found to be as potent a bronchodilator as theophylline and 5,000 times less potent than isoprenaline.[9]

Adhatoda vascia showed antiallergic and antiasthmatic properties in guinea pigs. A fraction containing the minor alkaloid vasicinol and 20 percent vasicine inhibited ovalbumin- and PAF-induced allergic reactions at a dose level of 5 mg per animal by inhalation and 2.5 $g \cdot kg^{-1}$ by intragastric administration.[10] *Adhatoda vasica* extract of flowers and leaves has been shown in guinea pigs to have an antitussive activity similar to codeine against coughing induced by irritant aerosols.[11]

A double-blind clinical trial was conducted on "Wintry," a product containing 25 mg of a mixture of vasicine and vasicinone per tablet, against placebo. One tablet was given thrice a day against the placebo for 4 weeks. An equal number of 30 patients of asthmatic bronchitis received the drug and the placebo, respectively. All patients were given 250 mg amoxicillin for the first week. Out of the 30 patients who received Wintry 21 showed improvement both clinically and on spirometer tests for lung function, 6 of the patients remained unchanged, the condition of 3 patients deteriorated. Of those on placebo, only 4 patients improved, whereas 10 remained unchanged and the condition of 16 patients deteriorated.[12]

The leaves of *Adhatoda vasica* are also commonly used to treat cold and are considered to be effective when administered at the first signs of the infection. Despite the long history of its use, there are no clinical trials to evaluate the full scope of the use of this plant, and this is an urgent requirement.

Despite a long safe history of the use of *Adhatoda vasica* in human beings, there has been concern on the possibility that vasicine exerts an abortifacient effect,[6] based on evidence from parenteral administration.[13]

An experimental study on rats,[14] on the possible abortive effect of oral administration of 325 mg·kg^{-1} per day of the leaf extract, produced no abortion in treated animals. Further, after an extensive review of the literature, it was concluded that there is no scientifically valid evidence for potentially harmful effects on human beings, including the effect during pregnancy.[15] Chronic toxicity studies in two species with vasicine hydrochloride at dose levels ranging from 2.5 to 20 mg·kg^{-1} body weight did not show any toxic effects. There was no difference in the body weight and the mortality of test animals and controls. Histopathology showed no abnormality of major organs.[16] Total extract of the plant, dissolved in water at 2-8 ml·kg^{-1} for 90 days, showed no toxicity.[17]

Albizzia lebbeck *Benth. (Family: Mimosaceae)*

Sanskrit: Sirish(a)	Tamil: Vagei
Hindi: Siris	English: East Indian Walnut Tree, Siris Tree

Albizzia lebbeck is a large deciduous, spreading tree found all over India, up to an elevation of 1,200 m. The bark, seeds, leaves, and flowers are used for medicinal purposes; however, the bark is considered in the classic literature as the best antidote to both plant and animal poisons. It is used both as a single drug and in combination with other drugs in the form of bark powder or decoction.[18] In Kerala, the bark powder, made into a paste, is rubbed on the body to soothe itching.[19]

The stem bark contains 7-11 percent condensed tannins; procyanidin B-2, procyanidin B-5, and procyanidin C-1: (-)-epicatechin; D-catechin; and isomers of leucocyanidin. Also present in the bark are friedelin, β- sitosterol, cardenolide, and anthraquinone glycosides.[20-22] Three saponins named albizziasaponin A, B, and C have also been isolated.[22] The flowers contain, approximately, 4 percent of an essential oil and several saponins lebbekanin A-H.[20,22]

The flower and bark decoction of *Albizzia lebbeck* has been studied experimentally for its general pharmacological properties, and especially for its antiasthmatic and antiallergic effect.[23] It has shown immunomodulatory activity and mast-cell stabilization apart from its ability to prevent allergen-induced bronchospasm.

In sensitized guinea pigs, the bark decoction acted as a shield against horse serum antigen,[23] whereas both the bark and the flower decoction protected against histamine-induced bronchospasm. The bark decoction had significant cromoglycate-like activity, such as action on the mast cells, and appeared to inhibit the early process of sensitization and synthesis of reaginic-type antibodies.[24,25] It reduced the secretion of macrophage migration inhibition factors.[25] *Albizzia lebbeck,* when administered simultaneously with histamine, reduces the release of catecholamine at a dose of 100 mg·kg^{-1} up to a maximum effective dose of 200 mg·kg^{-1} bodyweight of alcoholic extract.[26,27] Fractions of stem bark of *Albizzia lebbeck* also reduced the passive cutaneous anaphylaxis and mast-cell degranulation in rats.[28] Hot water and butanol extracts of the bark administered, once daily for 1 week, to mice that were previously immunized by sheep's red blood corpuscles, developed higher antibody titer that was comparable to the standard drug muramyl dipeptide (MDP).[29]

Bronchial Asthma

A few trials have been conducted with the bark of *Albizzia lebbeck* in bronchial asthma. A total of 60 patients were given 25 ml of the aqueous decoction, from 100 g of the bark, four times a day for 3 weeks. Excellent results were obtained in cases of not more than 2 years duration; however, in patients with a long history of the disease, the outcome was variable. The decoction was found to relieve difficulty in breathing, reduce cough, and increase the breath holding time, improve the vital capacity and forced respiratory volume in bronchitis. The saponins were considered to be the main active principle behind all these actions.[30]

In an open trial, 19 patients with bronchial asthma were given 30 ml decoction of *shirish* bark thrice daily for 6 weeks. There was significant fall in eosinophil count and the erythrocyte sedimentation rate ESR and increase in peak expiratory flow rate (PEFR). Nearly all patients experienced symptomatic relief. There was also highly significant effect based on a total of 12 subjective and objective parameters of bronchial asthma such as breathlessness, cough, paroxysmal attacks of dyspnea, wheezing, rhonchi, pulmonary function tests, etc. assessed in all patients before start of the trial and subsequently four times during and beyond treatment at 15-day intervals.[31]

The flowers have been tried out for tropical pulmonary eosinophilia.[32] See later in this chapter. Considering the results obtained so far, further trials need to be carried out with standardized material, controls, and larger patient numbers.

It has been reported that in the experience of Ayurvedic physicians no serious toxicity has been seen clinically.[24] In the clinical trial, using the flowers of *shirish,* no side effect or toxicity was seen.[32] LD_{50} in albino rats was found to be 2 $g \cdot kg^{-1}$ body weight and LD_0 0.4 $g \cdot kg^{-1}$. Rats that were given 25 $mg \cdot kg^{-1}$ of *Albizzia lebbeck* daily for 2 weeks showed no difference, from controls, in body weight, general behavior, and food intake. In addition, the mortality rate was similar in both groups.[24]

Boswellia serrata *Roxb. ex Coleb (Family: Burseraceae)*

In Ayurveda, *Boswellia serrata* (see Plate 2 in color gallery) has been used in a number of conditions. In respiratory tract conditions like cough, bronchitis, fever, and asthma it is used either by inhalation of the smoke or as a decoction.[33,34] When taken internally, it acts as a stimulant expectorant in pulmonary diseases.[35]

Research has shown that the gum resin of *Boswellia serrata* is useful in a number of inflammatory conditions in which leukotrienes play an important role in the causation and maintenance of diseases, such as inflammatory bowel diseases—Crohn's disease and ulcerative colitis,—rheumatism, asthma, and in the reduction of edema in certain kinds of brain tumor.[34] See Chapters 3, 8, and 13. In asthma, leukotrienes are the important mediators of inflammation, which cause bronchoconstriction, mucosal edema, enhance mucous secretion, and raise eosinophil levels. Therefore, leukotrienes have become important targets for potential antiasthmatic drugs.[36] The boswellic acids present in *Boswellia serrata* have been shown to inhibit leukotriene synthesis, and therefore are capable of playing a potentially useful role in the management of asthma.

In a double-blind placebo-controlled clinical trial, 80 patients of bronchial asthma were given either 300 mg of gum resin of *Boswellia serrata* or 300 mg lactose as a placebo thrice daily for 6 weeks. In the treated group, the mean duration of the disease was 9-15 years. Seventy percent of the treated group showed improvement in symptoms, such as difficulty in breathing, rhonchii, number of attacks, and lung function tests such as forced vital capacity, etc., [36] leading the authors to believe that further studies, with a standardized product, are required to confirm the initial results obtained.

Boswellia serrata is usually well tolerated; however, it can give rise to gastrointestinal side effects in a small percentage of patients. In the bronchial asthma trial, with 300 mg thrice daily, 2 out of 40 patients complained of stomach pain, nausea, and hyperacidity.[36] See also Chapter 3, section "*Boswellia serrata.*"

Curcuma longa *Linn. (Family: Zingiberaceae)*

Latin: *Curcuma domestica* Valeton	Hindi: Haldi
Sanskrit: Haridra	Tamil: Manjal
English: Turmeric	

Turmeric is a commonly used household remedy for cough and cold, taken mixed in hot milk. It is used, internally, in Ayurveda, to treat asthma, cold, cough, and fever,[37] usually along with other herbs and rarely ever alone.[38]

Curcumin, the main active principle and coloring matter in turmeric, has been shown to have a spasmolytic effect on various spasmogens.[39] Extracts of turmeric have been shown to have an antiallergic effect; the ethyl acetate extract being the most active in exerting anti-inflammatory and antiallergic effect.[40,41] In addition, the curcuminoids are considered to be very effective antiallergic components;[40] the activity of ethyl acetate extract and curcumin being owing to the inhibition of histamine release.[42]

Powdered rhizomes of *Curcuma longa* were given in increasing doses from 4 to 32 g daily for 15-45 days to 71 bronchitis patients,

13 bronchiestatis patients, 18 bronchial asthmatic patients, and 12 tropical eosinophilic patients. A significant relief in signs and symptoms was noticed in 11 out of 71 cases of bronchitis, 1 out of 13 cases of bronchiestatis, 5 out of 18 cases of bronchial asthma, and 6 out of 12 cases of tropical eosinophilia.[43]

Turmeric powder either as such or after frying in ghee—made from butter by heating until most of the water evaporates— was given in a dose of 6-12 g for 15-20 days to patients of asthma with differing "humoral vitiation" according to Ayurvedic criteria based on symptoms such as degree of dyspnea, phlegm, dryness of throat, rales, and ronchii. Sixty percent of the treated patients showed improvement with a decrease in the intensity of cough and dyspnea. In addition, there was a reduction in the amount of sputum. In this trial, the diagnosis was an Ayurvedic diagnosis, and there was variation in the dosage also.[38]

It would be worthwhile to conduct a trial to check the dosage requirements and the kind of clinical response that can be achieved considering the continued scientific support that turmeric receives from modern investigations.

For details on the safety of turmeric, a commonly used spice in Indian cooking, see Chapter 3. In the trial on patients with bronchial asthma, who were given 12 g·day^{-1} of turmeric powder, a few patients complained of dryness of mouth and throat, and a mild headache mitigated by the reduction in the dosage or changing the so-called "vehicle,"[38] which in Ayurveda, are hot water, milk or milk with clarified butter (ghee), used to aid in the absorption of the drug and in directing it to the required site.

Ocimum sanctum *Linn. (Family: Lamiaceae)*

Latin: *Ocimum tenuiflorum* Linn.	Hindi: Tulsi
Sanskrit: Tulasi	Tamil: Thulasi
English: Holy basil, Sacred basil	

Sacred to the Hindus, the holy basil is a small herb with an aromatic smell found throughout India and commonly cultivated in gardens and courtyards. There are two varieties of this herb: one with green stems called *Sri Tulasi* and the other with purple stems known as *Krishna Tulasi,* which is the preferred one in medicine. The leaves of the holy basil are a commonly used household remedy for cough, cold, bronchitis, and asthma. The leaves have the official status in the *Indian Herbal Pharmacopoeia,* 2002, for their expectorant properties.[44]

The leaves contain 0.4-0.8 percent of an essential oil containing eugenol and β-caryophyllene as major constituents.[44] In addition, the leaves contain tannins (4.6 percent); ursolic acid; several sterols, such as β-sitosterol, campesterol, sigmasterol; flavonoids, such as apigenin, luteolin, and their 7-glucuronides, molludistin, orientin;[44-46] and acids, such as gallic acid, caffeic acid, chlorogenic acid, and rosmarinic acid.[47]

Several phenolic compounds, isolated from fresh leaves and stems, exhibited antioxidant activity (e.g. apigenin, rosmarinic acid) and demonstrated COX-1 and COX-2 inhibitory activity (e.g., eugenol, apigenin, rosmarinic acid).[48] The alcoholic extract of *Ocimum sanctum* leaves was found to be protective against histamine and *Acacia arabica* pollen–induced asthma in guinea pigs in a dose-dependent fashion.[49] In addition, it acted as an inhibitor against histamine-induced spasm in guinea pig tracheal chain preparation.[49] A 50-percent alcoholic extract and volatile oil from fresh leaves inhibited histamine and acetyl choline–induced preconvulsive dyspnea in guinea pigs, but the extract from dried leaves did not contain these properties.[50,51]

All the trials with *Ocimum sanctum* are of preliminary nature and further trials are urgently needed with standardized preparations, larger patient numbers, and better methodology.

Asthma

In an open trial with 20 patients of asthma, 500 mg of *Ocimum sanctum* extract, made into tablets, was given thrice daily for 1 week. Relief was observed, within 3 days, in breathlessness and in vital capacity, but there was no change in the eosinophil count.[52] In another open trial, the leaves of *Ocimum sanctum* were tried in cases of bronchial asthma and stress-related hypertension, and were found to be highly effective in these cases. Unfortunately, more details are not available.[53]

Viral encephalitis

In a preliminary clinical trial, 16 patients with acute viral encephalitis were divided into two groups: one group of ten patients received steroids, whereas the remaining six patients were given dried aqueous extract from 2.5 g of fresh leaves four times daily. The crude extract of *Ocimum sanctum* was found to be more effective than steroids in the treatment of patients with viral encephalitis. In the steroid group two patients dropped out, six died, and two patients had residual paralysis, whereas in the *Ocimum sanctum* group one patient dropped out, one died, three recovered completely, and one had residual paralysis.[54]

The holy basil is generally considered a very safe drug, and many Indians often consume a few leaves as part of their daily ritual.[55] This habit is often cited as one reason for lower birth rates in men consuming holy basil leaves on a long-term basis, which may have some experimental evidence in the reversible antiandrogenic property of the leaves.[56] No side effects have been reported in the clinical trials.[46,52] Constipation was the only side effect, in one trial where doses ranging from 5 to 27 g were taken by 120 patients for 3 months.[55]

Piper longum *Linn. (Family: Piperaceae)*

Sanskrit: Pippali	Tamil: Tippali
Hindi: Pipli	English: Indian Long Pepper

Piper longum is a slender aromatic climber found throughout the hotter parts of India.[57] The roots, the stem, and more importantly the fruiting spikes are used for medicinal purposes.[58] *Piper longum* is a powerful stimulant and has been used for a long time for digestive and respiratory disorders. The fruits and stem are therefore often mixed with the ingredients of a stimulant soup called *"Tippili rasam"* in South India as a household remedy for cough and bronchial disorders. *Piper longum* has been mentioned in the *Caraka Samhita* as a prophylactic agent in asthma.[59] It is used in Ayurveda to treat cough, cold, asthma, bronchitis, laryngitis, gas, abdominal distention, and also arthritis and sciatica.[60,62] *Piper longum* is considered a rejuvenative drug for the lungs, and is used as a milk decoction to treat asthma.[60] The fruits have the official status in the *Indian Herbal Pharmacopoeia, 2002*, for their antiallergic, antiasthmatic, and hepatoprotective properties.[57]

The fruits contain 1 percent of an essential oil and 4-5 percent of the pungent principle piperine. Other minor components include piplartine and piperlongumine, and a low melting waxy alkaloid N-isobutyldeca-*trans*-2-*trans*-4-dienamide, piperidine alkaloids, a lignan, sesamin, terpenoids, and dihydrostigmasterol.[57]

The petroleum ether extract of the fruits acts as a respiratory stimulant at lower doses. However, with higher doses, it causes convulsions in several species of small animals.[61,62] Crude extracts as well as the alkaloid piplartine suppressed ciliary movements in the esophagus of frog; piplartine being more active than the aqueous or alcoholic extracts, suggesting that *Piper longum* may act by suppression of cough reflex.[63]

Piper longum fruit-milk extract reduced effectively passive cutaneous anaphylaxis in rats[64] and protected guinea pigs against antigen induced bronchospasm. However, there was no significant effect on the total quantity of histamine in various organs—lungs, trachea, and intestines or on the release of histamine on antigenic challenge.[65] In an experiment using rat lung perfusion in sensitized animals, the milk extract increased the rate of flow.[66] Piperine blocked the spasms induced by various spasmogens in isolated guinea pig and rabbit intestines, and decreased the rate of respiration.[67]

Bronchial asthma

There is also a special course of treatment in Ayurveda known as *Vardaman pippali* (*vardaman:* increasing; *pippali:* long pepper), which is given as a prophylactic in asthma. During this treatment, long pepper is given in increasing doses to reach a maximum for that age and then again reduced back to the original dosage. Three clinical studies have been conducted using this kind of regimen.

In a double-blind clinical study, 240 children suffering from bronchial asthma in the age group of neonates to 12 years were given 2-3 courses of the *Piper longum,* each course consisting of a gradually increasing dosage of *Piper longum* starting from a minimum of 1 g to reach a maximum of 30 g, and then a reduction of the dosage to the original dose. There was significant reduction in the frequency and severity of asthmatic attacks, with 80 percent of patients showing improvement, 17 percent no improvement, and 8 percent becoming worse.[68]

In another open study, 20 children (1-12 years) with asthma were administered *Piper longum* fruit powder in a gradually increasing dosage over a period of 5 weeks. Each child below 5 years received the 150 mg fruit powder in capsules, whereas a child above 5 years received 250 mg of the fruit powder in capsules. The dosage was one capsule per day in the first week, two in the second, three in the third, two in the fourth, and one in the fifth week. This regimen significantly reduced the severity and frequency of asthmatic attacks. There was no significant difference in the IgE values in six children. At the end of 1 year, 11 patients showed excellent response, 3 showed moderate response, whereas 3 out of 20 patients failed to show any satisfactory response. Three patients with a history of food allergy were able to consume the offending items after the treatment. There was excellent response to the drug and only one patient complained of nausea.[69]

In a preliminary study, a preparation of *Piper longum* with milk, known as *"Pippali kshira paka"*— made by boiling to dryness 40 g of long pepper in 500 ml of milk and 2 l of water—was given for 4 weeks in three divided daily doses to ten patients with bronchial asthma. The response was evaluated as good to moderate in eight patients.[70]

In another study using *"vardhaman pippali,"* in 60 patients with different respiratory disorders, the drug was found to exhibit good efficacy, and was found to be very effective in patients with bronchial asthma.[71]

The use of *Piper longum* fruits has been known for a long time, and is well tolerated in the dosages commonly used (250-500 mg thrice a day).[72] In the clinical trial on 20 children between the age group of 1 and 12 years, the tolerance to the drug was rated as excellent with only one patient complaining of nausea after the intake of drug.[69] Nausea was also noted in the trial on patients with bronchial asthma.[70] Toxicity studies in albino rats employing a milk extract of the fruit boiled in milk at 1 g·kg^{-1} did not cause any mortality.[72] Acute, subacute, and chronic toxicity studies showed no adverse effect.[72-74] In the treated animals there was a significant increase in the weight of lung and spleen, as compared to control animals.[74] No spermatotoxic effect was seen.[74]

Solanum xanthocarpum *Schrad. & Wendl.*
(*Family: Solanaceae*)

Latin: *Solanum surattense* Burm. f.	Hindi: Kateli
Sanskrit: Kantakari	Tamil: Kandankattiri
English: Yellow-Berried Nightshade	

Solanum xanthocarpum is a very spiny diffuse herb found throughout India. The drug consists of the dried whole plant, including leaves, stem, flowers, fruits, and root, and it has been used medicinally for a number of conditions since the time of Caraka and Sushruta.[75] However, it is best known for its use in respiratory disorders, helping to expectorate stubborn phlegm in productive cough, bronchitis, and asthma.[76] The plant is an official drug in the *Indian Herbal Pharmacopoeia* as an expectorant.[77]

The plant contains several steroidal alkaloids—0.2 percent solasodine, solamargine, β-solamargine, solasonine, and sterols, such as cycloartenol, norcarpesterol, cholesterol, and derivatives.[77]

Only a few studies have been carried out and these support the use of the drug in asthma. The glucoalkaloid and fatty acid fractions of *Solanum xanthocarpum* extracts cause liberation of histamine from the lung tissue, suggesting that the beneficial effect of the drug in bronchial asthma may be due to the removal of histamine from bronchial and lung tissue.[78,79] The glucoalkaloid and the alcoholic fraction at 2 mg·kg^{-1} ip also protected against antigen-induced bronchospasm; in sensitized guinea pigs the protection being estimated as 66.6-70.2 percent.[80] In addition, it has been suggested that the saponins from *Solanum xanthocarpum* may be inducing the formation of anti-allergic substances.[81]

The efficacy of *Solanum xanthocarpum* has been tried out in bronchial asthma.[82-86] Starting with a preliminary open study with 11 patients suffering from bronchial asthma and 4 patients suffering from nonspecific cough,[82] the next exploratory study had 60 patients with chronic obstructive airway disease,[83] and then *Solanum xanthocarpum* was given to 305 patients with chronic respiratory diseases. There were 250 cases of bronchial asthma, 43 of chronic bronchitis, and 12 cases were suffering from nonspecific unproductive cough. Patients were given whole plant powder in a dose of 1 g, two or three times a day for one month. Fifty percent of the patients showed complete relief of symptoms with no side effects. Complete relief was observed in 55-74 percent of patients with bronchial asthma—all cases of chronic bronchitis—and in seven cases of nonspecific unproductive cough. It was observed that the drug acted like an expectorant in the presence of phlegm, and it acted as an antitussive agent in the case of dry cough. [84]

In the trial of 93 patients with cough *(kasa)*, *Solanum xanthocarpum* was found effective in diminishing the intensity of cough and dyspnea in 50 percent of the cases using a total dose level of 60-200g of whole plant or root decoction, given in divided doses over a day for 15-20 days.[84] The dosages mentioned seemed highly excessive at first, but if taken together with the Hindi summary in the paper where decoction is mentioned and the next paper of the same author where patients were given 60-200 ml of decoction, the 60-200 g probably refers to 60-200 g of decoction and is indicated as such above. A few patients complained of mouth and throat dryness, and a feeling of warmth, which was reduced by lowering the dose.[85] According to *Selected Medicinal Plants of India,* dosage of *Solanum xanthocarpum* is 1-2 g of drug powder twice daily or 20-60 ml decoction twice daily.[75]

In an open exploratory trial, 44 patients with respiratory problems complaining of cough and dyspnea were given 60-120 ml of the whole plant or root decoction in a divided dosage with added honey for an average of 15-20 days. Diet was controlled and heavy food and salty and sour articles such as pickles were avoided. There was a washout period of 7 days when patients were given glucose capsules. If there was no improvement with the intake of glucose capsules, treatment with the drug decoction was started. Patients were divided into two groups of 21 and 23 based on symptoms as per Ayurvedic criteria. The drug was found to be more useful in the group of patients who had excessive phlegm, with 50 percent of them showing a reduction in the amount of phlegm. The doctors also felt that the root was more effective than the whole plant. The trial serves to give an indication of the utility of the drug and highlights the difficulty in correlating Ayurvedic concepts with modern terms. Side effects were similar to the earlier trial.[86] There is a need to hold further trials with larger numbers of patients, well-defined parameters, and with a standardized drug.

In an open trial, 16 patients with chronic bronchial asthma were treated with 300 mg tablets of *Solanum xanthocarpum* extract, 2-4 tablets being given thrice daily for 3 months. The improvement was graded as excellent in six, good in three, fair in two, and no improvement in five patients. The drug was evaluated as affording relief to 56 percent of the patients. No side effects were observed in patients even in those with diabetes, hypertension, and coronary heart disease.[87]

In another open trial, the effectiveness of a single dose of 300 mg of powdered whole plant of *Solanum xanthocarpum* or *Solanum trilobatum*—another plant drug commonly used especially in South India—was evaluated against the effectiveness of salbutamol 4 mg or deriphylline 200 mg (combination of theophylline and etiophylline). Pulmonary functions were assessed just before administration and again 2 hours after administration. Treatment with *Solanum xanthocarpum* or *Solanum. trilobatum* improved several parameters of pulmonary function significantly, although to a lesser extent when compared to deriphylline or salbutamol. The authors suggest that increased dosages may lead to effects comparable to standard drugs. No side effects were noted, both drugs being well tolerated.[88]

The studies emphasize the need to conduct further studies with a standardized drug to establish the dosage, the mechanism of action, and the usefulness of the drug in asthma.

In clinical trials using *Solanum xanthocarpum,* side effects have generally been observed only in a few patients and have been mild, involving dryness of the mouth and throat, and a feeling of warmth throughout the body, which disappeared on dose reduction.[85,86] In other studies, the drug was well tolerated and no adverse effects were observed.[87,88] In albino rats, the hot water extract of seeds showed toxicity at 200 mg·kg^{-1}.[77,89] In animal studies, the alkaloid solasodine has shown an antispermatogenic activity;[90] the relevance of these studies for human beings is yet to be established.

Terminalia belerica *Roxb. (Family: Combretaceae)*

The Sanskrit names of plants are very descriptive: usually evocative of either the appearance of the plant or its uses. Here the name *bibhitaka* or *vibhitaka* indicates that the regular use of this plant keeps one free from diseases. Fruits and oil from the plant have a number of uses: the pulp is analgesic; the unripe fruit is a laxative; and the fruit is a part of the three-fruit combination of *triphala,* which is a bowel tonic and a laxative. The ripe fruit is useful in diarrhea (see Chapter 3). It is also useful in asthma and cough, helping in reducing the bronchial inflammation. The pulp in honey is also used in eye diseases.[91] The fruit pericarp is the official drug in the *Indian Herbal Pharmacopoeia,* 2002, as an expectorant, a hypolipidemic, and a laxative.[92]

In an open exploratory clinical trial to evaluate the antitussive and antiasthmatic effect of *Terminalia belerica,* 93 patients, ages 1-79 years, were included in the trial after excluding 44 patients with tuberculosis. Among the patients included, 61 were suffering from cough *(kasa),* 12 from dyspnea *(swasa),* and 20 had both cough and dyspnea. The whole fruit, both rind and nut was powdered and administered in doses of 2-6 g thrice a day with water. No period of treatment is mentioned. The symptoms that were assessed were the following: cough (91), dyspnea (51), expectoration (58), pain in chest (29), wheezing (12), temperature (18), loss of weight (25), and loss of appetite (27). The evaluation revealed that 22 patients showed complete relief in symptoms, 27 had marked relief, 35 moderate relief, and 9 had no relief in symptoms. The clinical impression was that the drug has bronchodilatory, antitussive, and antiasthmatic effects.[93]

Terminalia belerica is generally considered safe in the doses used clinically. In the clinical trial reported above, the fruit powder was given in a dose of 2-6 g thrice a day with water; no adverse effects were noticed, except for abdominal disturbances, probably due to the laxative effect of the fruit.[93]

Tylophora indica *(Burm. f.) Merril (Family: Asclepiadaceae)*

Latin: *Tylophora asthmatica* Wight & Arn.	Hindi: Antamul
Sanskrit: Arkaparni, Anthrapachaka	Tamil: Nayppalai
English: Emetic swallow-wort, Indian, or Country ipecacuanha	

Tylophora indica is a perennial climber found throughout India, and more commonly in the eastern and southern parts of India, up to an elevation of 900 m. The leaves and roots, with emetic, expectorant, and antidysentric properties, are considered a substitute for ipecacuanha. The use of the plant was initially regional, confined only to areas where the plant grows. Later, interest in the plant grew through the work of Dr. Kotak and Dr. Shivpuri, who showed that consumption of just 3-6 leaves of *Tylophora indica* had prophylactic action lasting for several weeks, and the use of the plant became more widespread. The leaves are used as a household remedy for asthma, bronchitis, and whooping cough.[94,95]

The leaves contain several alkaloids (0.2-0.4 percent) of which tylophorine (0.1 percent) is the major alkaloid. In addition, there are sterols, α-amyrin, flavonoids, quercetin and kaempferol, tannins, glucose, calcium, salts, etc.[94,95]

Extracts and alkaloids from the leaves of *Tylophora indica* have been shown to have antiasthmatic, bronchodilatory, anti-inflammatory, antiallergic, and immune suppressive properties. The alcoholic extract and total alkaloids of *Tylophora indica* leaves have shown an antispasmodic effect in isolated tissues[96] and bronchodilation although inhibiting bronchoconstriction in guinea pig ileum.[97] Aqueous extract of *Tylophora indica* leaf powder[98] and tylophorine,[99] the major alkaloid, have shown an antiallergic effect and have modified the Schutz-Dale reaction in animals. In addition, the aqueous extract caused leucopenia indicating an immunosuppressive effect.[98] The antiallergic effects have been confirmed by lung perfusion experiments.[100] Tylophorine has also shown significant anti-inflammatory effect in several models of inflammation in rats.[101] In vitro, the total alkaloids ($0.1~\mu g \cdot ml^{-1}$) prevented the mast-cell degranulation produced by diazoxide at dosages similar to disodium cromoglycate.[102] *Tylophora indica* appears to stimulate phagocytic function[103,105] although inhibiting the humoral component of the immune system.[103] *Tylophora* alkaloids also inhibit cellular immune responses[104,105] when administered at any stage of the immune response.[104]

A preliminary clinical study on 56 patients with bronchial asthma and allergic rhinitis showed that there was a marked relief in 40-50 percent of the patients for a few weeks after ingestion of only 3-6 leaves, the dose being 1 fresh green leaf chewed and swallowed per day for 3 days. If the patient improved, no further leaves were given and the condition of the patient was monitored for 12 more weeks. Otherwise, leaf administration was continued for 3 more days, and in recalcitrant cases patients received leaves for 12 days. An initial observation was made that the magnitude of relief in symptoms experienced by the patients was dependent on the intensity of side effects like sore mouth, loss of taste, vomiting, etc.[106] This apparent correspondence between intensity of the side effects and the magnitude of reduction in symptoms was not borne out in subsequent trials.

Following these initial trials, further open and double-blind crossover trials were performed that too showed significant beneficial effects of *Tylophora indica* in asthma.[107-109]

In a double-blind study, 135 cases of bronchial asthma were included and categorized into three groups depending upon the kind of asthma as seasonal, irregular, and perennial. Patients were random-ized into each category and given either drug or placebo in two divided doses for 6 days. Of the 135 patients 71 were treated with dried-leaf powder of *Tylophora indica* and 64 with placebo. The drug consisted of shade-dried and powdered *Tylophora indica* leaf (200 mg), spinach leaf shade-dried and powdered (160 mg), and glucose (40 mg), whereas the placebo contained spinach leaf shade-dried and powdered, and glucose (340 mg) and ipecacuanha (60 mg). Improve-ment was assessed based on the reduction in signs and symptoms, reduction in the need for bronchodilators and steroids, and improve-ment in forced expiratory volume (FEV_1) and peak expiratory flow rate (PEFR). On evaluation it was found that the results were not sta-tistically different except in the perennial group where there was a significant response, as compared to the placebo group, at the end of the 2 weeks.[110] However, the question arises whether the use of ipeca-cuanha in the placebo group led to similar results being obtained in the drug and the placebo groups, since ipecacuanha is used as an expectorant.

The efficacy of *Tylophora indica* was evaluated in two cross-over double-blind studies, one against placebo and the other against stan-dard antiasthmatic drug containing ephedrine hydrochloride, theo-phylline, and phenobarbitone sodium. There was no significant difference in symptoms with the leaf compared to the standard asth-matic drug. In comparison with the placebo, the leaf showed a sustained rise in maximum breathing capacity, vital capacity, peak expiratory flow, and flow rate. There was also a significant reduction in nocturnal dyspnea.[111]

In a trial to evaluate the physiological basis of the therapeutic ef-fect of *Tylophora indica* in bronchial asthma patients, lung function tests, levels of 17-ketosteroids in urine, and absolute eosinophil levels were compared in 18 healthy and 11 bronchial asthma patients before and after the administration of *Tylophora*. Lung function tests included tidal volume, vital capacity, timed vital capacity, compli-ance, maximum ventilatory volume, and peak expiratory flow rate. Lung function tests were carried out in normal and asthmatic patients immediately after the intake of 10 mg isoprenaline and on the seventh day after two 100 mg capsules of *Tylophora* dried-leaf powder had been taken twice daily for 6 days. It was found that there was significant improvement in lung function tests in bronchial asthma patients. In addition, 17-ketosteroid levels increased and total eosinophil levels decreased as a result of *Tylophora indica (asthmatica)* intake.[112]

Allergic rhinitis

In another double-blind cross-over study, 50 allergic rhinitis patients were given either capsules of *Tylophora indica* (250 mg leaf powder) or a placebo (250 mg lactose). Patients received 1 capsule per day for 7 days. This was followed by a washout period of 5 days, then a cross over to the other capsules. Although *Tylophora* produced a significant reduction in the sneezing and nasal obstruction when compared to placebo, there was no significant difference between *Tylophora* and placebo regarding subjective feeling of nasal stuffiness, nasal smear, and response of nasal mucosa to antigen. The authors suggest that a higher dosage of 1 capsule twice a day for a longer period of a fortnight, after which the dose could be reduced, may be more effective.[113]

In clinical trials, where a fresh leaf of *Tylophora indica* was chewed, approximately 53-75 percent of patients reported side effects, such as nausea, lasting for a few hours. Sore mouth due to vesicant effect of the leaf and loss of taste for salt was for a longer duration and lasted up to 3-4 days after the last intake of leaf.[106,107] However, the frequency of side effects came down to 16.3 percent with the intake of the alcoholic extract of *Tylophora indica*. Risk-benefit analysis and the lasting relief obtained by very small doses were considered to compensate for the side effects seen.[108]

NOTES

1. Goyal HR. *Tamaka shwasa (bronchial asthma) a clinical study* (pp. 9-23, 31-32, 71). New Delhi: Central Council for Research in Ayurveda and Siddha, 1997.

2. Aulakh GS, Mahadevan G. Herbal drugs for asthma. *Indian Drugs* 26:593-599 (1989).

3. *The wealth of India, raw materials* (vol. 1, pp. 76-79). New Delhi: Publications and Information Directorate, CSIR, 1985.

4. Pandey G. *Dravyaguna vijnana* (vol. III, pp. 798-808) (materia medica—vegetable drugs). Varanasi: Krishnadas Academy, 2001.

5. *Selected medicinal plants of India. A monograph on identity, safety and clinical usage* (pp. 15-18). Bombay: Chemexcil. Basic Chemicals, Pharmaceuticals and Cosmetics Export Promotion Council, 1992.

6. *The Indian herbal pharmacopoeia* (rev. new edn., pp. 29-39). Mumbai: Indian Drug Manufacturers' Association, 2002.

7. Gupta OP, Sharma ML. Ray Ghatak BJ, Atal CK. Pharmacological investigations of vasicine and vasicinone—The alkaloids of *Adhatoda vasica. Indian J Med Res* 66:680-691 (1977).

8. Amin AH, Mehta DR. A bronchodilator alkaloid (vasicinone) from *Adhatoda vasica. Nature* 184:1317 (1959).

9. Bhide MB, Naik PY, Mahajani SS, Ghooi RB, Joshi RS. Pharmacological evaluation of vasicinone. *Bull Haffkine Institute* 2:6-11 (1974).

10. Müller A, Antus S, Bittinger M, Dorsch W, Kaas A, Kreher B, Neszmelyi A, Stuppner H, Wagner H. Chemistry and pharmacology of antiasthmatic plants *Galphimia glauca, Adhatoda vasica, Picrorhiza kurroa. Planta Med* 59 (suppl.):A586-A587 (1993).

11. Dhuley JN. Antitussive effect of *Adhatoda vasica* extract on mechanical or chemical stimulation–induced coughing in animals. *J Ethnopharmacol* 67:361-365 (1999).

12. Shah AC, Pajankar SP, Nabar ST, Trivedi AM, Deshmukh SN. A double blind study of "Wintry." A new bronchodilator in asthmatic bronchitis. *The Indian Practioner* 40:263-268 (1987).

13. Gupta AK, Tandon N. *Reviews on Indian medicinal plants* (vol. 1, pp. 257-287). New Delhi: Indian Council of Medical Research, 2004.

14. Burgos R, Forcelledo M, Wagner H, Müller A, Hancke J, Wikman G, Croxatto H. Non-abortive effect of *Adhatoda vasica* spissum leaf extract by oral administration in rats. *Phytomedicine* 4(2):145-149 (1997).

15. Claeson UP, Malmfors T, Wikman G, Bruhn JG. *Adhatoda vasica:* A critical review of ethnopharmacological and toxicological data. *J Ethnopharmacol* 72:1-20 (2000).

16. Pahwa GS, Zutshi U, Atal CK. Chronic toxicity studies with vasicine from *Adhatoda vasica* Ness in rats and monkeys. *Indian J Exp Biol* 25:467-470 (1987).

17. Farooq S, Pathak GK. Toxicity studies of total extract preparation of plant alkaloids in rats. *J Env Res* 9(1):7-11 (1999).

18. Pandey G. *Dravyaguna vijnana* (vol. III, pp. 480-490) (materia medica—vegetable drugs). Varanasi: Krishnadas Academy, 2001.

19. Moos SN. *Ayurvedic flora medica* (2nd edn., pp. 23-30). Kottayam: Vaidysarathy Press (P) Ltd, 1978.

20. *The wealth of India, raw materials* (vol.1, pp. 126-128). New Delhi: Publications and Information Directorate, CSIR, 1985.

21. *The wealth of India, raw materials* (first suppl. series, vol.1, pp. 36-37) New Delhi: National Institute of Science Communication, CSIR, 2000.

22. Une HD, Pal SC, Kature VS, Kasture SB. Phytochemical constituents and pharmacological profile of *Albizzia lebbeck. J Nat Remedies* 1(1):1-5 (2001).

23. Tripathi RM, Das PK. Studies on anti-asthmatic and anti-anaphylactic activity of *Albizzia lebbeck*. *Indian J Pharmacol* 9:189-194 (1977).

24. Tripathi RM, Sen PC, Das PK. Studies on the mechanism of *Albizzia lebbek*, an Indian indigenous drug, used in the treatment of atopic allergy. *J Ethnopharmacol* 1:385-396 (1979).

25. Tripathi RM, Sen PC, Das PK. Further studies on the mechanism of *Albizzia lebbek*, an Indian indigenous drug. *J Ethnopharmacol* 1:397-406 (1979).

26. Tripathi P, Tripathi YB, Dey PK, Tripathi SN. Release of catecholamines from the adrenal medulla by histamine and its prevention by *Albizzia lebbeck* in guinea pigs (letter to the editor). *Indian J Physiol Pharmacol* 27:176-178 (1983).

27. Tripathi P, Tripathi YB, Tripathi SN. Steroidogenic effect of *Albizzia lebbeck* Benth in guinea pigs. *Ancient Sci Life* 2:153-159 (1983).

28. Baruah CC, Gupta PP, Patnaik GK, Nath A, Kulshrestha DK, Dhawan BN. Anti-anaphylactic and mast cell stabilising activity of *Albizzia lebbeck* Benth. *Sirish. Indian Vet Med J* 21:127-132 (1997).

29. Barua CC, Gupta PP, Patnaik GK, Misra-Bhattacharya S, Goel RK, Kulshrestha DK, Dubey MP, Dhawan BN. Immunomodulatory effect of *Albizzia lebbeck*. *Pharm Biol* 38:161-166 (2000).

30. Tripathi SN, Shukla P, Mishra AK, Udupa KN. Experimental and clinical studies on adrenal function in bronchial asthma with special reference to the treatment with *Albizzia lebbeck*. *Quart J Surg Sci* 14:169-176 (1978).

31. Swamy GK, Bhattathiri PPN, Rao PV, Acharya MV, Bikshapathi T. Clincal evaluation of *sirisa twak kvatha* in the management of *tamaka shwasa* (bronchial asthma). *J Res Ayur Siddha* 18(1-2):21-27 (1997).

32. Shaw BP, Bera B. Treatment of tropical pulmonary eosinophilia with *shirisha* flower (*Albizzia lebbeck* Benth.) churna. *Nagarjun* 29(6):1-3 (1986).

33. Sharma PC, Yelne MB, Dennis TJ. *Database of medicinal plants used in Ayurveda* (vol. 1, pp. 404-417). New Delhi: Central Council for Research in Ayurveda and Siddha, 2000.

34. Ammon HPT. Ayurveda—Arzneimittel aus indischer Kultur. *Z Phytother* 22:136-142 (2001).

35. Nadkarni AK. *Dr KM Nadkarni's Indian materia medica* (vol. 1, pp. 211-212). Bombay: Popular Prakashan, 1976.

36. Gupta I, Gupta V, Parihar A, Gupta S, Lüdtke R, Safayhi H, Ammon HPT. Effects of *Boswellia serrata* gum resin in patients with bronchial asthma: Results of a double-blind, placebo-controlled, 6-week clinical study. *Eur J Med Res* 3:511-514 (1998).

37. Dash B. *Herbal treatment for asthma and bronchitis* (pp. 36-39). New Delhi: B. Jain Publishers (P) Ltd, 1988.

38. Jain JP, Bhatnagar LS, Parsai MR. Clinical trials of *haridra (Curcuma longa)* in cases of *tamak swasa* and *kasa*. *J Res Ind Med Yoga Homeo* 14:110-120 (1979).

39. Sinha M, Mukherjee BP, Sikdar S, Mukherjee B, Dasgupta SR. Further studies on the pharmacological properties of curcumin. *Indian J Pharm* 4:135 (1972).

40. Yano S, Terai M, Shimizu KL, Futagami Y, Horie S, Tsuchiya S, Ikegami F, Sekine T, Yamomoto Y et al. Antiallergic activity of extracts from *Curcuma longa*: Active components and mechanism of actions. *Phytomedicine* 3 (suppl.1):58 (1996).

41. Yano S, Terai M, Shimizu KL, Horie S, Futagami Y, Tsuchiya S, Ikegami F, Sekine T, Yamomoto Y, Fujimori H, Takamoto K, Saito K, Ueno K, Watanabe K. Antiallergic activity of *Curcuma longa* (I): Effectiveness of extracts containing curcuminoids. *Nat Med* 54:318-324 (2000).

42. Yano S, Terai M, Shimizu KL, Futagami Y, Horie S, Tsuchiya S, Ikegami F, Sekine T, Takamoto K, Saito K, Ueno K, Watanabe K. Antiallergic activity of *Curcuma longa* (II). Features of inhibitory actions on histamine release from mast cells. *Nat Med* 54:325-329 (2000).

43. Satyavati GV, Raina MK, Sharma M. Eds. *Medicinal plants of India* (vol. I, p. 315). New Delhi: Indian Council of Medical Research, 1976.

44. *Indian herbal pharmacopoeia* (rev. new edn., pp. 272-280). Mumbai: Indian Drug Manufacturers' Association, 2002.

45. Sharma PC, Yelne MB, Dennis TJ. *Database on Medicinal Plants used in Ayurveda* (vol. 2, pp. 500-530). New Delhi: Council for Research in Ayurveda and Siddha, 2001.

46. *WHO monographs on selected medicinal plants* (vol. 2, pp. 206-216). Geneva: World Health Organization, 2002.

47. Nörr H, Wagner H. New constituents from *Ocimum sanctum*. *Planta Med* 58:574 (1992).

48. Kelm MA, Nair MG, Strasburg GM, DeWitt DL. Antioxidant and cyclooxygenase inhibitory phenolic compounds from *Ocimum sanctum* Linn. *Phytomedicine* 7:7-13 (2000).

49. Palit G, Singh SP, Singh N, Kohli RP, Bhargava KP. An experimental evaluation of anti-asthmatic plant drugs from the ancient Ayurvedic medicine. *Aspects Allergy Immunol* 16:36-41 (1983).

50. Singh S, Agrawal SS. Anti-asthmatic and anti-inflammatory activity of *Ocimum sanctum* Linn. *J Res Edu Indian Med* 10(3):23-28 (1991).

51. Singh S, Agrawal SS. Anti-asthmatic and anti-inflammatory activity of *Ocimum sanctum* Linn. *Int J Pharmacognosy* 29:306-310 (1991).

52. Sharma G. [Antiasthmatic efficacy of *Ocimum sanctum*]. *Sachitra Ayurved* 35:665-668 (1983). Abstracted in *MAPA* 8306-2785.

53. Trivedi VP, Singh SK, Sharma SC, Singh N. *Seminar on Research in Ayurveda and Siddha* (p. 47). New Delhi: CCRAS, March 20-22,1995.

54. Das SK Chandra A, Agarwal SS, Singh N. *Ocimum sanctum (tulsi)* in the treatment of viral encephalitis (a preliminary clinical trial). *Antiseptic* 80:323-327 (1983).

55. *Selected medicinal plants of India. A monograph on identity, safety and clinical usage* (pp. 224-227). Bombay: Chemexcil. Basic Chemicals, Pharmaceuticals and Cosmetics Export Promotion Council, 1992.

56. Ahmed A, Ahamed RN, Aladakatti RH, Ghosesawar MG. Reversible antifertility effect of benzene extract of *Ocimum sanctum* on sperm parameters and fructose content in rats. *J Basic Clin Physiol Pharmacol* 13:51-59 (2002).

57. *Indian herbal pharmacopoeia* (rev. new edn., pp. 306-316). Mumbai: Indian Drug Manufacturers' Association, 2002.

58. Nadkarni AK. *Dr KM Nadkarni's Indian materia medica* (vol. 1, pp. 965-969). Bombay: Popular Prakashan, 1976.

59. *Caraka samhita,* ed. and trans. Sharma PV (1st edn., vol. II, p. 23, "Chikitsastanam," chapter 1, verse 32-35). Varanasi: Chaukhambha Orientalia, 1983.

60. Lad V, Frawley D. *The yoga of herbs* (pp. 180-182). Santa Fe, New Mexico: Lotus Press, 1986.

61 Kulshrestha VK, Srivastava RK, Singh N, Kohli RP. A study of central stimulant effect of *Piper longum. Indian J Pharmacol* 1(2):8 (1969).

62. Kulshrestha VK, Singh N, Srivastava RK, Rastogi SK, Kohli RP. Analysis of central stimulant activity of *Piper longum. J Res Indian Med* 6(1):17 (1971).

63. Banga SS, Garg LC, Atal CK. Effect of piplartine and crude extracts of *Piper longum* on the ciliary movements. *Indian J Pharmacy* 26:139-140 (1964).

64. Dahanukar SA, Zha A, Karandikar SM. Antiallergic activity of *Piper longum.`Indian J Pharmacol* 13:122 (1981).

65. Dahanukar SA, Karandikar SM. Evaluation of antiallergic activity of *Piper longum. Indian Drugs* 21:377-383 (1984).

66. Nayampalli SS, Nadkarni PM, Satoskar RS. Evaluation of antiallergic activity of *Piper longum* using rat lung perfusion. *Indian J Pharmacol* 13:90 (1981).

67. Neogi NC, Haldar RK, Rathor RS. Preliminary pharmacological studies on piperine. *J Res Indian Med* 6(1):24-29 (1971).

68. Fernandez A, Tavares A, Tavares F, Athavale VB. Asthma in children: A clinical controlled study of *Piper longum* in asthma. *Paediatr Clin India* 15:45-52 (1980).

69. Dahanukar SA, Karandikar SM, Desai M. Efficacy of *Piper longum* in childhood asthma. *India Drugs* 21:384-388 (1984).

70. Upadhay SD, Kansal CM, Pandey NN. Clinical evaluation of *pippali (Piper longum) Kshira Paka* on patients of bronchial asthma. A preliminary study. *Nagarjun* 25:256-258 (1982).

71. Anushman PS, Singh KP, Aasra KG. [Effect of *Vardhaman pippali (Piper longum)* in patients with respiratory disorders]. *Sachitra Ayurved* 37(1):47-49 (1984). Abstracted in *MAPA* 8406-2560.

72. *Selected medicinal plants of India. A monograph on identity, safety and clinical usage* (pp. 241-244). Bombay: Chemexcil. Basic Chemicals, Pharmaceuticals and Cosmetics Export Promotion Council, 1992.

73. Rege NN, Thatte UM, Dahanukar SA. Adaptogenic properties of six *rasayana* herbs used in Ayurvedic medicine. *Phytother Res* 13:275-291 (1999).

74. Shah AH, Al-Shareef AH, Ageel AM, Qureshi S. Toxicity studies in mice of common spices, *Cinnamomum zeylanicum* bark and *Piper longum* fruits. *Plant Foods Hum Nutr* 52:231-239 (1998).

75. *Selected medicinal plants of India. A monograph on identity, safety and clinical usage* (pp. 295-297). Bombay: Chemexcil. Basic Chemicals, Pharmaceuticals and Cosmetics Export Promotion Council, 1992.

76. Sivarajan VV, Balachandran I. *Ayurvedic Drugs and their plant sources* (pp. 211-213). New Delhi: Oxford and IBH Publishing Co Pvt Ltd, 1994.

77. *Indian herbal pharmacopoeia* (rev. new edn., pp. 402-410) Mumbai: Indian Drug Manufacturers' Association, 2002.

78. Gupta SS, Gupta NK. Effects of *Solanum xanthocarpum* and *Clerodendron serratum* on histamine release from tissues. *Indian J Med Sci* 21:795-799 (1967).

79. Gupta SS, Verma SCL, Singh C, Khandelwal P, Gupta NK. Chemical and pharmacological studies on *Solanum xanthocarpum (Kantakari). Indian J Med Res* 55:723-732 (1967).

80. Gupta SS, Rai M, Gupta NK. Histamine releasing effects of a few Indian medical plants used in bronchial asthma (letters to the editor). *Curr Sci* 36(2):42-43 (1967).

81. Gupta SS. Anti-allergic activity of plant saponins in relation to their histamine releasing anticholinesterase effects. *Indian J Physio Pharmacol* 14(2):95-101 (1970).

82. Sharma K, Puri AS, Sannd BN. Role of *kantkari (Solanum xanthocarpum)* in *shwas* and *kas*—bronchial asthma and non-specific cough. *J Res Ind Med* 6:200-201 (1971).

83. Bector NP, Puri AS. *Solanum xanthocarpum (kantakari)* in chronic bronchitis, bronchial asthma and non-specific cough (an experimental and clinical correlation). *J Assn Physicians India* 19:741-744 (1971).

84. Bector NP, Puri AS, Gupta RK. New approach to the treatment of some chronic respiratory diseases. *Indian J Med Res.* 59:739-742 (1971).

85. Jain JP. A clinical trial of *kantakari (Solanum xanthocarpum)* in cases of *kasa roga. J Res Ayur Siddha* 1:35-51 (1980).

86. Jain JP. A clinical trial of *kantakari (Solanum xanthocarpum)* in cases of *tamak swasa* (some respiratory diseases). *J Res Ayur Siddha* 1:447-460 (1980).

87. Pandya MM. Therapeutic value of *Solanum xanthocarpum (kantkari)* in bronchial asthma. *Sachitra Ayurved* 33:729-733 (1981).

88. Govindan S, Viswanathan S, Vijaysekaran V, Alagappan R. A pilot study on the clinical efficacy of *Solanum xanthocarpum* and *Solanum trilobatum. J Ethnopharmacol* 66:205-210 (1999).

89. Singh KK, Singh SP. Toxicity studies of *Solanum xanthocarpum* seeds in male albino rats. *J Res Edu Indian Med* 12:45-47 (1993).

90. Gupta RS, Dixit VP. Effects of short term treatment of solasodine on cauda epididymis in dogs. *Indian J Exp Biol* 40:169-173 (2002).

91. Gogte VM. *Ayurvedic pharmacology & therapeutic uses of medical plants* (pp. 438-440). Trans. SPARC, Mumbai: Bharatiya Vidya Bhavan, 2000.

92. *Indian herbal pharmacopoeia* (rev. new edn., pp. 429-438). Mumbai: Indian Drug Manufacturers' Association, 2002.

93. Trivedi VP, Nesamany SA, Sharma VK. A clinical study of the anti-tussive and anti-asthmatic effects of *Vibhitakphal churna (Teminalia belerica* Roxb.) in the cases of *kasa-swasa. J Res Ayur Siddha* III (1 & 2):1-8 (1982).

94. *The wealth of India, raw materials* (vol. X, pp. 398-399). New Delhi: Publications and Information Directorate, CSIR, 1976.

95. *Selected medicinal plants of India. A monograph on identity, safety and clinical usage* (pp. 333-336). Mumbai: Chemexcil. Basic Chemicals, Pharmaceuticals and Cosmetics Export Promotion Council, 1992.

96. Dhananjayan R, Gopalakrishnan C, Kameswaran L. Studies on the pharmacological effects of extracts and total alkaloids of *Tylophora indica. Indian J Pharmacol* 7(4):13-20 (1975).

97. Gupta SS. Pharmacological basis for the use of *Tylophora indica* in bronchial asthma. *Aspects Allergy Applied Immunol* 8:95-100 (1975).

98. Haranath PSRK, Shyamalakumari S. Experimental study on mode of action of *Tylophora asthamatica* in bronchial asthma. *Indian J Med Res* 63:661-670 (1975).

99. Gopalakrishnan C, Shankaranarayan D, Nazimudeen SK, Kameswaran L. Effect of tylophorine, a major alkaloid of *Tylophora indica,* on immunopathological and inflammatory reactions. *Indian J Med Res* 71:940-948 (1980).

100. Nayampalli SS, Sheth UK. Evaluation of the anti-allergic activity of *Tylophora indica* using rat lung perfusion. *Indian J Pharmacol* 11:229-232 (1979).

101. Gopalakrishnan C, Shankaranarayan D, Kameswaran L, Natarajan S. Pharmacological investigations of tylophorine, the major alkaloid of *Tylophora indica. Indian J Med Res.* 69:513-520 (1979).

102. Geetha VS, Viswanathan S, Kameswaran L. Comparison of total alkaloids of *Tylophora indica* and disodium cromoglycate in mast cell stabilisation. *Indian J Pharmacol* 13:199-201 (1981).

103. Atal CK, Sharma ML, Kaul A, Khajuria A. Immunomodulating agents of plant origin I. Preliminary screening. *J Ethnopharmacol* 18:133-141 (1986).

104. Ganguly T, Sainis KB. Inhibition of cellular immune responses by *Tylophora indica* in experimental models. *Phytomedicine* 8:348-355 (2001).

105. Ganguly .T, Badheka LP, Sainis KB. Immunomodulatory effect of *Tylophora indica* on Con A induced lymphoproliferation. *Phytomedicine* 8:431-437 (2001).

106. Shivpuri DN, Menon MPS, Prakash D. Preliminary studies in *Tylophora indica* in the treatment of asthma and allergic rhinitis. *J Assoc Physicians India* 16:9-15 (1968).

107. Shivpuri DN, Menon MPS, Prakash D. A cross-over double-blind study on *Tylophora indica* in the treatment of asthma and allergic rhinitis. *J Allergy* 43:145-150 (1969).

108. Shivpuri DN, Singhal SC, Prakash D. Treatment of asthma with an alcoholic extract of *Tylophora indica:* A crossover double-blind study. *Ann Allergy* 30:407-412 (1972).

109. Shivpuri DN, Agarwal MK. Effect of *Tylophora indica* on bronchial tolerance to inhalation challenges with specific allergens. *Ann Allergy* 31:87-94 (1973).

110. Gupta S, George P, Gupta V, Vinod R, Tandon, Sundaram KR. *Tylophora indica* in bronchial asthma- a double blind study. *Indian J Med Res* 69:981-989 (1979).

111. Thiruvengadam KV, Haranath K, Sudarsan S, Sekar TS, Rajagopal KR, Zacharian MGM, Devarajan TV. *Tylophora indica* in bronchial asthma. (A controlled comparison with a standard anti-asthmatic drug). *J Indian Med Assn* 71:172-176 (1980).

112. Gore KV, Rao AK, Guruswamy MN. Physiological studies with *Tylophora asthmatica* in bronchial asthma. *Indian J Med Res* 71:144-148 (1980).

113. Thiruvengadam KV, Kameswaran L, Ahmad B. *Tylophora indica* in allergic rhinitis. *J Indian Med Assn.* 76:181-184 (1981).

UPPER-RESPIRATORY TRACT INFECTIONS

The most common upper-respiratory tract infections (URTI) involving the nose, throat, sinuses, and larynx are the so-called common cold and influenza, both of which are viral infections. Common cold is characterized by a stuffy, runny nose, sore throat, headache, and fever. A number of plants have been used in Ayurveda to treat the URTIs; however, these have been little documented. At Banaras Hindu University in Varanasi and elsewhere, plants that stimulate the immune system have been studied for their potential in warding off URTI. Plants that have been experimented with are *Sida rhombifolia, Sida vernonicaefolia, Sida cordifolia,* and *Abutilon indicum* in combination, *Ocimum sanctum* and *Centella asiatica. Centella asiatica* is covered in Chapter 13.

Andrographis paniculata *(Burm. f.) Wall. ex Nees (Family: Acanthaceae)*

Sanskrit: Bhunimba, Kirata	Tamil: Nilavembu
Hindi: Kalmegh	English: The Creat

Andrographis paniculata (see Plate 3 in color gallery) is a small bitter herb found throughout India. All parts of the plant are used medicinally. The plant is best known as a bitter tonic and febrifuge useful in dysentery, cholera, consumption, influenza, bronchitis, swelling, and skin problems.[1] A tincture of the plant was useful in arresting the progression of the epidemic during outbreaks of influenza in India. It is considered efficacious in intermittent and remittent fevers.[2] The use of *kalmegh* as a bitter tonic and a hepatoprotective agent has been extensively investigated, as it is one of the most widely used plant in combination formulas for jaundice. See Chapter 4.

Clinical investigation using *Andrographis paniculata* in the prevention and treatment of cold, and the treatment of bronchitis, tonsillitis, and influenza, has been carried out in other parts of the world, notably in Sweden, where it has been in used for treatment of cold for the past 20 years, and also in Germany, Chile, Russia, and Thailand.

Andrographis paniculata extract and the diterpene lactone, andrographolide, from *Andrographis paniculata* have been the subject of numerous pharmacological investigations. The ethanolic extract[3] and andrographolide[4] have been shown to have antipyretic activity. In addition, andrographolide has been shown to have immunomodulatory,[5] anti-inflammatory,[6] and antiallergic[7] properties. The anti-inflammatory effect is possibly due to inhibition of expression of nitric oxide synthase in macrophages[8] and PAF-mediated inflammatory response.[9]

Common cold

In a placebo-controlled double-blind study, 1,200 mg of *Andrographis paniculata*'s dried extract containing 4 percent of andrographolides was evaluated against a placebo in 59 patients with common cold. Twelve 100 mg tablets of *Andrographis paniculata* were given to 33 patients, whereas 28 patients received similar-looking placebo tablets containing glucose for 4 days. On day 4, there was a significant reduction in the intensity of sore throat, tiredness, muscular ache, and the intensity of the disease in the drug-treated group but not in the placebo group.[10]

In another randomized placebo-controlled double-blind study, 50 patients with initial symptoms of common cold and sinusitis were included in the study and received either *Andrographis paniculata* or similar-looking placebo tablets. The preparation used in the study contained 85 mg of hydro-alcoholic extract standardized for andrographolide and deoxyandrographolide content and was taken in a dose of 4 tablets thrice daily for 5 days. Of the total patients, 67.5 percent in the drug group felt totally recovered compared to 36 percent in the placebo group. In the case of sick leave the drug group took 0.21 days of leave compared to 0.96 days in the placebo group.[11]

In a pilot double-blind study during winter to evaluate the potential preventive effects in common cold of *Andrographis paniculata*'s dried-extract tablets, 107 children around 18 years of age were recruited. Fifty-four students received two 100 mg tablets of *Andrographis paniculata* for 3 months, which had been standardized to contain 5.6 mg of andrographolide, whereas the other group with

53 students received 2 tablets containing 100 mg glucose. Students were evaluated weekly. There was no difference between the two groups in the number cases with cold in the first 2 months, but after the third month there was a significant decrease in the number of cases with cold in the drug-treated group, with 35 percent catching cold as compared to 62 percent in the placebo group.[12]

In a double-blind placebo-controlled study aimed at evaluating the effectiveness of the extract in reducing signs and symptoms of common cold, 158 patients were recruited who completed the study. The drug group of 79 patients received 1,200 mg·day^{-1} of *Andrographis paniculata* herb extract standardized to contain a minimum of 5 mg andrographolide and deoxyandrographolide, that is, four 100 mg tablets three times a day, and the placebo group with 79 patients received an equivalent amount of placebo tablets for a period of 5 days. After the second day of treatment, there was a significant decrease in the severity of exhaustion, sleeplessness, sore throat, and nasal secretion, whereas on day 4, there was a significant decrease in all symptoms in the *Andrographis paniculata* group—headache, earache, phlegm, and frequency and intensity of cough.[13]

Two other double-blind placebo-controlled trials, a pilot study with 46 patients and a phase-III study involving 179 patients with uncomplicated URTI, found that throat symptoms showed the most significant improvement.[14]

In a randomized double-blind comparative study in 152 adult patients with pharyngotonsilitis, the efficacy of the powdered leaves of *Andrographis paniculata* encapsulated in 250 mg and 500 mg capsules was evaluated against 325 mg paracetamol capsules in reducing the incidence of sore throat and fever. Patients were randomized and asked to take 3 capsules four times a day. After 3 days of treatment, the crude drug at 6 g·day^{-1} was found as effective as paracetamol in control of fever and sore throat after 7 days; clinical effects were not different in the three groups.[15] In an open study, treatment with standardized *Andrographis paniculata* showed reduction, within 48 hours, in the incidence of fever occurring with common cold.[16]

In two randomized double-blind-controlled clinical studies—a pilot study and a second study—*Andrographis paniculata* was evaluated against amantidine in an epidemic of influenza in Volgograd.

The pilot study involved 540 patients: 71 patients were on a combination drug Kan Jang consisting of 88.8 mg of *Androgaphis paniculata* and 10 mg of *Eleutherococcus senticosus*, whereas the control group was on an antiviral drug amantidine, paracetamol, and vitamin C. The Kan Jang therapy significantly reduced the occurrence of fever and clinical symptoms, such as headache, myalgia, and conjunctivitis, postinfluenza complications, and the number of days taken as sick leave was also reduced to 30.1 percent and 31.43 percent compared to 67.8 and 70.97 percent in the control group of the pilot and second study.[17]

The results of several trials on URTI in which a standardized extract of *Andrographis paniculata* has been used, with one exception, has been reviewed for safety and efficacy, which shows that there are only mild and infrequent reports of adverse events.[18] For other details see the Chapter 4 monograph *"Andrographis paniculata."*

NOTES

1. *The wealth of India, raw materials* (vol. 1, pp. 264-266). New Delhi: Publications and Information Directorate, CSIR,1985.

2. Nadkarni AK. *Dr KM Nadkarni's Indian materia medica* (vol. 1, pp. 101-103). Bombay: Popular Prakashan, 1976.

3. Vedavathy S, Rao KN. Antipyretic activity of six indigenous medicinal plants of Tirumala Hills, Andhra Pradesh, India. *J Ethnopharmacol* 33:193-196 (1991).

4. Madav S, Tripathi HC, Tandan, Mishra SK. Analgesic, antipyretic and antiulcerogenic effects of andrographolide. *Indian J Pharm Sci* 57:121-125 (1995).

5. Puri A, Saxena R, Saxena RP, Saxena KC, Srivastava V, Tandon JS. Immunostimulant agents from *Andrographis paniculata. J Nat Prod* 56:995-999 (1993).

6. Madav S,Tandan SK, Lal J, Tripathi HC. Anti-inflammatory activity of andrographolide. *Fitoterapia* 67:452-458 (1996).

7. Gupta PP, Tandon JS, Patnaik GK. Antiallergic activity of andrographolides isolated from *Andrographis paniculata* (Burm. f.) Wall. *Pharmacol Biol* 36:72-74 (1998).

8. Chiou WF, Lin JJ, Chen CF. Andrographolide suppresses the expression of inducible nitric oxide synthase in macrophage and restores the vasoconstriction in rat aorta treated with lipopolysaccharide. *Brit J Pharmacol* 125:327-334 (1998).

9. Amroyan E, Gabrielian E, Panossian A, Wikman G, Wagner H. Inhibitory effect of andrographolide on PAF-induced platelet aggregation. *Phytomedicine* 6:27-31 (1999).

10. Hancke J, Burgos R, Cáceres D, Wikman G. A double-blind study with a new monodrug Kan Jang: Decrease of symptoms and improvement in the recovery from common colds. *Phytother Res* 9:559-562 (1995).

11. Melchior J, Palm S, Wikman G. Controlled clinical study of standardized *Andrographis paniculata* extract in common cold—a pilot trial. *Phytomedicine* 3:315-318 (1996/1997).

12. Cáceres DD, Hancke JL, Burgos RA, Wikman GK. Prevention of common colds with *Andrographis paniculata* dried extract. A pilot double blind trial. *Phytomedicine* 4:101-104 (1997).

13. Cáceres DD, Hancke JL, Burgos RA, Sandberg F, Wikman GK. Use of visual analogue scale measurements (VAS) to assess the effectiveness of standardized *Andrographis paniculata* extract SHA-10 in reducing the symptoms of common cold. A randomized double blind placebo study. *Phytomedicine* 6:217-223 (1999).

14. Melichor J, Spasov AA, Ostrovskij OV, Bulanov AE, Wikman G. Double-blind, placebo-controlled pilot and phase III study of activity of standardized *Andrographis paniculata* Herba Nees extract fixed combination (Kan Jang) in the treatment of uncomplicated upper-respiratory tract infection. *Phytomedicine* 7:341-350 (2000).

15. Thamlikitkul V, Theerapong S, Boonroj P, Ekpalakorn W, Taechaiya S, Orn-Chom-Jan T, Pradipasena S, Timsard S, Dechatiwongse T, Chantrakul C, Punkrut W, Boontaeng N, Petcharoen S, Riewpaiboon W, Riewpaiboon A, Tenambergen ED. Efficacy of *Andrographis paniculata* Nees for pharyngotonsillitis in adults. *J Med Assoc Thai* 74:437-442 (1991).

16. Pharmacology Department of Sichuan Institute of Chinese Materia Medica. Primary study of the treatment of epidemic cold with *Andrographis paniculata* Nees A, B, C *Sichuan Communications on Chinese Trad Med Herbal Drugs* 1:21 (1975).

17. Kulichenko LL, Kireyeva LV, Malyshkina EN, Wikman G. A randomized, controlled study of Kan Jang versus amantadine in the treatment of influenza in Volgograd. *J Herbal Pharmacother* 3:77-93 (2003).

18. Coon JT, Ernst E. *Andrographis paniculata* in the treatment of upper respiratory tract infections: A systematic review of safety and efficacy. *Planta Med* 70:293-298 (2004).

OTHER PLANTS

In an open exploratory study, *Ocimum sanctum* was taken regularly by patients suffering from recurrent cold and URTI in the form of fresh leaves or decoction. It was found to prevent recurrent attacks presumably by stimulating the immune system. Similarly, in a study of 74 children subject to recurrent URTI, a four-herb combination of *Sida cordifolia, Abutilon indicum, Sida rhombifolia,* and *Sida vernonicaefolia* was found to have a highly significant effect in reducing the frequency of attacks after 12 months of intake, when compared to the pretreatment period.[1]

NOTE

1. Udupa KN. *Promotion of "Health for all" by Ayurveda and yoga* (pp. 81-82). Varanasi: The Tara Printing Works, 1985.

TROPICAL PULMONARY EOSINOPHILIA

Tropical pulmonary eosinophilia is a tropical disease found in India. It is characterized by cough, breathlessness, and high eosinophil levels of more than $2,000 \cdot cu \cdot mm^{-1}$.[1,2]

Albizzia lebbeck *Benth. (Family: Mimosaceae)*

In an open trial with 35 cases of tropical pulmonary eosinophilia (TPE), 17 patients were treated with 200 mg *Albizzia lebbeck (shirish)* flower twice daily for 6 weeks, with 82 percent showing excellent results, 12 percent good, and 6 percent showing poor response. No side effects or toxicity were observed.[1]

Ocimum sanctum *Linn. (Family: Laminaceae)*

A double-blind comparative clinical trial of *Ocimum sanctum* with diethyl carbamazine was conducted on 48 children with TPE. Patients were randomized into two groups—one receiving $200 \text{ mg} \cdot kg \cdot day^{-1}$ of *Ocimum sanctum* or $10 \text{ mg} \cdot kg \cdot day^{-1}$ diethyl carbamazine in three or four divided doses for 4 weeks. Both drugs were filled in identical capsules and the trial was conducted in a double-blind manner. *Ocimum sanctum* was found as effective as diethyl carbamazine in effecting clinical improvement and reduction of blood eosinophil levels, apart from producing similar improvement in radiological findings. Change in eosinophil levels was noticed in the second week of therapy when patients were examined and improvement in eosinophil levels continued when repeat measurements were carried out in the fourth week.[2,3]

Terminalia belerica *Roxb. (Family: Combretaceae)*

In a comparative trial of 37 children with cough, breathlessness, fever, chest pain, malaise, an eosinophil count of $2,000 \cdot cu \cdot mm^{-1}$, and more than 20 percent differential eosinophil count, 27 patients were given 20 mg$\cdot$kg^{-1} body weight of the kernel powder of *Terminalia belerica* in three divided doses, whereas ten patients received diethyl carbamazine (DEC) as a control drug. There was a significant reduction in the blood eosinophil count after 15 days that was completely normal after 4 weeks of treatment in comparison with DEC. Six-month follow-up showed that there were no relapses in the *Terminalia belerica* group, but there were relapses in the DEC-treated group.[3]

NOTES

1. Shaw BP, Bera B. Treatment of tropical pulmonary eosinophilia with shirisha flower (*Albizzia lebbeck* Benth.) churna. *Nagarjun* 29(6):1-3 (1986).

2. Jayasingh BK, Chaturvedi C, Tewari PV, Bhargava V. A double blind comparative trial of Ocimum sanctum Linn & diethylcarbamazine in tropical pulmonary eosinophilia. *Sachitra Ayurved* (March):654-661 (1987).

3. Sharma R, Chaturvedi C, Tewari PV. Management of tropical pulmonary eosinophilia in children with Ayurvedic drugs. *J Res Edu Indian Med* 6(1-2):11-17 (1987).

Chapter 6

Cardiovascular Drugs

Disorders of the cardiovascular system (heart, blood vessels, and blood circulation) are a major cause of morbidity and mortality in the world. With changing lifestyles and diet, as also with increased stress and pollution, cardiovascular diseases are reaching epidemic proportions not only in the developed world but also in the developing world. Plants have been used in Ayurveda for the treatment of heart disease or *Hrdroga,* as it is known in Sanskrit, both in the form of a single drug and in combination with other plants. There have been several plants that have been listed in ancient treatises as useful for heart problems since the time of Caraka and Sushruta—authors of the first Ayurvedic texts. Several reviews have been published considering the importance of the area. These include plants found useful in cardiovascular conditions,[1,2] which have been grouped under four categories depending upon their activity, such as cardioprotective plants that help in the management of ischemia and angina,[3] antiplatelet plants,[4] antihyperlipidemic plants,[5] and antihypertensive plants.[6,7] Many of these plants can be included in more than one category.

NOTES

1. Dwivedi S. Putative uses of cardiovascular friendly plants in preventive cardiology. *Ann Nat Acad Med Sci (India)* 32:159-175 (1997).
2. Dwivedi SD. Useful plants in cardiovascular ailments. *Nat Prod Radiance* 1(5):22-26 (2002).
3. Dwivedi S, Somani PN, Udupa KN. Indigenous drugs and ischaemic heart disease. *Arogya—J Health Sci* XIII:65-71 (1987).

doi:10.1300/5683_06

4. Dwivedi S, Amrita. Medicinal plants with antiplatelet activity. *Indian Drugs* 30:539-548 (1993).

5. Nayak S, Jain UK, Saraf A. Potent hypolipidemic herbal drugs: A review. *Sachitra Ayurved* 51:448-453 (1998).

6. Srimal RC, Shukla R. Recent research in India on indigenous plants for the treatment of hypertension. *Indian Drugs* 24:419-424 (1987).

7. Dwivedi S, Pachori SB, Amrita. Medicinal plants with hypotensive activity. *Indian Practitioner* XLVII:117-134 (1994).

CARDIOPROTECTIVE PLANTS

Of the few plants that have been studied, the best investigated is *Terminalia arjuna,* which has evoked considerable interest since the published report of a poor barber with ischemic heart disease (insufficient blood supply to the heart), owing to a heart block, who was relieved of his symptoms and was able to start work again. The barber was advised a milk decoction of *Terminalia arjuna* bark twice a day that relieved him of his symptoms.[1] Angina pectoris is characterized by pain in the chest due to coronary artery disease (CAD) or narrowing of the coronary arteries by deposition of fatty plaques on the wall of the arteries. In Ayurveda, factors causing heart disease and treatments for it have been described in the *Caraka Samhita.* The treatment of pain has also been included in it.[2] Acute chest pain with breathlessness is described in the *Sushruta Samhita.*[3] However, the different kinds of pain because of heart disease have been described in the *Astanga Hrdayam* of Vagbhata, *who also first advocated the use of Terminalia arjuna.*[4]

Terminalia arjuna *(Roxb.)* Wight & Arn. *(Family: Combretaceae)*

Sanskrit: Arjuna	Tamil: Vellamatta
Hindi: Arjuna	

Terminalia arjuna (see Plate 6 in color gallery)is a large evergreen tree found throughout India, especially near waterways. It is also grown for its shade. The smooth pink-gray stem bark has been used as a medicine for hundreds of years since 700 BC. Mentioned in the *Caraka* and *Sushruta Samhita* for the treatment of skin conditions, ulcers, fractures, uterine problems, and urinary disorders,[5] the use of *Terminalia arjuna* in heart diseases was mentioned for the first time in the *Astanga Hrdayam* of Vagbhata.[6] Its use as a cardiotonic in heart problems, especially in the form of a milk decoction, was advocated by another well-known physician of ancient times known as Cakradatta or Cakrapanidatta.[7]

Constituents isolated from *Terminalia arjuna* bark include the following components: tannins; several triterpenoid genins and glycosides, including arjunic acid, arjunolic acid, terminic acid, arjungenin, arjunolitin, arjunetin, arjunglycosides I, II, III and friedelin; flavonoids, such as arjunolone and baicalein; phenolic acids, such as ellagic acid; leucoanthocyanidins, for example leucocyanidin and leucodelphinidin; phytosterols (β-sitosterol); and large amounts of calcium salts.[5,8]

Early pharmacological studies using the total extract of *Terminalia arjuna* showed cardiotonic activity, increasing the force of contraction in frogs[9] and in dogs.[10] In a study to investigate the mechanism of action, it was found that the aqueous portion of the alcoholic extract exhibited a lowering of blood pressure and heart rate (bradycardia), which was centrally mediated,[11] whereas another study showed that *Terminalia arjuna* had a depressant action at higher concentration because of its peripheral action.[12] A significant positive inotropic effect was also shown in rat atria by the aqueous extract,[13] which has been attributed to the release of noradrenaline from the sympathetic nerve endings, that is by an action on β_1-adrenoreceptors, although the extract caused a relaxation of vascular smooth muscle, which was not mediated by β_2 adrenoreceptors.[14] Depending upon the solvent used for extraction, the extract is enriched in compounds possessing either positive or negative inotropic action.[11,13,14]

In isoproterenol ischemia in rats, *Terminalia arjuna* showed prostaglandin E_2 (PGE_2)-like activity inducing coronary vasodilation and hypotension.[15] The aqueous extract also enhanced coronary flow in isolated perfused rabbit heart preparation.[16] Powdered bark has been shown in rats to prevent oxidative stress associated with ischemic reperfusion injury.[17] In addition, arjunolic acid, a triterpene from the bark, has been shown to exert a protective effect against damage caused by isoproterenol-induced myocardial necrosis.[18] *Terminalia arjuna* also has potent antioxidant activity[19] and has a favorable effect on coronary risk factors such as hyperlipidemia, lowering cholesterol levels in rabbits fed a high-fat diet.[20-25] The lipid-lowering effect has been shown to occur through inhibition of cholesterol biosynthesis in the liver and increased excretion of bile acid. There is also an increased activity of the enzyme responsible for lipid metabolism in the body—plasma lecithin, cholesterol acytransferase activity, and stimulation of the receptor responsible for the destruction of low-density lipoprotein.[26] *Terminalia arjuna* bark 50 percent methanolic extract, at a dose level of 250 and 500 mg·kg^{-1}, reversed the abnormal platelet adhesiveness and the incidence of ECG abnormalities in hypercholesterolemic rabbits,[27] and at the same dose level improved the endothelial function.[28]

A number of studies have investigated the use of *Terminalia arjuna;* most of them have been in the area of angina and ischemic heart disease, one in congestive heart failure, a few cases of ventricular arrhythmias, in its antioxidant capacity and in the control of hyperlipidemia. One of the first studies that triggered interest in the use of *Terminalia arjuna* was conducted in 1951.[29]

Angina pectoris

In an open trial, 25 patients with angina pectoris were given 500 mg of *Terminalia arjuna* bark extract twice a day in addition to their usual antianginal drugs for 3 months. When evaluated at the end of 1 and 3 months, respectively, it was found that the exercise tolerance increased and the treadmill grading had significantly improved. There was, however, no reduction in the consumption of antianginal drugs and the drug was well tolerated and no side effects were observed.[30] Details are not available regarding the extraction solvent used for preparation of the bark extract.

In another open trial with 15 stable and 5 unstable angina patients, *Terminalia arjuna* was given for 3 months, at the end of which, in the stable angina group, there was a significant improvement in angina, decrease in blood pressure, and improvement in exercise tolerance increased as indicated by the delay in onset of angina on a treadmill test. In unstable angina patients, there was only an insignificant change in anginal frequency. No adverse effects were seen on liver and kidney functions.[31]

In another open trial, 29 patients with angina pectoris were administered 600 mg of *Terminalia arjuna* bark powder. In 17 Tread Mill Test (TMT) positive cases, improvement seen was evaluated as 20.3, 57, and 67 percent reduction of symptoms after 20, 40, and 60 days of treatment, whereas in TMT negative cases greater improvement was seen with 30.4, 47, and 68 percent reduction of symptoms, respectively.[32]

In a double-blind placebo-controlled cross-over study, 58 male patients with chronic stable angina NYHA class II-III, who showed provocable ischemia on exercise, were given 500 mg of *Terminalia arjuna* 90 percent alcohol extract 8 hourly, isosorbide nitrate 40 mg daily, or a matching placebo for 1 week each after a wash-out period of 3 days in a randomized double-blind cross-over fashion. All patients were evaluated clinically at the end of each week of therapy apart from biochemical and treadmill exercise evaluation. Patients on *Terminalia arjuna* extract showed improvement both in clinical parameters and exercise tolerance, which was similar to isosorbide mononitrate when compared to placebo.[33]

Congestive heart failure

Properly evaluated plants can be useful in the long-term treatment of chronic heart failure (inadequate heart function causing insufficient supply of oxygen and nutrients to the lungs and extremities). In an early study ten patients with congestive heart failure, who were classified as being in NYHA Class I (one patient), Class II (five patients), and Class III (four patients), were given 4 g of powdered *Terminalia arjuna* bark twice a day before food for 1 month, which caused a significant diuresis ($p < 0.01$). All patients showed improvement in their functional class, breathlessness, and overall feeling of well-being and comfort. In addition, there was a fall in both systolic and diastolic blood pressure.[34]

In a double-blind placebo-controlled study, 12 patients with severe refractory heart failure, NYHA Class IV, were given either 500 mg of *Terminalia arjuna* bark extract 8 hourly or a matching placebo for 2 weeks each as an adjuvant, in addition to the patients' intake of digoxin, diuretics, ACE-inhibitors, vasodilators, and potassium supplementation. After 2 weeks there was a wash-out period for 2 weeks, before the cross-over preparation was administered. All patients experienced breathlessness during rest period or after minimal activity. Baseline evaluation was carried out for both clinical and laboratory parameters, in addition to an echocardiogram at the start of the trial, after *Terminalia arjuna* and placebo treatment. There was an improvement in dyspnea, fatigue, edema, and the walking distance when patients were on *arjuna* therapy. At the end of 4 months nine patients had improved to Class II, whereas three patients had improved to Class III. In the second open phase of the trial all patients were continued on *arjuna* therapy (500 mg every 8 hours) for about 2 years in addition to their other drugs (flexible diuretic, vasodilator, and digitalis), and patients continued to show improvement in signs and symptoms, exercise tolerance, NYHA class, and quality of life.[35]

Coronary artery disease

In two cases of ventricular premature contractions associated with coronary artery disease, *Terminalia arjuna* powder 500 mg was given thrice a day, and ventricular premature contractions disappeared in both cases.[36]

In an open study, ten patients of postmyocardial infarction angina (post-heart attack chest pain) and two patients of ischemic cardiomyopathy (disease of the heart muscle causing weakened force of contraction) were treated with 500 mg of *Terminalia arjuna* stem bark powder 8-hourly for 3 months in addition to the conventional treatment of nitrates, aspirin, and/or calcium channel blockers. Another group of 12 patients with postmyocardial infarction angina, who were only on conventional treatment, served as controls. Both groups showed a significant reduction in anginal frequency; however, only the *Terminalia arjuna* group showed a significant reduction in left ventricular ejection fraction and reduction in left ventricular mass, as shown by echocardiogram. In addition, two patients with cardiomyopathy showed improvement in coronary heart failure from NYHA Class III to Class I. No side effects on the kidney, liver, and blood were seen.[37]

Lipid lowering in coronary heart disease

In an open trial, 51 cases with coronary heart disease (CHD) were treated with 500 mg of *Terminalia arjuna* bark powder filled in capsules and given 2 capsules twice daily with milk for 4 months. There was a significant regulation of blood pressure and lipid profile in these patients. Patients got considerable symptomatic relief with improvement in breathlessness, palpitation, and chest pain after 1 month of treatment and there was significant normalization at 4 months.[38]

In a randomized open trial, 105 patients with CHD were matched for age and disease status and then randomized into three groups. One group received placebo capsules, one group received 400 IU of vitamin E, and the third group received 500 mg capsules of *Arjuna* bark powder. Lipid and lipid peroxide levels were determined after 30 days of intake. There was no significant change in lipid levels in groups receiving placebo and Vitamin E, whereas in the *arjuna* group there was a significant decrease in total cholesterol and LDL cholesterol. In addition, there was a significant reduction in lipid peroxide levels in both vitamin E and *arjuna* groups.[39]

Terminalia arjuna is well tolerated in the usual dosages of 1-2 g used in clinical trials and considered optimum for the treatment of coronary artery disease (CAD).[30, 40] Side effects seen are mild—gas tritis, headache, constipation, abdominal discomfort, body ache, nausea, and insomnia— and only in a few patients.[33,35] No organ toxicity in liver and kidney,[37] and no metabolic toxicity has been reported in patients taking *Terminalia arjuna* for 24 months.[35] In vitro studies have shown that methanol and acetone extracts of *Terminalia arjuna* show an antimutagenic activity.[41]

Inula racemosa *Hook f. (Family: Asteraceae)*

Sanskrit: Pushkara	Hindi: Pushkaramoola, pokharmoola

Inula racemosa is a tall stout herb growing up to 1.5 m in the north-western Himalayas from 1,500 to 4,200 m elevation.[42] The roots are prized in Ayurveda for their expectorant action in cough and also in breathlessness and chest pain. It is described in the *Caraka Samhita* as the best drug for precordial pain[43] and also mentioned in several other formulae, both as a single drug and in combination with other drugs for the treatment of heart disease. It is also used internally for the treatment of tuberculosis and externally for skin problems.

Roots of *Inula racemosa* contain 10 percent inulin and 1.3 percent of an essential oil, which contains several lactones, chiefly alantolactone and isoalantolactone.[42,44]

Inula racemosa has been shown to have a protective effect on experimental myocardial infarction in rats when compared to a control group.[45] In addition, it has also been shown to have a negative inotropic and chronotropic effect in frog heart.[46]

Based on the high regard accorded to *Inula racemosa* by Caraka in relieving chest pain, it was tried out in a small number of patients with ischemic heart disease complaining of chest pain and ST-segment depression shown in the ECG on exertion. In an open study, nine patients with ischemic heart disease were treated with 3 g of *Inula racemosa* root powder taken 90 minutes before testing. At this dosage it prevented postexercise ST depression in all cases, leading the authors to conclude that the results were comparable to nitroglycerine with enhanced improvement seen with *Inula racemosa*.[47]

In an earlier trial with *Commiphora mukul* in cases of ischemic heart disease, it was found that patients continued to have precordial pain for periods ranging from 3 to 9 months, despite the intake of guggul, and requiring the additional use of nitroglycerine to control pain.[48] Therefore, *Inula racemosa*, which is considered the drug of choice to control chest pain, was added. In an initial trial, a combination of *Inula racemosa* with *Commiphora mukul* gum in the ratio of 1:1 was tried on 50 patients with ischemic heart disease at 6 g per day in three divided doses for 4 months. At the end of the trial period, five patients had recovered and had no precordial pain, and the serum cholesterol and ECG were within normal limits. A total of 40 patients showed varying degrees of improvement such as reduction in precordial pain and ECG or serum cholesterol levels although five patients did not show any improvement at all. A longer treatment period was expected to yield the desired results.[49]

Thus, two studies have been published by the same institution—one in which 150 patients[50] were enrolled and the other with 200 patients.[51] All patients had precordial pain relieved with nitroglycerine and showed breathlessness and changes in the ST-segment depression and T-wave in the ECG after exercise, which is characteristic of myocardial ischemia. Patients were recruited for the trial and given 6-8 g of the 1:1 combination of the drug for a period of 6 months. Cholesterol, triglycerides, and total lipids showed significant fall from the first month onwards. [50] At the end of the trial period, of the 200 patients, 25 percent (52 out of 200) had a normal ECG, 59 percent showed improvement in ECG, 25 percent (50 out of 200) had no precordial pain, and 69.2 percent patients (110 out of 159) had no dyspnea.[51]

To further improve patient comfort, two further combinations were tried out. In the first combination *Bacopa monnieri* plant juice, which has an anxiolytic effect, made from an equal quantity by weight was added to equal amounts of the powders of *Inula racemosa* and *Commiphora mukul* and made into 500 mg pills; 12 such pills were given to 50 patients in divided doses for a period of 6 months and ECG taken for 45 patients. After 6 months, 8 out of 45 patients had no precordial pain and both ECG and lipid levels were normal; 60 percent (30 out of 45) of the patients showed improvement in chest pain, in ECG, and serum lipid levels, 8 out of 45 patients improved with relief only in precordial pain but not in lipid levels or ECG, whereas two patients showed no improvement.[52]

In the second combination, in addition to *Inula racemosa* and *Commiphora mukul, Centella asiatica* and *Hypericum perforatum* were added to allay anxiety and depression in 406 patients with one or more risk factors for CHD. The formulation consisted of 500 mg of total extracts per capsule combined in the following ratio: each 20 mg of the combination contained *Inula racemosa* root extract—3 mg·kg^{-1}; the gum resin of *Commiphora mukul* —7 mg·kg^{-1}; *Centella asiatica* whole plant extract—8 mg·kg^{-1}; and *Hypericum perforatum* leaf extract—2 mg·kg^{-1}. The drug combination was administered in a dose of 20 mg·kg^{-1} in divided doses for 6 months. A control group consisting of 57 males and 28 females were kept on placebo. The drug-treated group showed significant improvement in nervousness, sleeplessness, tremors, irritability, and fatigue. In addition, there was a decrease in both diastolic and systolic blood pressure, correction in total cholesterol, and increase in HDL-cholesterol ratio in the treated group, but not in the placebo group.[53]

Larger doses of *Inula racemosa* have a laxative effect.[54] In a 1:1 combination with *Commiphora mukul* it showed no adverse effect when given to 250 patients with CHD to assess the effect on body composition.[55]

NOTES

1. Udupa KN. Scope of use of *Terminalia arjuna* in ischaemic heart disease. *Ann Natl Acad Indian Med* 1(1):54-58 (1986).

2. *Caraka Samhita,* ed. and trans. Sharma PV (vol. II, pp. 429-434, "Chikitsasthanam," chapter 26, verse 70-96). Varanasi: Chaukambha Orientalia. 1983.

3. *Susrutha samhita,* ed. and trans. Bhishagratna KL (vol. III, 4th edn., p. 263, "Uttara-tantra," chapter 42, verse 67-68). Varanasi: Chowkhamba Sanskrit Series Office, 1991.

4. Vagbhata, *Astanga Hrdayam,* ed. and trans. Srikantha Murthy KR (pp. 274-280, "Chikitsasthanam," chapter VI, verse 25-59). Varanasi: Krishnadas Academy, 1995.

5. Kumar S, Prabhakar YS. On the ethnomedical significance of Arjun tree, *Terminalia arjuna* (Roxb.) Wight & Arnot. *J Ethnopharmacol* 20:173-190 (1987).

6. Vagbhata, *Astanga Hridya,* ed. and trans. Srikantha Murthy KR (vol. II, 2nd edn., p. 279, "Chikitsasthana," chapter VI, verse 53-54a). Varanasi: Krishnadas Academy, 1995.

7. Cakrapanidatta, *Cakradatta,* ed. and trans. Sharma PV (1st edn., p 280, "Hrdroga," verses 14-17). Varanasi: Chaukhambha Orientalia, 1994.

8. Tripathi VK, Singh B, Tripathi RC, Upadhay RK, Pandey VB. *Terminalia arjuna:* Its present status. A review. *Oriental J Chem* 12(1):1-16 (1996).

9. Ghosh BN. School of tropical medicine, Calcutta: Personal Communication, 1953. Quoted in Chopra RN, Chopra IC, Handa KL, Kapur LD. *Chopra's Indigenous drugs of India* (2nd edn., pp. 421-424). Calcutta: Academic Publishers, 1958.

10. Gupta LP, Sen SP, Udupa KN. Pharmacognostical and pharmacological studies in *Terminalia arjuna. J Res Indian Med Yoga Homeopath* 11(4):16-24 (1976).

11. Singh N, Kapur KK, Singh SP, Shanker K, Sinha JN, Kohli RP. Mechanism of cardiovascular action of *Terminalia arjuna. Planta Med* 45:102-104 (1982).

12. Srivastava RD, Dwivedi S, Sreenivasan KK, Chandrasekhar CN. Cardiovascular effects of *Terminalia* species of plants. *Indian Drugs* 29:144-149 (1992).

13. Radhakrishnan R, Wadsworth RM, Gray AI. *Terminalia arjuna,* an Ayurvedic cardiotonic increases contractile force of rat isolated atria. *Phytother Res* 7:266-268 (1993).

14. Karamsetty M, Ferrie TJ, Kane KA, Gray AI. Effects of an aqueous extract of *Terminalia arjuna* on isolated rat atria and thoracic aorta. *Phytother Res* 9:575-578 (1995).

15. Dwivedi S, Chansouria JPN. Somani PN, Udupa KN. Influence of certain indigenous drugs on PGE$_2$ like activity in the ischaemic rabbit aorta. *Indian Drugs* 24:378-382 (1987).

16. Bhatia J, Bhattacharya SK, Mahajan P, Dwivedi S. Experimental evaluation of cardiovascular and cardioprotective effects of *Terminalia arjuna*. *Indian J Pharmacol* 31:57 (1999).

17. Gauthaman K, Maulik M, Kumari R, Manchanda SC, Dinda AK, Maulik SK. Effect of chronic treatment with bark of *Terminalia arjuna:* A study on the isolated ischemic-reperfused rat heart. *J Ethnopharmacol* 75:197-201 (2001).

18. Sumitra M, Manikandan P, Kumar DA, Arulselvan N, Balakrishna K, Manohar BM, Puvanakrishnan R. Experimental myocardial necrosis in rats: Role of arjunolic acid on platelet aggregation, coagulation and antioxidant status. *Mol Cell Biochem* 224:135-142 (2001).

19. Munasinghe J, Seneviratne CK, Thabrew MI, Abeysekara A. Antiradical and antilipidperoxidative effects of some plant extracts used by Sri Lankan traditional practioners for cardioprotection. *Phytother Res* 15:519-523 (2001).

20. Tiwari AK, Gode JD, Dubey GP. A comparative study between *Terminalia arjuna* and cholestryamine. Effect of certain lipids and lipoproteins in hypercholesterolemic rabbits. *Indian Drugs* 26:664-667 (1989).

21. Tiwari AK, Gode JD, Dubey GP. Effect of *Terminalia arjuna* on lipid profiles of rabbits fed hypercholesterolemic diet. *Int J Crude Drug Res* 28:43-47 (1990).

22. Pathak SR, Upadhyaya L, Singh RH, Dubey GP, Udupa KN. Effect of *Terminalia arjuna* W&A on autocoidal lipid profiles in rabbits. *Indian Drugs* 27:221-227 (1990).

23. Shaila HP, Udupa SL, Udupa AL, Nair NS. Effect of *Terminalia arjuna* in experimental hyperlipidemia in rabbits. *Int J Pharmacog* 35:126-129 (1997).

24. Shaila HP, Udupa SL, Udupa AL. Hypolipidemic effect of *Terminalia arjuna* in cholesterol fed rabbits. *Fitoterapia* 68:405-409 (1997).

25. Ram A, Lauria P, Gupta R, Kumar P, Sharma VN. Hypocholesterolaemic effects of *Terminalia arjuna* tree bark. *J Ethnopharmacol* 55:165-169 (1997).

26. Khanna AK, Chander R, Kapoor NK. *Terminalia arjuna:* An Ayurvedic cardiotonic regulates lipid metabolism in hyperlipaemic rats. *Phytother Res* 10:663-665 (1996).

27. Chatterjee S. Effect of *Terminalia arjuna* on abnormal platelet reactivity in hypercholesterolaemic rabbits. *Indian Drugs* 37:135-138 (2000).

28. Chatterjee S. *Terminalia arjuna* improves endothelial vasodilator function in cholesterol-fed rabbits. *Indian Drugs* 37:433-436 (2000).

29. Colbawala HM. An evaluation of the cardiotonic and other properties of *Terminalia arjuna*. *Indian Heart J* 3:205-230 (1951).

30. Jain V, Poonia A, Agarwal RP, Panwar RB, Kochar DK, Mishra SN. Effect of *Terminalia arjuna* in patients of angina pectoris (a clinical trial). *Indian Med Gazz* 26(2):56-59 (1992).

31. Dwivedi S, Agarwal MP. Antianginal and cardioprotective effects of *Terminalia arjuna,* an indigenous drug, in coronary artery disease. *J Assoc Physicians India* 42:287-289 (1994).

32. Saxena S, Trivedi VP. A clinico-pharmacological assessment of arjuna *(Terminalia arjuna)* powder in *Hridvikar* (angina pectoris) (p. 195). New Delhi: National Symposium on Ancient Indian Science, Engineering & Technology Interfaced with the Modern Knowledge, December 14-15, 2001.

33. Bharani A, Ganguli A, Mathur LK, Jamra Y, Raman PG. Efficacy of *Terminalia arjuna* in chronic stable angina: A double-blind, placebo-controlled, cross-over study comparing *Terminalia arjuna* with isosorbide mononitrate. *Indian Heart J* 54:170-175 (2002).

34. Verma SK, Bordia A. Effect of *Terminalia arjuna* bark *(arjun chhal)* in patients of congestive heart failure and hypertension. *J Res Edu Ind Med* VII(4):31-36(1988).

35. Bharani A, Ganguly A, Bhargava KD. Salutary effect of *Terminalia arjuna* in patients with severe refractory heart failure. *Int J Cardiol* 49:191-199 (1995).

36. Dwivedi S, Avasthi R, Mahajan S. Role of *Terminalia arjuna* in ventricular tachyarrythmias. *Indian Practioner* XLVII:523- 525 (1994).

37. Dwivedi S, Jauhari R. Beneficial effects of *Terminalia arjuna* in coronary artery disease. *Indian Heart J* 49:507-510 (1997).

38. Tripathi VK, Singh B, Jha RN, Pandey VB, Udupa KN. Studies on *Arjuna* in coronary heart disease. *J Res Ayur Siddha* 21(1-2):37- 40 (2000).

39. Gupta R, Singhal S, Goyle A, Sharma VN. Antioxidant and hypocholesterolaemic effects of *Terminalia arjuna* tree bark powder: A randomised placebo controlled trial. *J Assoc Physicians India* 49:231-235 (2001).

40. Dwivedi SD. Useful plants in cardiovascular ailments. *Nat Prod Radiance* 1(5):22-26 (2002).

41. Kaur K, Arora S, Kumar S, Nagpal A. Antimutagenic activities of acetone and methanol fractions of *Terminalia arjuna. Food Chem Toxicol* 40:1475-1482 (2002).

42. Satyavati GV, Gupta AK, Tandon N (eds.). *Medicinal plants of India* (vol. 2, pp. 72-80). New Delhi: Indian Council of Medical Research, 1987.

43. *Caraka Samhita,* ed. and trans. Sharma PV (vol. 1, pp.168-172, "Sutrasthanam," chapter 25, verse 40). Varanasi: Chaukamba Orientalia, 1981.

44. *The wealth of India, raw materials* (vol. V, pp. 236-237). New Delhi: Publications and Information Directorate, CSIR, 1959.

45. Patel V, Banu N, Ohja JK et al. Effect of indigenous drug *(pushkarmula)* on experimentally induced myocardial infarction in rats. *Act Nerv Super* Suppl 3:387-394 (1982).

46. Tripathi YB, Tripathi P, Upadhyay BN. Assessment of adrenergic beta-blocking activity of *Inula racemosa. J Ethnopharmacol* 23:3-9 (1988).

47. Tripathi SN, Upadhyaya BN, Gupta VK. Beneficial effect of *Inula racemosa (Pushkarmoola)* in angina pectoris: A preliminary report (letter to the editor). *Indian J Physio Pharmacol* 28:73-75 (1984).

48. Upadhyaya BN, Tripathi SN, Dwivedi LD. Hypochpolesterolaemic and hypolipidaemic action of gum *guggulu* in patients of coronary heart disease. *J Res Ind Med Yoga Homeo* 11(2):1-8 (1976).

49. Tripathi SN, Upadhyay BN, Sharma SD, Gupta VK, Tripathi YB. Role of *pushkara guggulu* in the management of ischaemic heart disease. *Ancient Sci Life* 4:9-19 (1984).

50. Singh R, Singh RP, Batliwala PG, Upadhyay BN, Tripathi SN. *Puskara-guggulu* an antianginal and hypolipidemic agent in coronary heart disease (CHD). *J Res Ayur Siddha* XII (1-2):1-18 (1990).

51. Singh RP, Singh R, Ram P, Batliwala PG. Use of *pushkar-guggul*, an indigenous antiischemic combination, in the management of ischemic heart disease. *Int J Pharmacog* 31:147-160 (1993).

52. Sharma SD, Upadhyay BN, Tripathi SN. A new Ayurvedic compound for the management of ischaemic heart disease *(Hrdroga)*. *Ancient Sci Life* V:161-167 (1986).

53. Dubey GP, Agarwal A, Dixit SP, Pathak SR. Individuals at risk of coronary heart disease (CHD), its prevention and management by an indigenous compound. *Ancient Sci Life* XIIX:48-57 (2000).

54. *Selected medicinal plants of India. A monograph on identity, safety and clinical usage* (pp. 188-189). Mumbai: Chemexcil. Basic Chemicals, Pharmaceuticals and Cosmetics Export Promotion Council, 1992.

55. Dubey GP, Singh S, Mishra AK. Effect of *Pushkar-guggulu* on body composition in CHD cases. *Sem Res Ayurveda and Siddha*. New Delhi: CCRAS, March 20-22, 1995.

HYPOLIPIDEMIC PLANTS

Lipid levels are considered to be a risk factor for several diseases, including heart problems. Over 50 plants are used in Ayurveda to lower lipid levels.[1] The etiopathology of obesity and associated lipid disorders have been described in a very comprehensive manner in the *Sushruta Samhita*,[2] and its parallel to modern theories of the development of atherosclerosis was noticed by Dr. Satyavati and Dr. Dwarakanath in the 1960s.[3]

Commiphora wightii *(Arn.) Bhandari* *(Family: Burseraceae)*

Latin: *Commiphora mukul* Engl, *Balsamodendron mukul* Hook ex Stocks

Sanskrit: Guggul, Devadhoopa

Hindi: Guggulu, guggul

Tamil: Maishaki Gukkal

English: Indian Bdellium

Commiphora wightii, better known in the literature as *Commiphora mukul* (see Plate 7 in color gallery), is a small to medium-sized tree found in the arid regions of India. It is cultivated in Rajasthan and Gujarat. The tree has a papery bark, and when an incision is made in the bark, a thin yellow gum oozes out, quickly solidifies, and is collected and purified. This gum resin has been used medicinally for a long time in Ayurveda, spanning several hundred years. It was first mentioned in the *Atharva veda,* then in the first texts of Ayurveda, the *Caraka Samhita,* and *Sushruta Samhita,* and later in numerous other texts, for its effectiveness on the heart, obesity, and diabetes.[4] Scientific investigation on *Commiphora wightii* has centered mainly on the anti-inflammatory effect and its hypolipidemic effect, for which it is an official drug in the *Indian Herbal Pharmacopoeia,* 2002.[5]

In *Sushruta Samhita,* there is a description of the changes that occur in cases of obesity, which remarkably parallels the modern interpretation of the etiology and pathogenesis of atherosclerosis.[6,7] The *Sushruta Samhita* also deals with the treatment of obesity and of lipid disorders, and the consequences associated with the various conditions. However, the age of the resin is considered to play an important role in the kind of effect produced—an old sample being useful in reducing body weight and lipid levels, whereas a new sample of the gum can have the reverse effect.[7] The crude gum also needs to be purified, as described in ancient texts, by boiling in a decoction of *triphala* (equal quantities of *Terminalia chebula, Terminalia belerica,* and *Emblica officinalis*) in order to free it from side effects such as skin rashes, diarrhea, irregular menstruation, restlessness, and hiccup.[7]

The gum resin has a complex composition with approximately 0.4 percent of an essential oil containing myrecene, dimyrecene, several steroids, Z- and E-guggulsterones, considered important for the hypolipidemic properties, and guggulsterols I-VI. Sesamin and cholesterol are found as well.[4,5]

The cholesterol-lowering properties of the crude gum resin and various fractions have been studied extensively over the years. The first report in 1966 showed that the crude gum could protect cholesterol-fed rabbits against atherosclerosis and also significantly reduce serum cholesterol levels in hypercholesterolemic rabbits,[8] apart from a reduction in the body weight of the treated animals.[9] The hypocholesterolemic effect has been shown by other workers in several species of experimental animals.[7,10] The activity has been found to be in the steroid fraction, especially in the two ketonic steroids Z- and E-guggulsterones.[11] The two guggulsterones have also been shown to inhibit platelet aggregation.[12]

Several theories have been propounded to explain the hypolipidemic activity of the gum resin. Guggulsterone exhibits potent antioxidant activity[13] and reversed myocardial necrosis induced by isoproterenol in rats.[14] The gum resin[15,16] and Z- guggulsterone[17] have been shown to stimulate the thyroid, and the gum has also been shown to induce triidothyronine production.[18] In addition, Z-guggulsterone acts as an Bile Acid Receptor (BAR) antagonist[19] and also as an antagonist of farnesoid X receptor FXR;[20] this may contribute to the cholesterol-lowering activity of the guggulsterones and of the gum resin.

Several trials have been conducted on the gum resin of *Commiphora mukul,* the so-called fraction A, and on guggulipid, which is the standardized ethyl acetate fraction of *Commiphora mukul* containing 2.5 percent guggulsterones developed at the Central Drug Research Institute, Lucknow, India.

Gum guggul

In preliminary open clinical trials, *guggul* was given in doses of 12-16 g per day to 22 patients with hypercholesterolemia associated with disorders such as obesity, ischemic heart disease, hypertension, etc. for a period of 12 weeks. At the end of the treatment period, it was observed that there was a fall in cholesterol levels by 33 percent in 96 percent of the cases, fall in triglycerides by 32.7 percent in 88 percent cases, decrease in free fatty acids by 62 percent, and decrease in serum phospholipids by 40 percent. In addition, there was a decrease in the body weight of ten patients by 1.4 kg every month.[8]

Gum *guggul* was also tried on 12 patients with elevated lipid levels—9 patients were obese, 2 had ischemic heart disease, and 1 patient had cerebral thrombosis. Treatment with *guggul* lowered the serum turbidity and prolonged the coagulation time.[21]

Other trials with gum *guggul* were held on patients with obesity/hyperlipidemia at several centers and confirmed the significant lowering of not only the serum cholesterol level, triglycerides, and total lipids but also of nonesterified fatty acids.[22-25] Two of these trials also compared the efficacy of Fraction A with gum *guggul*.[22,23] A significant increase in HDL cholesterol has also been reported apart from lowering of other lipid parameters.[26]

Fraction A

Petroleum ether extraction of *guggul* led to three fractions named A, B, and C, of which fraction A was found to have the maximum lipid-lowering action in chicks[27] and therefore was subjected to clinical trials. In a clinical study with 44 patients, fraction A was compared with clofibrate and an experimental drug from Ciba. In 20 patients 0.5 g fraction A was given twice a day for periods varying from 6 to 34 weeks. In the trial, patients were randomly assigned to receive one of the drugs. On analysis, fraction A was found to lower the serum levels of total lipids, triglycerides, cholesterol, phospholipids, and beta lipoprotein. In addition, the lowering of triglycerides was best in fraction A of *guggul*. Side effects observed with fraction A were hiccups (1 patient), diarrhea (3 patients), and restlessness and apprehension (1 patient).[28]

In a long-term study, 41 cases of hyperlipoproteinemia were treated with 0.5 g of fraction A thrice daily for 75 weeks with 10 cases on 2 g·day^{-1} of clofibrate also for 75 weeks serving as a comparative control. The reduction seen with fraction A was statistically significant for the entire treatment period. The reduction of cholesterol was 26.2 percent with *guggul* as against 31.5 percent with clofibrate, whereas for triglycerides the reduction for *guggul* was 36.5 percent as against 33.3 percent for clofibrate. Side effects such as diarrhea were seen in five patients.[29]

This was also borne out in a clinical study on 40 obese, 40 hypercholesterolemic, and 40 hyperlipemic patients. The effect of gum *guggul* 2 g thrice daily or fraction 'A' 0.5 g twice daily was studied. Fraction A was able to significantly reduce the serum cholesterol and serum lipids in 21 days, in a manner similar to clofibrate.[23]

In another double-blind cross-over study with fraction A, again with a dose of 1.5 g·day^{-1} for 4 weeks at a time, in 48 hypercholesterolemic patients with a mean level of 280 mg percent of cholesterol brought about a significant reduction of total cholesterol, total lipids, and triglycerides.[30]

Studies on human beings and on experimental animals to elucidate the mechanism of action of fraction A showed that there was mobilization of cholesterol from the tissues, a decrease in its synthesis, and increased excretion of cholesterol leading to a fall in cholesterol levels.[31]

Guggulipid

Guggulipid is the standardized ethyl acetate extract of gum *guggul.* It has been suggested that the hypolipidemic effect of guggulipid is dependent upon the etiology of the disease with nondiabetic hyperlipidemic patients being benefited with significant lowering of cholesterol, triglycerides, total lipids, and beta lipoprotein, whereas no such effect was seen in diabetic patients.[32]

In a phase I safety study, 400 mg guggulipid administered thrice a day for 4 weeks to 21 patients of primary hyperlipidemia was shown to be without any adverse effect on liver function, blood sugar, blood urea, hematological parameters, and ECG. There was also a significant lowering of cholesterol and/or triglycerides in 15 patients at the end of 4 weeks.[33]

In a comparative cross-over trial, guggulipid (500 mg every 8 hours) was evaluated against clofibrate (500 mg every 8 hours) in 30 patients of primary hyperlipidemia and judged to have better hypolipidemic activity than clofibrate.[34] A dosage of 500 mg of guggulipid was given thrice a day for 6 weeks to evaluate its usefulness in 22 patients of primary hyperlipidemia. The serum cholesterol levels were significantly lowered in 59 percent of patients, the effect beginning to be seen after 2 weeks and reaching a maximum in 4-6 weeks. The fall in cholesterol levels and triglycerides was 24.5 and 27 percent, respectively. There was a return to pretreatment values within 6 weeks of stopping the drug. The drug was well tolerated.[35]

In 25 patients with nephrotic syndrome, 75 mg three times a day of guggulipid was given for 12 weeks. HDL cholesterol levels increased after 8 weeks, although significant changes in the electrocardiogram were seen only after 12 weeks of therapy.[36]

In a randomized double-blind trial in 61 patients with hypercholes-terolemia, 31 on guggulipid and 30 on placebo, patients were given 50 mg of guggulipid or placebo capsules for 24 weeks along with a diet rich in fruits and vegetables. Guggulipid decreased the total cho-lesterol, LDL cholesterol, triglycerides, and total cholesterol/high-density lipoprotein cholesterol ratio by approximately 11-12 percent with no changes being observed in the placebo group. Lipid perox-ides also decreased by about 33 percent in the guggulipid group, whereas the placebo group remained unchanged. The HDL choles-terol level was unchanged in both groups. After a wash-out period of another 12 weeks, changes in lipoproteins were again reversed in the guggulipid group, with no changes being observed in the placebo group. The overall impression was that the combined effect of diet and guggulipid was equal to that of modern drugs.[37]

In another randomized-controlled trial[38] guggulipid was given in two dose levels three times a day of 1,000 mg and 2,000 mg or match-ing placebo in 103 cases of hyperlipidemia for 8 weeks. It was found that there was an increase in LDL cholesterol in both 1,000 mg as well as 2,000 mg dosage groups when compared to placebo where there was a decrease. It appears that there was no favorable effect on lipid levels. The dose given is much above the dosage for guggulipid, although standard doses were also tried out. In addition, six patients on guggulipid showed skin rashes reduced by prior processing of the gum to remove impurities.[9] Skin rashes are also encountered when larger doses are used. The age of the resin is considered to play an im-portant role on lipid-lowering activity levels and needs to be taken into consideration.[7]

Coronary artery disease

In an exploratory trial, gum *guggul* fraction A was given at a dose of 500 mg twice a day to both healthy subjects and coronary artery patients. In healthy subjects, it produced a 22-percent increase in se-rum fibrinolytic activity within 24 hours of administration, whereas it increased to 40 percent after 30 days. In coronary artery patients, it was found that the serum fibrinolytic activity increased by 19 percent after 24 hours and reached 33 percent after 30 days. A reduction in the platelet adhesive index by 19 and 16 percent in healthy controls and in patients, respectively, was also seen.[39]

In another study, of the 42 patients with coronary artery disease, only 21 patients were given 1.5 g of *Commiphora mukul* every day, whereas the remaining patients were not. It was found that patients receiving the drug showed reduction of euglobin lysis time and increase in fibrinolytic activity, whereas controls did not show any change in these parameters. There was no significant change in platelet aggregation.[40]

Ischemic heart disease

In a trial, 135 patients with ischemic heart disease and symptoms of precordial pain, dyspnea on effort, history of angina, or previous history of myocardial infarction were included. Of these, 110 patients served as the treatment group, and 25 patients were kept as the control group. The clinical profile and changes in serum lipids were evaluated at monthly intervals for the various parameters, whereas ECG was evaluated before and after treatment. Purified *guggul* powder was given in a dose of 8 g·day^{-1} for 3 months. There was a fall in lipid parameters comparable to clofibrate. Precordial pain and dyspnea also improved and grades I and II patients became absolutely free of the symptoms. Patients of grade III and IV also showed improvement. There was a reduction in weight of an average of 1 kg·month^{-1}. ECG changes were seen in seven cases with improvement in S-T segment depression and inversion of T-wave in patients of long-standing ischemia.[41]

Side effects associated with *guggul* are generally gastrointestinal in nature, reduced by purification of the resin and seen more often with larger dosages.[4] These include diarrhea, skin rashes, headache, irregular menstruation, and restlessness.[7] It has been shown not to have acute, subacute, and chronic toxicity in rats, dogs, and monkeys. Since it increases menstrual discharge it is not to be taken during pregnancy.[5] *Guggul* inhibits platelet aggregation,[12] and is probably best avoided with other blood thinning agents. Guggulipid given at a dose level of 400 mg thrice a day for 4 weeks showed no adverse effect on liver function, blood sugar, blood urea, and hematological parameters.[33]

Considering the variable nature of the preparation used in the different trials, it would be useful to conduct trials with well-defined material, along with dosage studies. It would be important to take into account the age of the resin, since old resin is said to have a beneficial effect on obesity as mentioned in the *Sushruta Samhita.*[7,42] Thus, it would be necessary to identify components that may be responsible for having a reverse effect of increasing lipid levels.

Trigonella foenum-graecum *Linn. (Family: Fabaceae)*

Sanskrit: Methika	Tamil: Vendium
Hindi: Methi	English: Fenugreek

See Chapter 11 for an introduction to fenugreek. Fenugreek seeds have been shown to reduce lipid levels in a number of experimental animals such as rats, dogs, and rabbits.[43-50] There was significant reduction of serum cholesterol levels ($p < 0.00005$) in both normal (42 percent) and hypercholesterolemic (58 percent) rats on feeding with a diet of 50 percent *Trigonella foenum-graecum* seeds.[43] The saponin fraction that interacts with the bile salts has been shown to reduce cholesterol levels in rats.[45,46] In rats the ethanol extract contains hypocholesterolemic constituents like saponins, which led to a 18-26 percent reduction in plasma cholesterol.[46] In dogs the lipid extract had no effect on cholesterol levels, but the fiber-rich (53.9 percent) and saponin- containing (4.8 percent) defatted portion showed significant reduction of cholesterol levels in normal and in hypercholesterolemic dogs.[48] A principle isolated from the aqueous extract showed hypoglycemic, hypocholesterolemic, and hypotriacylglycerolemic activities in hyperlipidemic rabbits.[49] Different levels of fenugreek and extracts were tried on rabbits both in normal animals and those pretreated with a high fat diet. Plasma cholesterol levels were reduced in both groups; however, reduction in triglyceride levels was seen only in the high fat diet group when animals were treated with 30 percent of diet enriched with seed powder or extracts; changes in cholesterol, triglycerides, and LDL cholesterol were seen. There was no change in HDL cholesterol but the ratio of HDL to LDL changes favorably.[50]

Clinical studies have demonstrated the beneficial effect of fenugreek seeds in hyperlipidemic patients and in diabetic patients. For trials on diabetic patients see Chapter 11, "Antidiabetic agents."

In an open exploratory trial 10 hyperlipidemic patients were given isocaloric diets with or without the addition of 100 g of debitterized fenugreek powder for 20 days. Patients receiving a diet with added fenugreek showed significant reduction in total serum cholesterol, LDL, VDL cholesterol, and triglyceride levels. HDL cholesterol did not change but ratios with respect to total cholesterol and LDL and VLDL showed a favorable change.[51]

In patients with mild to moderate hypercholesterolemia,[52] fenugreek seeds were able to reduce cholesterol levels. In another open trial, 20 hypercholesterolemic patients, ages 50-65 years, were given germinated fenugreek seeds powder in packets of 12.5 g and 18 g to incorporate daily one packet into any food of their choice for 1 month. It was found that fasting blood levels taken one day before the start of the trial and after the treatment period of 1 month showed significant reduction of total cholesterol and LDL levels at the 18 g dose level, although there was a hypolipidemic effect at both levels. No significant change in HDL, VLDL, and triglyceride levels was seen in any of the patients. Germination was found to bring about definite changes in the soluble fiber content of the seeds.[53]

In a single blind trial with placebo control, 18 hypercholesterolemic patients were divided into three groups and were given 50 g packets of defatted deodorized fenugreek seed powder (FG), 50 g placebo powder, or 25 g placebo powder plus 25 g FG powder to be taken orally before lunch and dinner for 20 days. Lipid profiles were checked with fasting blood samples on 0, 10, and 20 days. Significant changes in total cholesterol, triglycerides, and VLDL levels were seen in both the fenugreek groups as compared to placebo.[54]

The safety of fenugreek is covered in Chapter 11 "Antidiabetic agents."

NOTES

1. Nayak S, Jain UK, Saraf A. Potent hypolipidemic herbal drugs: A review. *Sachitra Ayurved* 51:448-453 (1998).

2. *Sushruta samhita,* trans. Bhishagratna KL (vol. 1, 4th edn., pp.135-137, "Sutrasthana," chapter 15, verse 32). Varanasi: Chowkhamba Sanskrit Series Office, 1991.

3. Satyavati GV. Gum *Guggul (Commiphora mukul)*: The success story of an ancient insight leading to a modern discovery. *Ind J Med Res* 87:327-335 (1988).

4. *Selected medicinal plants of India. A monograph on identity, safety and clinical usage* (pp. 103-107). Bombay: Chemexcil, Basic Chemicals, Pharmaceuticals and Cosmetics Export Promotion Council, 1992.

5. *The Indian herbal pharmacopoeia* (rev. new edn., pp. 134-143). Mumbai: Indian Drug Manufacturers' Association, 2002.

6. *Sushruta samhita,* trans. Bhishagratna KL (vol. 1, 4th edn., pp. 135-137, "Sutrasthana," chapter 15, verse 32). Varanasi: Chowkhamba Sanskrit Series Office, 1991.

7. Satyavati GV. Gum *guggul (Commiphora mukul)*: The success story of an ancient insight leading to a modern discovery. *Ind J Med Res* 87:327-335 (1988).

8. Satyavati GV. Effect of an indigenous drug on disorders of lipid metabolism with special reference to atherosclerosis and obesity *(medoroga)*. MD thesis (Ayurveda), Varanasi: Banaras Hindu University, 1966.

9. Satyavati GV, Dwarakanath C, Tripathi SN. Experimental studies on the hypocholesterolemic effect of *Commiphora mukul* Engl. *(Guggul)*. *Indian J Med Res* 57:1950-1962 (1969).

10. Satyavati GV, Raina MK, Sharma M. (eds.). *Medicinal plants of India* (vol. 1, pp. 269-276). New Delhi: Indian Council of Medical Research, 1976.

11. Kapoor NK, Nityanand S. Effect of *guggul* steroids on cholesterol biosynthesis in rats. *Ind J Biochem Biophys* 15:77 (1978).

12. Mester L, Mester M, Nityanand S. Inhibition of platelet aggregation by "*guggulu*" steroids. *Planta Med* 37:367-369 (1979).

13. Singh K, Chander R, Kapoor NK. Guggulsterone, a potent hypolipidaemic, prevents oxidation of low density lipoprotein. *Phytother Res* 11:291-294 (1997).

14. Kaul S, Kapoor NK. Reversal of changes of lipid peroxide, xanthine oxidase and superoxide dismutase by cardio-protective drugs in isoproterenol induced myocardial necrosis in rats. *Indian J Exp Biol* 27:625-627 (1989).

15. Singh AK, Prasad GC, Tripathi SN. *In vitro* studies on thyrogenic effect of *Commiphora mukul (guggulu)*. *Ancient Sci Life* 2(1):23-28 (1982).

16. Singh AK, Tripathi SN, Prasad GC. Response of *Commiphora mukul (guggulu)* on melatonin induced hypothyroidism. *Ancient Sci Life* III (2):85-90 (1983).

17. Tripathi YB, Tripathi P, Malhotra OP, Tripathi SN. Thyroid stimulatory action of Z-guggulsterone: Mechanism of action. *Planta Med* 54:271-277 (1988).

18. Panda S, Kar A. *Gugulu (Commiphora mukul)* induces triiodothyronine production: Possible involvement of lipid peroxidation. *Life Sci* 65:137-141 (1999).

19. Wu J, Xia C, Meier J, Li S, Hu X, Lala DS. The hypolipidemic natural product guggulsterone acts as an antagonist of the bile acid receptor. *Mol Endocrinol* 16:1590-1597 (2002).

20. Urizar NL, Liverman AB, Dodds DT, Silva FV, Ordentlich P, Yan Y, Gonzalez FJ, Heyman RA, Mangelsdorf DJ, Moore DD. A natural product that lowers cholesterol as an antagonist ligand for FXR. *Science* 296:1703-1706 (2002).

21. Tripathi SN, Shastri VVS, Satyavati GV. Experimental and clinical studies on the effect of *Guggulu (Commiphora mukul)* in hyperlipaemia and thrombosis. *J Res Indian Med* 2(2):10 (1968).

22. Kuppurajan K, Rajagopalan SS, Rao TK, Vijayalakshmi AN, Dwarakanath C. Effect of *guggulu (Commiphora mukul* Engl.) on serum lipids in obese subjects. *J Res Ind Med* 8:1-8 (1973).

23 Kuppurajan K, Rajagopalan SS, Rao KT, Sitaraman R. Effect of *guggulu (Commiphora mukul* Engl.) on serum lipids in obese, hypercholesterolemic and hyperlipemic cases . *J Assoc Physicians India* 26:367- 373 (1978).

24. Keerti Sharma, Puri AS, Sharma R, Prakash S. Effect of gum *guggulu* on serum lipids in obese subjects. *J Res Indian Med Yoga Homeo* 11:132-134 (1976).

25. Jain AP. Clinical assessment of the value of *Commiphora mukul (guggul)* in obesity and hyperlipidemia. *ICMR Bull* 10:83-84 (1980).

26. Verma SK, Bordia A. Effect of *Commiphora mukul* (gum *guggul*) in patients of hyperlipidemia with special reference to HDL cholesterol. *Indian J Med Res* 87:356-360 (1988).

27. Mehta VL, Malhotra CL, Kalrah NS. The effect of various fractions of gum *guggul* on experimentally produced hypercholesteraemia in chicks. *Indian J Physiol Pharmacol* 12:91-95 (1968).

28. Malhotra SC, Ahuja MMS. Comparative hypolipidaemic effectiveness of gum *guggul (Commiphora mukul)* fraction A, ethyl-p-chlorophenoxyisobutyrate and Ciba-1347-Su. *Indian J Med Res* 59:1621-1632 (1971).

29. Malhotra SC, Ahuja MMS, Sundaram KR. Long term clinical studies on the hypolipidemic effect of *Commiphora mukul (guggulu)* and Clofibrate. *Indian J Med Res* 65:390-395 (1977).

30. Kotiyal JP, Bisht DB, Singh DS. Double blind cross-over trial of gum *guggulu (Commiphora mukul)* Fraction A in hypercholesterolemia. *J Res Indian Med Yoga Homeo* 14:11-16 (1979).

31. Malhotra C. Pharmacological and clinical studies on the effects of *Commiphora mukul (Guggulu)* and clofibrate on certain aspects of lipid metabolism. PhD thesis, New Delhi: All India Institute of Medical Sciences, 1973.

32. Das PK, Dasgupta G, Mishra AK. Clinical studies on medicinal plants of India. In Dhawan BN (ed.), *Current research on medicinal plants of India* (p. 72). New Delhi: Indian National Science Academy, 1986, quoting Satoskar RS, *Ann Rep*. Bombay: Dept of Pharmacol, Seth GS Medical College, 1983.

33. Agarwal RC, Singh SP, Saran RK, Das SK, Sinha N, Asthana OP, Gupta PC, Nityanand S, Dhawan BN, Agarwal SS. Clinical trial of gugulipid—A new hypolipidemic agent of plant origin in primary hyperlipidemia. *Indian J Med Res* 84:626-634 (1986).

34. Baldwa VS, Gupta ML. Effect of *Commiphora mukul* (gugulipid) and clofibrate on lipid profile in hyperlipidemia. A comparative cross over study. *Rajasthan Med J* 24(3):90-92 (1985).

35. Gopal K, Saran RK, Nityanand, Gupta PP, Hasan M, Das M, Sinha N, Agarwal SS. Clinical trial of ethyl acetate extract of gum *gugulu* (gugulipid) in primary hyperlipidemia. *J Assoc Physicians India* 34(4):249-251 (1986).

36. Beg M, Afzaal S, Akhter N. Hypolipidemic and cardioprotective effectiveness of guglip in patients of nephrotic syndrome. *Indian Med Gazette* 132 (2):35-38 (1998).

37. Singh RB, Niaz MA, Ghosh S. Hypolipidemic and antioxidant effects of *Commiphora mukul* as an adjunct to dietary therapy in patients with hypercholesterolemia. *Cardiovasc Drug Ther* 8:659-664 (1994).

38. Szapary PO, Wolfe ML, Bloedon LT, Cucchiara AJ, DerMarderosian AH, Cirigliano MD, Rader DJ. Guggulipid for the treatment of hypercholesterolemia: A randomized controlled trial. *JAMA* 290:765-772 (2003).

39. Bordia A, Chuttani SK. Effect of gum *guggulu* on fibrinolysis and platelet adhesiveness in coronary heart disease. *Indian J Med Res* 70:992-996 (1979).

40. Baldwa VS, Sharma RC, Ranka PC, Chittora MD. Effect of *Commiphora mukul (guggul)* on fibrinolytic activity and platelet aggregation in coronary artery disease. *Rajasthan Med J* 19:84-86 (1980).

41. Upadhyay BN, Tripathi YB, Tripathi SN. Primary and secondary prevention of ischaemic heart disease by *guggulu (C. mukul)*. *J Res Edu Ind Med* 1(1):51-59 (1982).

42. *Sushruta samhita,* trans. Bhishagratna KL (vol. 2, 4th edn., pp. 314-315, "Chikitsasthana," chapter 5, verse 44). Varanasi: Chowkhamba Sanskrit Series Office, 1991.

43. Singhal PC, Gupta RK, Joshi LD. Hypocholesterolaemic effect of *Trigonella foenum-graecum (methi)*. *Curr Sci* 51:136-137 (1982).

44. Sharma RD. Hypocholesterolemic activity of fenugreek *(T. foenum graecum)*: An experimental study in rats. *Nutr Rep Int* 30:221-232 (1984).

45. Sharma RD. An evaluation of hypocholesterolemic factor in fenugreek seeds *(T. foenum graecum)* in rats. *Nutr Rep Int* 33:669-677 (1986).

46. Stark A, Madar Z. The effect of an ethanol extract derived from fenugreek *(Trigonella foenum-graecum)* on bile acid absorption and chlolesterol levels in rats. *Br J Nutr* 69:277-287 (1993).

47. Khosla P, Gupta DD, Nagpal RK. Effect of *Trigonella foenum-graecum* (fenugreek) on serum lipids in normal and diabetic rats. *Indian J Pharmacol* 27:89-93 (1995).

48. Valette G, Sauvaire Y, Baccou JC, Ribes G. Hypercholesterolaemic effect of fenugreek seeds in dogs. *Atherosclerosis* 50:105-111 (1984).

49. Puri D, Prabhu KM, Murthy PS. Hypocholesterolemic effect of the hypoglycemic principle of fenugreek *(Trigonella foenum-graecum)* seeds. *Indian J Clin Biochem* 9:13-16 (1994).

50. Al-Habori M, Al-Aghbari AM, Al-Mamary M. Effects of fenugreek seeds and its extracts on plasma lipid profiles: A study on rabbits. *Phytother Res* 12:572-575 (1998).

51. Sharma RD, Raghuram TC, Rao VD. Hypolipidaemic effect of fenugreek seeds. A clinical study. *Phytother Res* 5:145-147 (1991).

52. Singh RB, Niaz MA, Rastogi V, Singh N, Postiglione A, Rastogi SS. Hypolipidemic and antioxidant effects of fenugreek seeds and triphala as adjuncts to dietary therapy in patients with mild to moderate hypercholesterolemia. *Perfusion* 11:124-130 (1998).

53. Sowmya P, Rajyalakshmi P. Hypocholesterolemic effect of germinated fenugreek seeds in human subjects. *Plant Foods Human Nutr* 53:359-365 (1999).

54. Prasanna M. Hypolipidemic effect of fenugreek: A clinical study. *Indian J Pharmacol* 32:34-36 (2000).

OTHER HYPOLIPIDEMIC PLANTS

Emblica officinalis *Gaertn. (Family: Euphorbiaceae)*

The use of the fruits of *Emblica officinalis* (see Plate 1 in color gallery) in the treatment of acidity, gastritis, dyspepsia, and acid peptic ulcer has already been dealt with in Chapter 3, "Gastrointestinal agents." Experiments on small animals, notably rabbits, have shown that fruits of *Emblica* have a beneficial effect on cholesterol levels in atherosclerosis[1-3] in the serum, aorta, and liver.[4] Rabbits that were made hypercholesterolemic by cholesterol feeding and a fat-rich diet were then fed 5 ml·kg^{-1} body weight of fresh *Emblica officinalis* juice per day for 60 days. Serum cholesterol fell by 82 percent, triglycerides by 66 percent, phospholipids by 77 percent, and LDL levels by 90 percent. In addition, tissue lipid levels and aortic plaques showed reduction.[5] Flavonoids from *Emblica* have been shown to exert a very potent hypolipidemic and hypoglycemic effect in rats[6] by reducing synthesis and increasing the degradation of cholesterol.[7]

In an open study, supplementation of the diet of normal and hypercholesterolemic men aged 35-55 years with *Emblica officinalis* for 28 days showed that both groups of subjects showed a decrease in cholesterol levels, which rose to initial values 2 weeks after the withdrawal of supplementation.[8] Further studies need to be carried out.

See Chapter 3, "Gastrointestinal agents" for safety of *Emblica officinalis.*

NOTES

1. Mishra M, Pathak UN, Khan AB. *Emblica officinalis* Gaertn and serum cholesterol level in experimental rabbits. *Br J Exp Pathol* 62:526-528 (1981).

2. Thakur CP, Mandal K. Effect of *Emblica officinalis* on cholesterol-induced atherosclerosis in rabbits. *Indian J Med Res* 79:142-146 (1984).

3. Thakur CP, Thakur B, Singh S, Sinha PK, Sinha SK. The Ayurvedic medicines *haritaki, amala* and *bahira* reduce cholesterol-induced atherosclerosis in rabbits. *Int J Cardiol* 21:167-175 (1988).

4. Thakur CP. *Emblica officinalis* reduces serum, aortic and hepatic cholesterol in rabbits. *Experientia* 41:423-424 (1985).

5. Mathur R, Sharma A, Dixit VP, Varma M. Hypolipidemic effect of fruit juice of *Emblica officinalis* in cholesterol-fed rabbits. *J Ethnopharmacol* 50:61-68 (1996).

6. Anita L, Vijayalakshmi NR. Beneficial effects of flavonoids from *Sesamum indicum, Emblica officinalis* and *Momordica charantia. Phytother Res* 14:592-595 (2000).

7. Anila A, Vijayalakshmi NR. Flavonoids from *Emblica officinalis* and *Mangifera indica*—Effectiveness for dyslipidemia. *J Ethnopharmacol* 79:81-87 (2002).

8. Jacob A, Pandey M, Kapoor S, Saroja R. Effect of the Indian gooseberry *(amla)* on serum cholesterol levels in men aged 35-55 years. *Eur J Clin Nutr* 42:939-944 (1988).

ANTIHYPERTENSIVE PLANTS

Plants are not the first line of treatment for hypertension; however, the use of *Rauwolfia serpentina* led to the isolation of reserpine as an antihypertensive, which has now fallen into disuse because of the side effects of the molecule. Nonetheless, the search for possible herbs for treatment of hypertension continues.

Coleus forskohlii *Briq. (Family: Lamiaceae)*

Latin: *Coleus barbatus* Benth.	Hindi: Gurmal
Sanskrit: Makandi, Mayini	English: Kaffir Potato

Coleus forskohlii is a perennial herb, which is found throughout India in the plains and in the subtropical Himalayan region. Other species of *Coleus* are used in Ayurveda,[1] and there is a divided opinion on this species being mentioned in the traditional texts. The drug with the Sanskrit name *Makandi* is mentioned in various texts starting from about 1340 AD with the *Raj Nighantu* and it being equated with *Coleus forskohlii.*[2] It is used by tribals externally for skin problems, boils, eczema, cough, and as a tonic. The plant has tuberous roots that are used as a vegetable and also used medicinally. A labdane diterpene, coleonol, better known as forskolin, was isolated from the roots and shown to have antihypertensive and positive inotropic effect. Forskolin has been shown to have significant hypotensive activity in anesthetized cats and rats and also in hypertensive rats because of the relaxation of vascular smooth muscle.[3,4,5]

In an exploratory trial, 14 patients with hypertension were treated with 100-200 mg of *Coleus forskohlii* root powder taken thrice a day. Out of 14 patients, 13 responded to the treatment within 4-15 days.[6] Another pilot study revealed that using ethanolic extract of *Coleus forskohlii* in 23 patients at a dose of 165 mg extract per capsule taken thrice a day for 3 weeks brought down both systolic and diastolic blood pressure. Therefore, the group was increased and 37 patients were divided into two groups: the first group of 28 patients received 1 capsule thrice a day and the other group of 9 patients with blood pressure levels of 190 mm systolic and 100 mm diastolic received 2 capsules thrice a day for 6 weeks. The blood pressure fell continuously for 5 weeks after which no further fall was seen. There was also decrease in serum cholesterol, creatinine, and in blood urea. It was estimated that most patients required 15 mg·day^{-1} of coleonol (forskolin) to be present in the extract, although patients with higher blood pressure required 30 mg·day^{-1}. The drug was well tolerated and no major side effects were observed.[7] The results obtained warrant further studies with controls and larger patient numbers.

Coleus forskohlii roots are eaten in North India for the treatment of cough.[1] In the clinical trial using standardized extract of roots no major side effects were seen.[7]

NOTES

1. Valdés III LJ, Mislankar SG, Paul AG. *Coleus barbatus (C forskohlii)* (Lamiaceae) and the potential new drug Forskolin (Coleonol). *Econ Bot* 41:474-483 (1987).

2. Shah V. *Coleus forskohlii* (Willd.) Briq—An overview. In Handa SS, Kaul MK (eds.). *Supplement to cultivation and utilization of medicinal plants* (pp. 385-411). Jammu Tawi: Regional Research Laboratory, 1996.

3. Dubey MP, Srimal RC, Patnaik GK, Dhawan BN. Hypotensive and spasmolytic activities of coleonol, active principle of *Coleus forskohlii* Briq. *Indian J Pharmacol* 6:15-16 (1975).

4. Dubey MP, Srimal RC, Nityanand S, Dhawan BN. Pharmacological studies on coleonol, a hypotensive diterpene from *Coleus forskohlii*. *J Ethnopharmacol* 3:1-13 (1981).

5. Lidner E, Dohadwalla AN, Bhattacharya BK. Positive inotropic and blood pressure lowering activity of a diterpene derivative isolated from *Coleus forskohli: Forskolin. Arzneimittel Forschung* 28:284-289 (1978).

6. Kansal CM, Srivastava SP, Dubey CB, Tandon JS. *Nagarjun* 3:56 (1978), quoted in Dubey CB, Srimal RC, Tandon JS. Clinical evaluation of ethanolic extract of Coleus *forskohli* in hypertensive patients. *Sachitra Ayurved* 49:931-936 (1997).

7. Dubey CB, Srimal RC, Tandon JS. Clinical evaluation of ethanolic extract of Coleus *forskohli* in hypertensive patients. *Sachitra Ayurved* 49:931-936 (1997).

VENOUS DISORDERS

There are two kinds of veins that help return blood to the heart—the superficial veins, which constitute 10 percent, and deep-seated veins, which constitute 90 percent. The superficial veins have valves that if not working can lead to stagnation of blood, pain in the legs, twisted contorted veins, and edema. Inadequate return of blood is termed venous insufficiency, which can lead to varicosity of veins or varicose veins. This can stem from lack of movement either because of the sedentary nature of work involving sitting at the desk or from professions involving long hours of standing.[1]

Centella asiatica *(Linn.) Urban. (Family: Apiaceae)*

Latin: *Hydrocotyle asiatica* Linn.	Tamil: Vallarai
Sanskrit: Mandukaparni	English: Indian Pennywort
Hindi: Brahma Manduki	

Centella asiatica (see Plate 8 in color gallery) is a slender, creeping herb found in moist areas. The plant and the leaves are used medicinally for a variety of conditions. However, *Centella asiatica* is best known in India as a mental rejuvenator *(medhya rasayana)* or memory tonic for reducing mental fatigue and improving mental clarity. For details see Chapter 12, "Central nervous system agents." It has also been used extensively for improving skin conditions of varied etiology and for healing of wounds and ulcers, both internally and externally. See Chapter 9 for its effect on wound healing. It is traditionally used for improving blood circulation and reduction of edema stemming from debility.[2,3]

The major chemical constituents are the triterpenoid saponins— madecassoside and asiaticoside— and their aglycones—asiatic acid and madecassic acid. Several other saponins including brahmoside and brahminoside, triterpenoid acids, and an alkaloid hydrocotyline have been isolated.[4]

Scientific studies based on clinical and pharmacological data have shown that it is useful in venous hypertension, venous insufficiency, and in varicose veins since it is useful in lowering levels of lysosomal enzymes that are considered responsible for valvular damage.[5] The triterpene glycoside, asiaticoside, has been shown to hasten wound healing by increasing collagen I synthesis.[6] Most of the trials have been conducted with the total triterpene fraction (TTFCA) or the titrated extract of *Centella asiatica* (TECA) containing 30 percent asiatic acid, 30 percent madecassic acid, and 40 percent asiaticoside; however, a lipid preparation with *Centella asiatica* as major component has been recommended for capillary fragility.[7]

Extracts of *Centella asiatica* showed a positive effect on mucopolysaccharide metabolism when tried on patients with varicose veins. Basal levels of uronic acids and lysosomal enzymes are elevated in varicose vein patients, which indicate an increased mucopolysaccharide turnover in these patients. Treatment with 60 mg·day^{-1} for 3 months of the active triterpenic fraction led to lowering of elevated values of uronic acid and lysosomal enzymes resulting in improved vein tonicity, vein dispensability, and decrease in subjective complaints in 80 percent patients with venous insufficiency of the lower limbs.[8]

In a single-blind placebo-controlled trial, 89 patients with venous hypertension microangiopathy were treated with *Centella asiatica* extract. It was found that there was significant difference from the placebo of all the parameters tested,[9] so that it was possible to distinguish between 60 and 120 mg daily.[10] Several models have been used to test the effect of *Centella asiatica* extract at two different dosage levels against placebo in venous hypertension and are reported in the October 2001 issue of *Angiology*.[11] Symptoms of venous hypertension such as ankle edema, pain and cramps, tiredness, and restless lower extremities improved in the treated groups on 30 and 60 mg of *Centella asiatica* extract (TTFCA) thrice a day.[12]

In another study, 10 normal subjects, 22 with moderate superficial venous hypertension, and 12 with postphlebitic limbs and severe hypertension were studied first for 2 weeks without treatment and then after administering 60 mg *Centella asiatica* extract thręe times a day for 2 weeks. There was also improvement in capillary permeability in patients both with moderate superficial venous hypertension and severe venous hypertension having ankle and foot edema in the evening.[13]

In a double-blind placebo-controlled trial, 94 patients with chronic venous insufficiency were administered either 60 or 120 mg per day of *Centella asiatica* extract (TECA) for 8 weeks. There was improvement in the feeling of heaviness in the limbs, edema, and in vein dispensability in the treated group, although vein dispensability increased in the placebo group.[14]

The trials have been conducted using special extract or combinations of isolated components. It would be useful to study the effect of standardized plant material or simpler whole extracts to extend the scope of usage.

Centella asiatica is generally considered safe and has a low degree of toxicity. It is traditionally considered a vegetable and consumed as food. No adverse reactions have been reported in doses commonly used. No mortality has been reported in mice up to 5 g·kg^{-1} body weight.[15]

NOTES

1. Schlenger R. Volkskrankheit Venenleiden. Funktion und Erkrankungen des Venensystems. *Deutsche Apoth Ztg* 133:3202-3206 (1993).

2. Nadkarni AK. *Dr KM Nadkarni's Indian materia medica* (vol. I, pp. 662-666). Bombay: Popular Prakashan, 1976.

3. Gogte VM. *Ayurvedic pharmacology and therapeutic uses of medicinal plants* (pp. 466-468). Trans. SPARC, Mumbai: Bharatiya Vidya Bhavan, 2000.

4. *Indian herbal pharmacopoeia* (rev. new edn., pp.123-133). Mumbai: Indian Drug Manufacturers' Association, 2002.

5. Tyler VE. *Herbs of choice: The therapeutic use of phytomedicinals* (pp. 111-112). New York Pharmaceutical Products Press, 1994.

6. Bonte M, Dumas M, Chaudagne C, Meybeck A. Influence of asiatic acid, madecassic acid and asiaticoside on human collagen I synthesis. *Planta Medica* 60:133-135 (1994).

7. Anon. The therapeutic index. Addendum (p. 19). Madras: The Indian Medical Practioners' Co-operative Pharmacy and Stores (no year given).

8. Arpaia MR, Ferrone R, Amritano M, Nappo C, Leonardo G, del Guercio R. Effect of *Centella asiatica* extract on mucopolysaccharide metabolism in subjects with varicose veins. *Int J Clin Pharmacol Res* 10:229-233 (1990).

9. Belcaro, et al. Efficacy of Centellase in the treatment of venous hypertension evaluated by a combined microcirculatory model. *Curr Ther Res* 46:1015 (1989)

10. Incandela L, Belacaro G, De Sanctis MT, Cesarone MR, Griffin M, Ippolito E, Bucci M, Cacchio M. Total triterpenic fraction of *Centella asiatica* in the treatment of venous hypertension: A clinical prospective, randomized trial using a combined microcirculatory model. *Angiology* 52 (suppl. 2):S61-67 (2001).

11. *Angiology* 52 (suppl.) (2001).

12. Belcaro GV, Rulo A, Grimaldi R. Capillary infiltration and ankle edema in patients with venous hypertension treated with TTFCA. *Angiology* 41:12-18 (1990).

13. Belcaro GV, Grimaldi R, Guidi G. Improvement of capillary permeablility in patients with venous hypertension after treatment with TTFCA. *Angiology* 41:533-540 (1990).

14. Pointel JP, Boccalon H, Cloarec M, Ledevehat C, Joubert M. Titrated extract of *Centella asiatica* (TECA) in the treatment of venous insufficiency of the lower limbs. *Angiology* 38:46-50 (1987).

15. *Selected medicinal plants of India. A monograph on identity, safety and clinical usage* (pp. 83-86). Bombay: Chemexcil Basic Chemicals, Pharmaceuticals and Cosmetics Export Promotion Council, 1992.

Chapter 7

Urinary Tract Drugs

In Ayurveda, plants have been used to maintain the proper functioning of the kidneys and the urinary tract. The various disease conditions of the kidneys and the urinary tract described in Ayurveda have their closest equivalents in modern parlance to urinary tract infections *(mutra kricchara),* urinary stones *(asmari)* and obstructive uropathies *(mutragatha).*

DIURETICS

Diuretics remove excess water from the body by increasing urinary excretion. This is useful in conditions like high blood pressure, heart failure, glaucoma, edema, nephrotic syndrome, and liver cirrhosis.[1] *Mutra virechanya dravya* is the Ayurvedic equivalent of diuretics.[2] Over 150 plants have been reported to be diuretics.[3] Plants like *Boerhaavia diffusa* and *Tribulus terrestris* are rich in potassium. The herbal diuretics in Ayurveda are considered mild and nontoxic. However, only a few of them have been investigated to some degree and further long-term studies are required.

Boerhaavia diffusa *Linn. (Family: Nyctaginaceae)*

Latin name: *Boerhaavia repens* Linn.	Hindi: Biskhafra
Sanskrit: Punarnava English: Spreading hogweed	Tamil: Mukkarete

Boerhaavia diffusa is a spreading plant with a thick perennial root found growing throughout India up to an altitude of 2,000 m. Both the whole plant and the root have been used in medicine for a variety of conditions; however, it is most widely used in Ayurveda for treating renal and urinary problems. The tender shoots are eaten as a vegetable. The plant has traditionally been used to reduce edema associated with kidney, heart, gastrointestinal tract disorders, and general debility. In addition, it is a cardiotonic, has laxative and diuretic activity, is useful in fever, and acts as a rejuvenative or *rasayana*. It has both diuretic and anti-inflammatory properties and therefore is useful in inflammatory renal diseases.[4] The plant has an official status in the *Indian Herbal Pharmacopoeia*, 2002, as a diuretic and hepato-protective agent.[5] It has been used to treat edema and ascites resulting from early cirrhosis of the liver and in chronic peritonitis. See Chapter 4, "Hepatoprotective agents."

Boerhaavia diffusa contains an antifibrinolytic glycoside—punarnavoside, alkaloids, rotenoids (boeravinones A, B, C, D, E), lignans (liridoderdin, syringaresinol mono β-D-glucoside), flavones, ursolic acid, sterols (β-sitosterol), boeravine, β-ecdysone, hypoxanthine 9-L-arabinofuranoside, and potassium salts.[4,5]

Pharmacological studies have shown that the plant has both diuretic[6] and anti-inflammatory activities[6,7] with maximum activity being seen in samples collected during the rainy season.[4] When the various parts of the plant were tested, it was found that the extracts of leaves and roots showed significantly more anti-inflammatory and diuretic activities as compared to the whole plant.[8] In addition, the alkaloidal fraction has been shown to have immunomodulatory activity.[9] *Punarnava* has also been found useful in acute pyelonephritis in albino rats,[10] and has been found to exhibit a diuretic effect equivalent to furosemide.[11]

The initial trials were more exploratory in nature with very few patients, inadequate inclusion criteria, and lack of objective end points, which, however, served to give a clinical impression of the nature of the drug. The first trial included 5 cases of parenchymatous nephritis along with 19 cases of dropsy and jaundice, which were treated with *Boerhaavia diffusa*. It was found that the increase in urine output was accompanied by a decrease in the albumin content, and a decrease in specific gravity of the urine.[12] Clinical trials to evaluate the diuretic effect of *Boerhaavia diffusa* were also conducted in 34 patients suffering from edema and dropsy because of varied causes using liquid extracts derived from both the dry and fresh plant and found that they were equally effective in the reduction of edema.[13]

A total of 22 patients diagnosed with nephrotic syndrome were randomly allocated to one of two groups and treated with either *punarnava* crude drug—as powder or in the form of decoction— or steroids and diuretics in the control group. There were several dropouts and only 15 patients completed the trial—12 in the drug group and 3 in the control group. Of the 12 patients who completed the trial 4 patients were relieved and 7 improved, whereas 1 patient showed deterioration. In the control group, two patients were relieved, whereas one improved. It was observed that the treatment with *punarnava* induced a slow and prolonged diuresis, and patients had relief in edema and a decrease in albuminuria with increase in protein levels.[14]

In an open trial, 40 patients with nephrotic syndrome presenting edema, burning micturition, and albumin in urea were treated with three 500 mg capsules of fresh powder of *Boerhaavia diffusa* given thrice a day for 1 month. It was found that there was an increase in serum protein level and a reduction in urinary protein excretion in patients. Of the 27 patients who were severely anemic before the start of the trial 6 came into the normal range. There was a moderate decrease in blood urea and a significant reduction in serum creatinine concentration, whereas serum protein levels showed an increase. Levels of serum sodium and potassium showed only marginal changes and the final level depended on the initial values, the diet, and the primary condition of the patients. The level of immunoglobulins also tended to become normal.[11]

The aerial parts of *Boerhaavia diffusa* are eaten as a vegetable and the plant is well tolerated, although it may show a laxative effect in some patients.[15] The drug may cause vomiting in larger doses because of its emetic properties.[5,16] The acute oral toxicity of a lyophilized decoction and juice of fresh leaves showed no toxicity in mice up to 5 $g \cdot kg^{-1}$.[17] The alcoholic extract of whole plant did not show any toxicity in mice up to an oral dose of 2 g·kg^{-1}.[18] No teratogenic effect was seen in experimental animals.[19]

Further trials are needed with standardized drug, dosage studies, objective parameters, and larger patient numbers since the early studies have served to give an impression of the clinical utility of the drug.

Tribulus terrestris *Linn. (Family: Zygophyllaceae)*

Sanskrit: Gokshura	Tamil: Nerunji
Hindi: Gokhru	English: Puncture Vine, Land Calotrops

Tribulus terrestris is an annual herb found growing throughout India up to an altitude of 5,400 m. The plant has bright yellow flowers appearing after the rains, followed shortly by prickly fruits, which are medicinally important. The fruits are best known in Ayurveda for their diuretic action, and are thus considered helpful in burning micturition, chronic cystitis, and in expelling renal and urinary calculi.[20] The fruits are also used as an aphrodisiac for promoting strength and in heart problems.[21] The dried ripe fruits have the official status in the *Indian Herbal Pharmacopoeia,* 2002, as a diuretic and an antiurolithiatic agent.[22]

The fruits contain several steroidal saponins such as terrestrosins A, B, C, D, E; alkaloids; sterols such as β-sitosterol, campesterol, stigmasterol; flavonoids; cinnamic acid derivative (terrestiamide); tannins; and fixed oil. The saponins in the leaves and roots have a high hemolytic index, but are absent in the stems and seeds.[20,22]

Studies conducted in several experimental animals have shown diuretic activity.[23-25]

In an open trial, 75 patients with mild to moderate hypertension (140-179 mm Hg systolic and 90-109 mm Hg diastolic) were divided into three groups of 25 each. Two groups of 25 each, apparently under same conditions, were treated with 3 g·kg^{-1} in three divided doses of aqueous extract of *Tribulus terrestris.* Group A received the whole-plant extract, group B the fruit extract, whereas the control group of 25 patients was given a similar dose of lactose for 4 weeks.

Patients were assessed at the end of every week both for the presenting symptoms of headache, giddiness, insomnia, etc. and objective parameters such as systolic and diastolic blood pressure, and also urinary volume, pulse rate, and serum cholesterol. Both drug-treated groups showed a significant fall in both diastolic and systolic blood pressure, whereas there was no significant change in the placebo group. There was maximum improvement in headache and giddiness in group A (whole-plant extract), whereas group B (fruit extract) showed improvement in palpitation and swelling.[26]

It has been reported that the drug causes toxicity in sheep in Australia and in South Africa. It has been suggested that this is due to the presence of the alkaloids harmane and norharmane that accumulate in the body, as a result of which the animals stagger.[27] In an experiment in India in which 4 lb of fresh *Tribulus terrestris* was given to goats and sheep and 8 lbs to calves, no toxic effect was observed during the observation period of 1 month. Similarly during daily feeding of 1 kg plant juice for 8 days to calves and sheep, no toxicity was seen.[28] Some toxicity has also been reported in mice. However, it is considered a safe drug in man.[29] No side effects were reported in the trial for use as an antihypertensive.[26] In a clinical trial conducted on 406 patients using the saponin of *Tribulus terrestris* over a long period, no toxic effects were seen on blood picture, liver, and kidney.[30]

NOTES

1. BMA. *The British Medical Association illustrated medical dictionary* (p. 177). London: Dorling Kindersley, 2002.

2. Singh RG. Herbal diuretic therapy: A promise for modern physicians. *J Res Edu Indian Med* 9(2):109-112 (1990).

3. Seth UK, Sethy VH. Indigenous diuretics. In Udupa KN, Chaturvedi GN, Tripathi SN (eds.), *Advances in research in Indian medicine* (pp. 1-54). Varanasi: Banaras Hindu University, 1970.

4. *The wealth of India, raw materials* (vol. 2, pp. 174-176). New Delhi: Publications and Information Directorate, CSIR, 1988.

5. *Indian Herbal Pharmacopoeia* (rev. new edn. pp. 88-97). Mumbai: Indian Drug Manufacturer's Association, 2002.

6. Singh RH, Udupa KN. Studies on the indigenous drug *punarnava*. Part III. Experimental and pharmacological studies. *J Res Indian Med* 7(3):17-27 (1972).

7. Bhalla TN, Gupta MB, Bhargava KP. Anti-inflammatory activity of *Boerhaavia diffusa* L. *J Res Indian Med* 6(1):11-15 (1971).

8. Mudgal V. Comparative studies on the anti-inflammatory and diuretic action with different parts of the plant *Boerhaavia diffusa* Linn. *(Punarnava). J Res Indian Med* 9(2):57-59 (1974).

9. Mungantiwar AA, Nair AM, Shinde UA, Dikshit VJ, Saraf MN, Thakur VS, Sainis KB. Studies on the immunomodulatory effects of *Boerhaavia diffusa* alkaloidal fraction. *J Ethnopharmacol* 65:125-131 (1999).

10. Singh A, Singh RH, Singh RG, Misra N, Vrat S, Prakash M, Singh N. Effect of *Boerhaavia diffusa* Linn. *(Punarnava)* in acute pyelonephritis in albino rats. *Indian Drugs* 26(1):10-13 (1988).

11. Singh RP, Shukla KP, Pandey BL, Singh RG, Usha, Singh RH. Recent approach in clinical and experimental evaluation of diuretic action of *punarnava (B. diffusa)* with special reference to nephrotic syndrome. *J Res Edu Indian Med* 11(1):29-36 (1992).

12. Basu BB. Therapeutic uses of *Boerhaavia diffusa* Linn. *Indian Med Gazz* 56:308-310 (1921).

13. Chopra RN, Ghosh S, Dey P, Ghosh PN. Pharmacology and therapeutics of *Boerhaavia diffusa (Punarnava). Indian Med Gazz* 58:203-208 (1923).

14. Singh RH, Udupa KN. Studies on the Indian indigenous drug, *punarnava* (*Boerhaavia diffusa* Linn.) Part IV. Preliminary controlled clinical trial in nephrotic syndrome. *J Res Indian Med* 7(3):28-33 (1972).

15. *Selected medicinal plants of India. A monograph on identity, safety and clinical usage* (pp. 56-59). Bombay: Chemexcil. Basic Chemicals, Pharmaceuticals and Cosmetics Export Promotion Council, 1992.

16. Nadkarni AK. *Dr KM Nadkarni's Indian materia medica* (vol. 1, pp. 202-207). Bombay: Popular Praksahan, 1976.

17. Hiruma-Lima CA, Graciosa JS, Bighetti EJ, Germonśen Robineou L, Souza Brito AR. The juice of fresh leaves of *Boerhaavia diffusa* L *(Nyctaginaceae)* markedly reduces pain in mice. *J Ethnopharmacol* 71:267-274 (2000).

18. Chandan BK, Sharma AK, Anand KK. *Boerhaavia diffusa:* a study of its hepatoprotective activity. *J Ethnopharmacol* 31:299-307 (1991).

19. Singh A, Singh RG, Singh RH, Mishra N, Singh N. An experimental evaluation of possible teratogenic potential of *Boerhaavia diffusa* in albino rats. *Planta Med* 57:315-316 (1991).

20. *The wealth of India, raw materials* (vol. X, pp. 283-284). New Delhi: Publications and Information Directorate, CSIR, 1976.

21. Sivarajan VV, Balachandran I. *Ayurvedic drugs and their plant sources* (pp. 155-157). New Delhi: Oxford and IBH Publishing Co Pvt. Ltd., 1994.

22. *Indian Herbal Pharmacopoeia* (rev. new edn., pp. 459-466). Mumbai: Indian Drug Manufacturers' Association, 2002.

23. Kumari GS, Iyer GY. Preliminary studies on the diuretic effects of *Hygrophila spinosa* and *Tribulus terrestris. Indian J Med Res* 55:714-716 (1967).

24. Singh RC, Sisodia CS. Effect of *Tribulus terrestris* fruit extracts on chloride and creatinine renal clearances in dogs. *Indian J Physiol Pharmacol* 15:93-96 (1971).

25. Singh RG, Singh RP, Usha Shukla KP, Singh P. Experimental evaluation of diuretic action of herbal drug *Tribulus terrestris* Linn on albino rats. *J Res Edu Indian Med* 10(1):19-21 (1991).

26. Murthy AR, Dubey SD, Tripathi K. Anti-hypertensive effect of *Gokshura* (*Tribulus terrestris* Linn). A clinical study. *Ancient Sci Life* XIX:139-145 (2000).

27. Bourke CA, Stevens GR, Carrigan MJ. Locomotor effects in sheep of alkaloids identified in Australian *Tribulus terrestris*. *Aus Vet J* 69(7):163-165 (1992).

28. Sastry MS. Toxicity of *Tribulus terrestris* L. *Agric Res* 4(1):54 (1964).

29. *Selected medicinal plants of India. A monograph on identity, safety and clinical usage* (pp. 323-326). Bombay: Chemexcil. Basic Chemicals, Pharmaceuticals and Cosmetics Export Promotion Council, 1992.

30. Bowen W, Long'en M, Tongku L. Clinical observation on 406 cases of angina pectoris of coronary heart disease treated with saponin of *Tribulus terrestris*. *Chin J Integ Trad West Med* 10(2):85-87 (1990).

PLANTS FOR URINARY TRACT DISORDERS

Crataeva nurvala *Buch.-Ham (Family: Capparidaceae)*

Latin: *Crataeva = Crateva. Crataeva magna* (Lour) DC, *C. religiosa* var. *nurvala* (Buch.-Ham.) Hook.f. & Thom.

Sanskrit: Varuna   Hindi: Varun

Tamil: Maralingam

Crataeva nurvala (see Plate 9 in color gallery) is a deciduous tree found throughout India, well known for its handsome foliage and beautiful cream-colored flowers. The ash-gray stem bark is used in Ayurveda for treating urinary disorders both as a single drug and also in combination with other drugs. Thus, it has been used for the treatment of urinary stones, for benign prostatic hypertrophy (BPH), and for treating urinary infections. It is also used to improve appetite and is used both internally and externally to treat rheumatism. However, it is best known for its action on urinary calculi and it has an official status in the *Indian Herbal Pharmacopoeia*, 2002, as an anti-urolithiatic drug.[1]

The major constituent is the triterpene lupeol (0.6 percent), which has been shown to have antilithotriptic activity. Other constituents are the alkaloids (cadabicine, cadabicine diacetate, and cadabicine dimethyl ether), minor flavonoids [(-)-catechin, (-)-epicatechin 5-glucoside, and (-)-epiafzelechin], sterols (diosgenin, β-sitosterol, β-sitosterol acetate, lupeol acetate, α-spinosterol acetate, α-taraxasterol, 3-epilupeol, lupenone), triterpenes (betulinic acid, friedelin, varunol), flavonoids (rutin, quercetin), and the isothiocyanate glucoside—glucocapparin.[1,2]

Benign prostatic enlargement

The equivalent of benign prostatic enlargement or enlargement of the prostate gland leading to difficulty in passing urine is known as *mutragranthi* in Ayurveda (*mutra:* urine; *granthi:* knot or block). *Crataeva nurvala* is considered useful in *mutragatha* or various obstructive conditions of the urinary tract.[2]

The bladder function of ten dogs was studied using flow cystometry after treatment with *Crataeva nurvala* for 40 days, which showed a hypertonic effect against the initial values.[3] The ethanolic extract of *Crataeva nurvala* has shown anti-inflammatory activity in carrageenin-induced edema in experimental animals.[4] The petroleum ether extract of the stem bark has shown anti-inflammatory activity in acute, subacute, and chronic models of inflammation.[5] In addition, lupeol was shown to exhibit anti-inflammatory effect.[6,7]

In an open study on 30 patients with prostatic hypertrophy and resultant hypotonic bladder, 50 ml stem-bark decoction (prepared by boiling 1 part stem bark with 16 parts water, reducing to one-fourth and filtering) was given twice a day to patients and the bladder function examined using cystometric studies. It was found that patients experienced improvement in bladder tone with consequent relief in symptoms such as frequency of urination, incontinence, pain, and retention of urine. The force in expulsion of urine was also found to increase. In patients exhibiting hypotonia and atonia after prostectomy, the decoction was found to increase bladder tone, whereas improvements were also seen in neurogenic bladder. The residual volume of urine decreases significantly.[3]

In an open study with 56 patients with enlarged prostate, 50 were on drug while 6 patients and 10 healthy subjects served as control. A total of 50 patients were treated daily with freshly prepared decoction of *Crataeva nurvala* stem bark as described above, dose in Indian measures of 4-6 tolas twice a day (5 tolas = 2 fluid ozs.) for a period of 6 months. Major presenting symptoms were retention of urine, dribbling, frequent micturition and burning, and difficulty in passing urine. Most patients had mild renal insufficiency. The status of patients was evaluated after 3-4 weeks, 3 months, and 6 months of therapy. Seventy percent of patients had complete relief in symptoms at the end of 6 months, whereas the remaining patients had considerable relief. Initially 56 percent of patients showed hypotonia, 36 percent showed hypertonia, and a mere 8 percent were normotonic. However, at the end of 6 months, 75 percent of patients were normotonic with normal residual urine, whereas 25 percent were hypotonic with residual urine below 50 cc. The action of the drug was considered significant when compared to the small control group. This has been ascribed to the action on the bladder musculature and to its anti-inflammatory activity.[4]

Urinary stones

Stones in the urinary tract are termed *asmari* in Ayurveda (*asmam:* stone; *ari:* enemy; or enemy in the form of stone). There are different kinds of stones described in Ayurveda and comparison of the Ayurvedic descriptions with Western literature suggests that they correspond to differences in chemical composition.[2]

Decoction[4, 8] of *Crataeva nurvala* and extract [9,10] reduced significantly weight of stones in experimental animals. In calcium oxalate lithiasis, treatment with the decoction elevated levels of the oxalate-synthesizing liver enzyme glycolic oxidase and lowered the deposition of stone-forming constituents in the kidney. In addition, partial reversal of magnesium excretion prevented stone formation, since lower levels of magnesium tend to increase oxalate deposition.[8] The pentacyclic triterpene lupeol has been shown to possess antiurolithiatic properties in albino rats at a dose level of 50 mg·kg^{-1}. Animals treated with lupeol showed reduced tendency to form stones, and very small stones were dissolved or flushed out.[11] Lupeol (25 mg·kg^{-1} body weight) has been shown to reduce renal excretion of calcium oxalate and also to reduce renal tubular damage as seen by lowered levels of several urinary marker enzymes, which indicate renal tissue damage.[12] In addition, lupeol has antioxidant activity, which contributes to its protective action against calculosis.[13]

In an open trial, 46 patients with urinary stone were treated with 50 ml of stem-bark decoction of *Crataeva nurvala* administered twice a day for varying periods. It was found that 28 patients were spontaneously able to pass the stone in 1-47 weeks, whereas 18 patients had considerable relief in symptoms. The average time for passing the stones was 16 weeks for all except two patients who needed 36 and 47 weeks. The process of expulsion of the stone may be both due to the action of the drug in reducing the stone size and its action on the smooth muscle.[3]

A study of urinary electrolytes after 1 month of treatment with *C. nurvala* was found to alter the relative proportion of urinary electrolytes involved in calculus formation. Excretion of urinary calcium was greatly reduced, although that of sodium and magnesium was significantly increased. In addition, crystalurea was found reduced in 75 percent of patients.[3]

Another trial was carried out with 55 patients (calcium oxalate stones) in group A, 15 patients (calcium phosphate nephrolithiasis) in group B, and a control group (20 subjects). The decoction of the stem bark was given to patients for 12 weeks resulting in considerable reduction in pain (70.90 percent in group A; 73.33 percent in group B), and dysuria (63.63 percent in group A; 53.84 percent in group B), whereas some patients experienced radiological reduction in the size of stones (33.33 percent in group A; 35.72 percent in group B).[14]

Urinary infection

Urinary tract infection (UTI) is a very commonly found condition, and is generally of bacterial origin. Based on symptoms, UTI has been correlated with *mutrakrichhra vyadhi* in Ayurveda. Symptoms include discomfort associated with urination.[15]

In vitro studies showed that *Crataeva nurvala* extract showed antibacterial activity against strains causing urinary infections.[16]

In an open trial, *Crataeva nurvala* decoction was given to patients suffering from urinary tract infection for 4 weeks. There was relief in symptoms and absence of pus cells together with negative cultures in some patients; however, 68 percent continued to test positive for infection even while experiencing relief of symptoms.[3]

In a study, 84 patients with UTI were treated with stem-bark decoction of *Crataeva nurvala*. Of the 84 patients 55 percent had complete relief and 40 percent showed improvement.[17]

Thus *Crataeva nurvala* has several useful properties for urinary tract disorders combined together in one drug and deserves further studies to fully exploit its properties.

The decoction of stem and root bark are well tolerated.[18]

NOTES

1. *Indian herbal pharmacopoeia* (rev. new edn., pp. 153-160). Mumbai: Indian Drug Manufacturers' Association, 2002.

2. Prabhakar YS, Suresh Kumar D. *Crataeva nurvala:* An Ayurvedic remedy for urological disorders. *Br J Phytother* 4(3):103-109 (1997).

3. Deshpande PJ, Sahu M, Kumar P. *Crataeva nurvala* Hook and Forst. *(varuna)*—The Ayurvedic drug of choice in urinary disorders. *Indian J Med Res* 76 (suppl. December):46-53 (1982).

4. *Effects of varuna (Crataeva nurvala Buch.-Ham.) in enlarged prostate, associated urinary disorders* (pp. 37-39, 8-29). New Delhi: Central Council for Research in Ayurveda and Siddha, Ministry of Health & Family Welfare, Government of India, 1987.

5. Das PK, Rathor RS, Lal R, Tripathi RM, Biswas M. Anti-inflammatory and antiarthritic activity of *varuna*. *J Res Indian Med* 9:9-16 (1974).

6. Singh S, Bani S, Singh GB, Gupta BD, Banerjee SK, Singh B. Anti inflammatory activity of lupeol. *Fitoterapia* 68:9-16 (1997).

7. Geetha T, Varalakshmi P. Anti-inflammatory activity of lupeol and lupeol linoleate in adjuvant-induced arthritis. *Fitoterapia* LXIX:13-19 (1998).

8. Varalakshmi P, Shamila Y, Latha E. Effect of *Crataeva nurvala* in experimental urolithiasis. *J Ethnopharmacol* 28:313-321 (1990).

9. Anand R, Patnaik GK, Jain P, Kulshreshtha DK, Srimal RC, Dhawan BN. Anti-urolithiatic activity of *Crataeva nurvala* in albino rats. *Indian J Pharmacol* 22:23-24 (1990).

10. Anand R, Patnaik GK, Kulshreshtha DK, Mehrotra BN, Srimal RC, Dhawan BN. Anti-urolithiatic activity of *Crataeva nurvala* ethanolic extract on rats. *Fitoterapia* 64:345-350 (1993).

11. Anand R, Patnaik GK, Kulshreshta DK, Dhawan BN. Anti-urolithiatic activity of lupeol, the active constituent isolated from *Crataeva nurvala*. *Phytother Res* 8:417-421(1994).

12. Malini MM, Baskar R, Varalakshmi P. Effect of lupeol, a pentacyclic triterpene, on urinary enzymes in hyperoxaluric rats. *Jpn J Med Sci Biol* 48:211-220 (1995).

13. Baskar R, Meenalakshmi Malini M, Varalakshmi P, Balakrishna K, Bhima Rao R. Effect of lupeol isolated from *Crataeva nurvala* stem bark against free radical induced toxicity on experimental urolithiasis. *Fitoterapia* 67:121-125 (1996).

14. Singh RG, Usha, Kapoor S. Evaluation of the antilithic properties of *varun (Crataeva nurvala)*: An indigenous drug. *J Res Edu Indian Med* 10(2):35-39 (1991).

15. Reddy RG. Combating UTI in Ayurveda. *Express Pharma Pulse* (August 9):21 (2001).

16. Chandra S, Gupta CP. Antibacterial activity of medicinal plant *Crataeva nurvala* (bark) against bacterial strains causing urinary tract infection. *Asian J Chem* 13:1181-1186 (2001).

17. Kumar P, Singh LM, Deshpande PJ. Clinical study with *Crataeva nurvala* in urinary tract infection. *J Sci Res Plants Med* 3(2&3):75-79 (1982).

18. *Selected medicinal plants of India. A monograph on identity, safety and clinical usage* (pp. 108-111). Bombay: Chemexcil. Basic Chemicals, Pharmaceuticals and Cosmetics Export Promotion Council, 1992.

Emblica officinalis

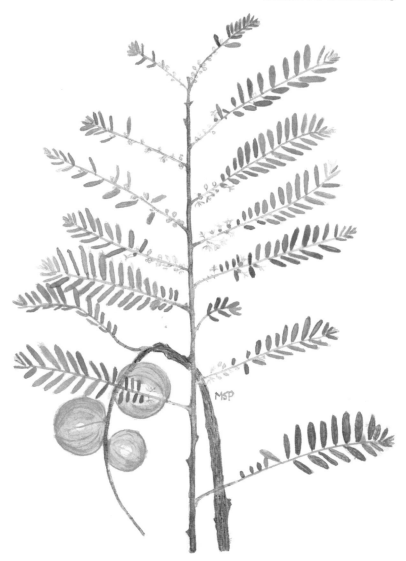

PLATE 1. Illustration of *Emblica officinalis*.

Boswellia serrata

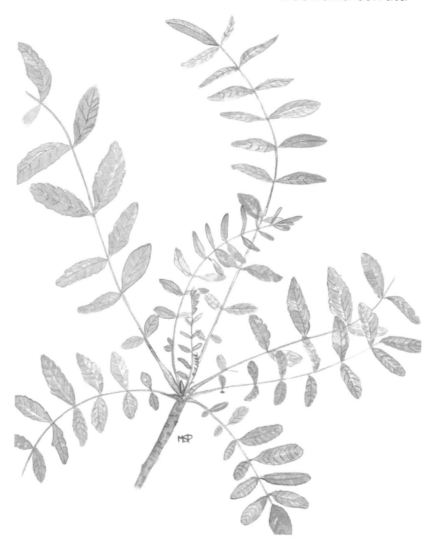

PLATE 2. Illustration of *Boswellia serrata*.

Andrographis paniculata

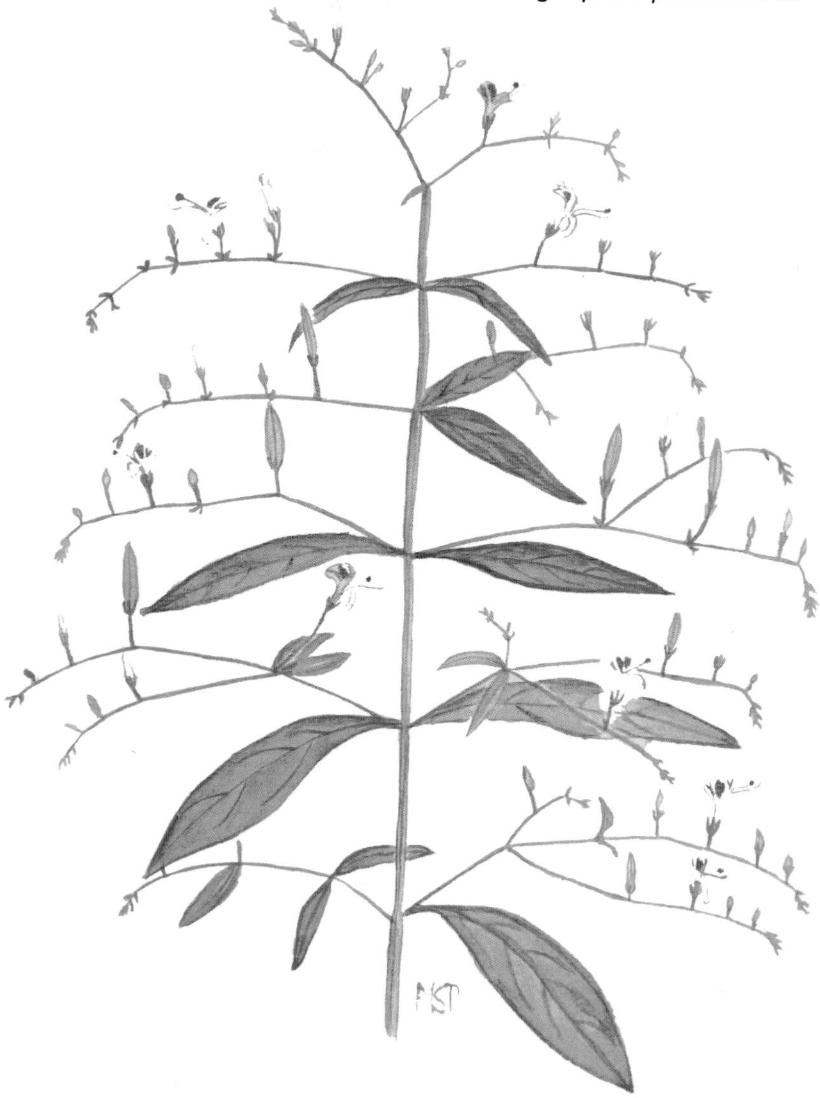

PLATE 3. Illustration of *Andrographis paniculata*.

Tinospora cordifolia

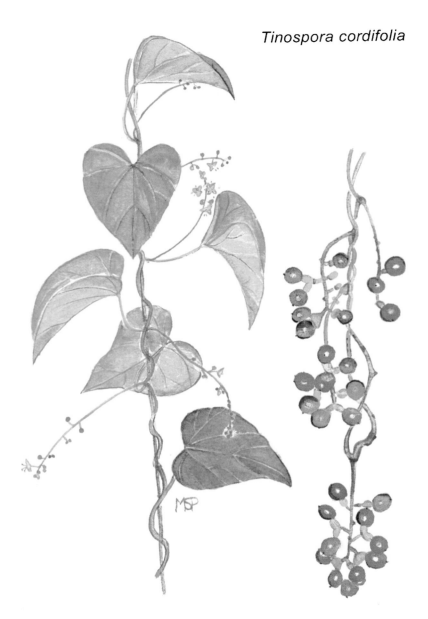

PLATE 4. Illustration of *Tinospora cordifolia*.

Phyllanthus amarus

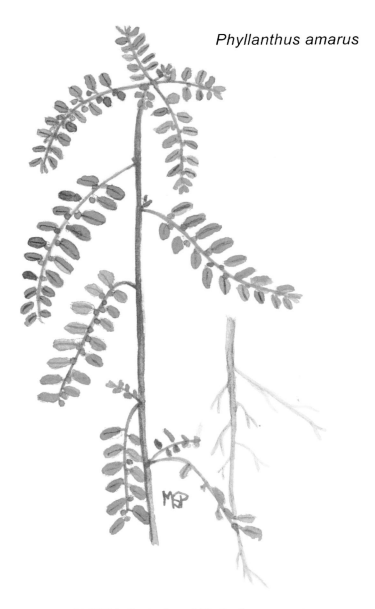

PLATE 5. Illustration of *Phyllanthus amarus*.

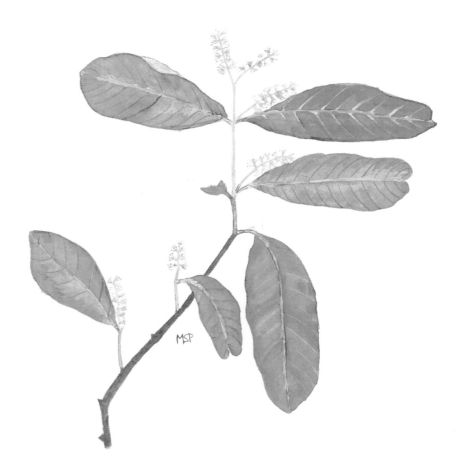

PLATE 6. Illustration of *Terminalia arjuna*.

Commiphora wightii

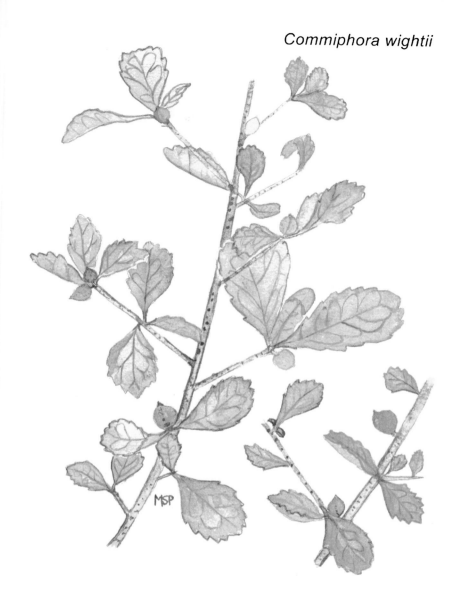

PLATE 7. Illustration of *Commiphora wightii*.

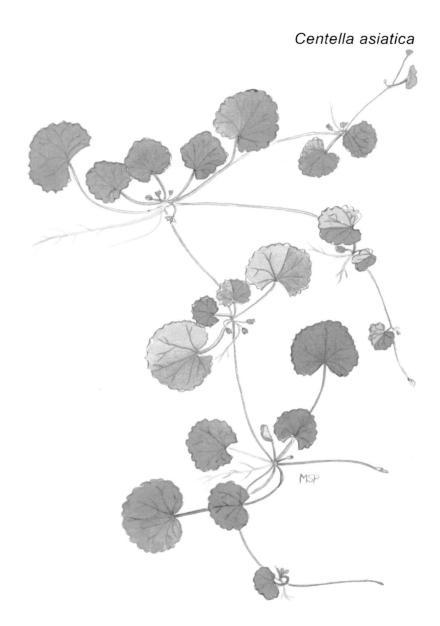

PLATE 8. Illustration of *Centella asiatica*.

Crataeva nurvala

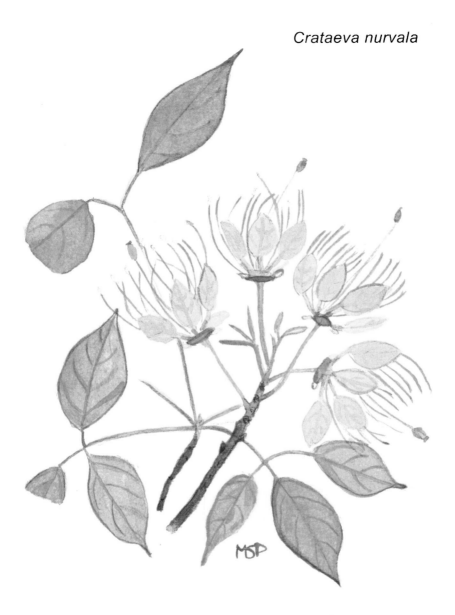

PLATE 9. Illustration of *Crataeva nurvala*.

Cissus quadrangularis

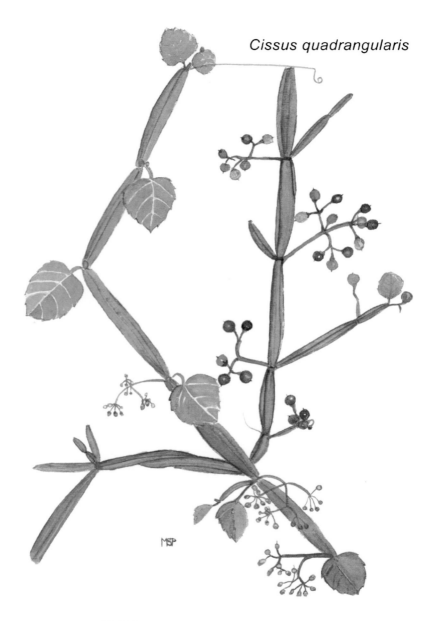

PLATE 10. Illustration of *Cissus quadrangularis*.

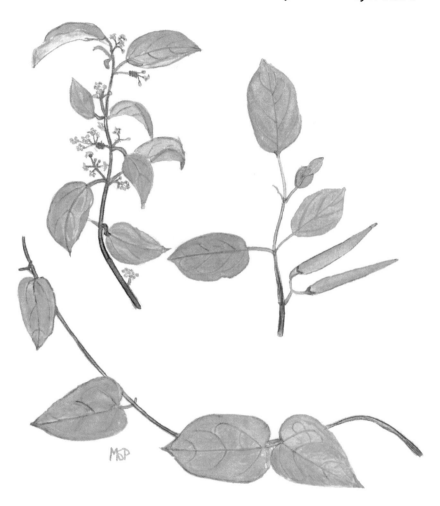

PLATE 11. Illustration of *Gymnema sylvestre*.

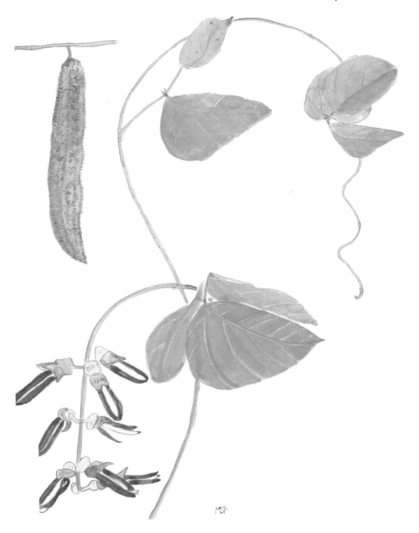

PLATE 12. Illustration of *Mucuna pruriens*.

Chapter 8

Antirheumatic Agents

Inflammatory disorders, including arthritis and rheumatism, are a major cause of suffering in the world. In Ayurveda, several plants have been used to treat inflammation, rheumatism, and arthritis. Traditionally, these are used in combination for treatment, rather than as single drugs. Pharmacological testing has been carried out, and over 69 plants have shown encouraging activity as anti-inflammatory agents, while 27 have shown definite anti-inflammatory activity. Of these, seven have been clinically studied: *Boswellia serrata, Commiphora mukul, Curcuma longa, Semecarpus anacardium, Tinospora cordifolia, Vitex negundo, Withania somnifera,* and *Zingiber officinale.*

RHEUMATOID ARTHRITIS

Inflammation of the joints, or arthritis, covers many kinds of disorders characterized by pain, swelling, and stiffness of the joints, of which the most common is rheumatoid arthritis, afflicting 2-3 percent of the population. It is a chronic disorder affecting fingers, wrists, toes, and other areas of the body. It is still not certain as what causes the disease. According to modern medicine, various factors, including infection and autoimmune disorders, are considered to play a major role in causing this disease.

In Ayurveda, poor digestion is considered the root cause of all disease. An impaired digestion leads to the formation of *ama,* which gets deposited at various locations, such as the joints, leading to pain

doi:10.1300/5683_08

and swelling of the joints. The disease entity *amavata* described by Caraka corresponds most closely to rheumatoid arthritis, and attempts have been made to verify this concept of the cause of this disease owing to faulty digestion by treating patients with digestive stimulants such as ginger, which aid digestion and absorption. See under *Zingiber officinale* in this chapter.

Boswellia serrata *Roxb. ex Coleb. (Family: Burseraceae)*

Boswellia serrata (see Plate 2 in color gallery) gum resin contains the pentacyclic triterpene acids—boswellic acids—that have been shown to be powerful inhibitors of leukotrienes, which play a major role in the cause and perseverance of inflammation in diseases such as arthritis, asthma, ulcerative colitis, Crohn's disease, etc. In addition, it also inhibits the enzyme elastase and the enzyme C-3 convertase of the complement system; these have been summarized in Chapter 3, "Gastrointestinal agents."

Details of the clinical studies were taken from abstracts, interviews, and reports of conferences, since there are few published papers. The first trials were exploratory in nature and were conducted on 20 patients,[1] and then later extended to cover a total of 175 patients[2] in the age group of 10-50 years, who had been suffering for the past 1-6 years from various musculoskeletal rheumatic disorders of moderate to severe intensity, including rheumatoid arthritis and ankylosing spondylitis, and who had earlier been treated with various antirheumatic drugs. Of the 175 patients, 122 were either bedridden or incapacitated from doing normal work and suffered from morning stiffness. These patients showed relief in presenting symptoms 2-4 weeks after starting the treatment. When 17 of these patients were put on placebo, symptoms recurred within 10 days. Out of the remaining 53 patients, 35 showed good results, whereas 18 did not show any appreciable response within a week of starting the treatment. None of the patients complained of any side effects.

In an open and double-blind cross-over study at the Government Medical College, Patiala, India, 30 patients were selected based on the criteria enumerated by the American Rheumatic Association and were treated with 200 mg of Boswellic acids thrice daily for 8 weeks.

The arthritic score—which determines the severity of rheumatic complaints—the erythrocyte sedimentation rate (ESR), and the rheumatoid factor were checked after 14 days. Supplementary analgesics such as diclofenac sodium were required for the first 2 weeks but could be stopped subsequently. There was significant improvement in morning stiffness, tenderness, and swelling of various joints and in restored function. Significant improvements were also seen in the ESR and the arthritic score. In long-term studies of more than a year, the acceptability of the drug was found to be good with no side effects seen.[3,4] Similar results were observed in 60 patients.[5]

Patients with long-standing rheumatoid arthritis showing inflammatory activity despite medication were included in two placebo-controlled studies and the results were evaluated for 81 patients: 39 on the drug and 42 on placebo. Joint swelling, joint pain, ESR, C- reactive protein as indicator of inflammation, morning stiffness, patients' estimation of pain, their general condition, as well as the use of anti-inflammatory drugs were evaluated before therapy, and after 6 and 12 weeks. There was marked improvement in all the investigated parameters in the *Boswellia* group as compared to the placebo group.[6]

In a published survey of a number of open and placebo-controlled trials in 260 patients with rheumatoid arthritis, the effect of administration of special extracts of *Boswellia serrata* H15 consisting of 400 mg tablets given as a dosage of 3 tablets twice or thrice daily was evaluated by using different approaches in the different trials. The basis for evaluation included joint swelling, pain, ESR, morning stiffness, additional anti-inflammatory drugs required, side effects and tolerance to therapy. It was found that the drug produced a significant reduction in swelling, pain, and morning stiffness. In addition, ESR was reduced and patients could reduce the intake of NSAIDS with the added advantage of improved health and well-being.[7]

In another double-blind pilot study, where 78 patients were recruited in 4 centers, the results of 37 patients available at one center has been published, which concludes that treatment with H15 did not show any measurable difference when compared with placebo, and further studies with larger patients numbers are required.[8] However, it is interesting that patients received a high dose (3,600 mg), much above that used in earlier positive trials. Further studies including dose-searching studies need to be carried out.

Information on safety on *Boswellia serrata* is covered in Chapter 3, "Gastrointestinal agents."

Commiphora wightii *(Arn.) Bhandari (Family: Burseraceae)*

Latin: *Commiphora mukul* Engl, *Balsamodendron mukul* Hook ex Stocks	
Sanskrit: *Guggul,* Devadhoopa	Hindi: Guggulu, *Guggul*
Tamil: Maishaki Gukkal	English: Indian Bdellium

Commiphora mukul (Commiphora wightii) (see Plate 7 in color gallery) is better known for its hypolipidemic effect as a result of the scientific work carried out on it, but in Ayurveda, several combination preparations of the purified gum resin of the tree with other herbs are used for the treatment of rheumatic disorders. More details regarding the plant, purification, and other aspects of its chemistry are available in Chapter 6.

A number of studies have been carried out to establish the anti-inflammatory activity of gum *guggul.* The gum resin has been shown to exhibit anti-inflammatory activity[9-11] comparable to hydrocortisone and butazolidine,[9] and partially comparable to indomethacin and dexamethasone in experimental animals, the activity being seen in the acidic fraction of the resin.[12] The steroidal component of fraction A, obtained by petroleum ether extraction of the resin, showed a pronounced antiarthritic effect, better than phenylbutazone and comparable to hydrocortisone[13] and hydrocortisoneacetate.[14] In rheumatism, produced by using killed mycobacterial adjuvant in experimental animals, *Commiphora mukul* gum fraction A was found to be as effective as phenylbutazone and ibuprofen in reducing joints swelling.[15] The aqueous extract of gum *guggul* showed significant anti-inflammatory activity reducing maximal and total edema response in carrageenan-induced rat paw edema.[16] Gum *guggul* lipid extract was evaluated in both acute and chronic models of inflammation and was found active only in Freund's adjuvant-induced model; however, the doses used, that is 250 mg·kg^{-1}, caused considerable morbidity and morality in infected animals but not in the healthy ones.[17]

Rheumatoid arthritis

Very few clinical studies have been carried out on *Commiphora mukul* as a single drug for rheumatism, and these have been of a preliminary nature. Dose-requirement studies carried out with purified *guggul,* on 35 patients suffering from rheumatoid arthritis, assessed it to be a digestive and an analgesic agent based on its antirheumatic activity and its action on the ESR. Also to be evaluated were the side effects and the potential development of drug resistance.[18]

In another open study, purified *guggul* was given to 30 patients with rheumatoid arthritis. It was found that 66.66 percent of patients showed complete remission of the disease, 23.33 percent showed major improvement, and 10 percent showed minor improvement. The impression was that the drug had anti-inflammatory and analgesic properties.[19]

The petroleum ether extract known as fraction A was tried on human beings and found to have an anti-inflammatory effect at 500 mg·kg·day^{-1}.[20] In a randomized double-blind trial with 60 patients with confirmed rheumatoid arthritis, the disease modifying potential of gum *guggul* (group A) 500 mg capsules and a proprietary preparation known as Rhumayog with gold (group B) was tried against Auranofin (group C), which has been a standard drug in the therapy of chronic polyarthritis and psoriatic polyarthritis. It was found that the disease-modifying effect was seen in both group A taking *guggul* and group C taking Auronofin with statistically significant improvement in Ritchie index, degree of morning stiffness, and platelet aggregation; however, therapy with Auronofin is accompanied by many side effects such as diarrhea, skin eruptions, kidney damage, etc., and must be constantly monitored by a doctor.[21]

Osteoarthritis

Osteoarthritis is a common disease of the weight-bearing joints. The cartilage lining the joints degenerates due to wear and tear resulting in pain, stiffness, and sometimes loss of function. In Ayurveda,

this is called *sandhigatavata*. In another trial, 30 osteoarthritis patients with a score of 2 or more on the Kellegren-Lawrence scale, for
at least one knee, were included in the trial. A dosage of 500 mg capsule of *Commiphora mukul* concentrated extract was given thrice a
day together with food for 1 month after which there was a significant
improvement in both primary and secondary outcome measures, and
there was continued improvement in the primary outcome measure at
the 2-month marker and also on further follow-up. No side effects
were observed, and it was concluded that *Commiphora mukul* was a
relatively safe drug to reduce symptoms of osteoarthritis.[22]

Spondylosis and sciatica

In open trials, the effect of purified *guggul* (4 g·day^{-1} in three divided doses) for 21 days has also been tried out in patients of cervical
spondylosis (affecting joints between vertebrae in the neck) and ankylosing spondylitis (affecting spinal vertebrae and the sacrosiliac
joints). A total of 22 patients took part in the cervical spondylosis
trial and 17 in the ankylosing spondylitis trial. The effect of purified
guggul alone was compared with the effect of a preparation of fresh
Vitex negundo leaves fried in oil and applied externally for 15 minutes,
and that of the combined effect of *guggul* and the fried-leaf preparation in a few patients in the three groups. The combination offered
greater symptomatic relief in both cervical spondylosis and ankylosing spondylitis; however, pain relief was better with *guggul*.[23,24] The
response to *guggul* was poor in patients with ankylosing spondylitis.
In patients with sciatica (pain along the sciatic nerve affecting but-
tocks and thighs, and sometimes extending down the leg and the
foot), when *guggul* was administered along with *katibasti* treatment
(soaking the area with hot oil for 15-40 minutes), it was found to be
very effective.[25]

Plant combinations

The clinical effects of combinations of *guggul* with ginger *(sunthi)*
in rheumatoid arthritis, and the clinical effects of combinations of
guggul with other herbs like *Dalbergia lanceolaria* and *Semecarpus
anacardium* in osteoarthritis, frozen shoulder, and sciatica have been

studied and found to be more effective than the individual herbs alone.[26]

Considering the importance of *Commiphora mukul* in the treatment of rheumatic disorders in Ayurveda, there is a paucity of clinical data to emphasize its importance. In addition, the age of the resin, composition of the drug, and its efficacy profile in different rheumatic conditions needs to be worked out. Further, experimental studies to find out the mechanism of action of the drug are also required.

Information on the safety of *guggul* is covered in Chapter 6, "Cardiovascular drugs."

Curcuma longa *L. (Family: Zingiberaceae)*

Latin: Curcuma domestica Valeton	Hindi: Haldi
Sanskrit: Haridra	Tamil: Manjal
English: Turmeric	

Turmeric has been used internally[27] and externally[28] for its anti-inflammatory properties since the time of Caraka and Susrutha. Turmeric has traditionally been used in India for a variety of ailments, including digestion due to its choleretic activity—see Chapter 3, "Gastrointestinal agents"—and for the management of asthma—see Chapter 5, "Respiratory tract drugs." The other important properties that have been scientifically investigated include its antioxidant, anticancer, immunostimulant, and antiviral properties. The rhizome is an official drug in the *Indian Herbal Pharmacopoeia,* 2002, for its anti-inflammatory, stomachic, and tonic properties.[29]

Other aspects of turmeric, including distribution and chemical constituents, are covered in Chapter 3, where it is first discussed. The pharmacology of turmeric has been extensively reviewed,[30-36] and turmeric has been shown to possess anti-inflammatory properties in the various models, including acute, subacute, and chronic models of inflammation. In an experimental study, examination of petroleum ether, alcoholic extract, and aqueous extract of turmeric showed that the aqueous extract was the most active when administered intraperitoneally in an acute model. The essential oil and the curcumins are considered to be among the active constituents showing anti-inflammatory activity. Administration via the intraperitoneal route produces better anti-inflammatory activity when compared to the oral administration of the crude drug powder, owing to the poor absorption of curcumin.[31] However, the serum concentration, extent of absorption, and bioavailability of curcumin can be increased severalfold by coadministration of curcumin with piperine, which is a bioavailability enhancer. Thus, in human volunteers when 2 g curcumin was coadministered with 20 mg of piperine there was a 2,000 percent increase in bioavailability of curcumin.[37]

Curcumin has been shown to inhibit a number of different molecules involved in inflammation.[36] It has been shown to inhibit prostaglandin synthesis,[38] cyclooxygenase,[39] and lipoxygenase.[40] Curcumin is also a natural inhibitor of the COX-2 enzyme. Drugs showing COX-2 inhibition are currently being advocated by pharmaceutical companies because of their relative lack of side effects on the gastrointestinal system. Curcumin has been shown to inhibit the release of both COX-1 and COX-2 enzymes; with better inhibition of the COX-2 enzyme.[41] The relatively weaker action on COX-1 reflects the better GI tolerance of curcumin.

In a randomized double-blind placebo-controlled study in dogs with osteoarthritis of the canine elbow, or hip, an extract of *Curcuma longa (domestica)* and *Curcuma xanthorrhiza* or placebo was given twice daily for 8 weeks. The test preparation was received by 25 dogs, whereas 29 received the placebo. Although there was no difference in the peak vertical force, the overall assessment of the efficacy of the investigators was statistically significant; the owner's assessment was short of statistical significance.[42]

There have been no reported trials using the whole drug. However, curcumin has been tried out in studies with small numbers of patients of rheumatoid arthritis. Considering the potential of the drug, further clinical studies are required.

In a double-blind, cross-over short-term study for 2 weeks, the antirheumatic activity of 1,200 mg·day^{-1} curcumin was evaluated against 300 mg·day^{-1} of phenylbutazone in 18 patients with rheumatoid arthritis. There was significant improvement in morning stiffness, walking time, and swelling of the joints after 2 weeks of oral curcumin therapy. Neither any side effects nor any change in grip strength, articular index, or ESR was observed in either of the two groups ascribed to the short period of administration.[43] In a continuation of the same trial, the number of patients was increased to 31 and the dose levels were increased to 1,800-2,100 $mg \cdot day^{-1}$ and given for longer periods of 5-6 weeks;[30] however, more details are not available. There was significant improvement in all patients.

Similarly, not much detail is available regarding the effect of 1,500 $mg \cdot day^{-1}$ curcumin on patients with osteoarthritis for 4-6 weeks, apart from the reported subjective improvement by the few patients on whom it was tried.[30]

In a double-blind study the effect of 400 mg of oral curcumin given thrice a day for 6 days to patients with postoperative inflammation (hernia or hydrocele) was studied along with oral antibiotic—ampicillin. Phenylbutazone 100 mg given thrice a day served as the reference drug. Parameters evaluated were spermatic cord edema and tenderness, postoperative pain, and tenderness, which were added to arrive at a total intensity scale. Curcumin was found to significantly reduce the total intensity score (2.38) as compared to placebo (1.0), which was comparable to the effect seen with phenylbutazone (1.57).[44]

Further clinical studies are needed to arrive at the utility of turmeric and curcumin in different conditions; the safety of turmeric and curcumin is covered in Chapter 3.

Semecarpus anacardium *Linn. f (Family: Anacardiaceae)*

Sanskrit: Bhallataka	English: Marking nut, Oriental cashew
Hindi: Bhilawa	Tamil: Senkottei

Semecarpus anacardium is a medium-sized, deciduous tree found throughout the hotter parts of India and in the outer Himalayas.[45] The official part of the plant is the fruit, and the fruit is a very powerful drug belonging to the group of toxic materials used in

Ayurveda. Therefore, it is used only after processing to make it suitable for consumption. After processing it is considered a rejuvenative *(rasayana)* with very powerful antiaging effects. The oil from the fruit and the juice from the bark of the tree have vesicant action said to affect sensitive people even at a distance, so that people are often afraid even to approach the tree.[46] The Sanskrit name *bhallataka* is derived from *bhalla* or spear. It is also one of the most heat-generating herbs used in Ayurveda, and therefore called *agni* or *analla,* in Sanskrit, which denotes fire. Because of this heat-producing property, there are restrictions for its use in hot weather: by pregnant women, the elderly, and the very young. Its use is also contraindicated in people of a *pitta* constitution, that is, those people who already have a lot of "heat" in their body. In addition, the drug is often administered with milk, clarified butter, or with butter products that are considered to mitigate the heating effects of the drug. Thus it is a drug that is to be taken only under supervision of a competent doctor using carefully processed, detoxified material.[47] The English name "marking nut" refers to the use of the black vesicant oil present in the fruit for marking clothes by washermen.[45] When used appropriately *bhallataka* helps in a number of disease conditions, including digestive disorders, piles, rheumatism, and cancer.

The fruits contain anacardic acid, aromatic amines, and about 32 percent of vesicant oil—the major constituent of which was termed bhilwanol and later shown to be a mixture of phenolic compounds consisting of more than seven carboxylic acids. Also present are numerous biflavonoids—including tetrahydroamentoflavone, tetrahydrorobustaflavone, and galluflavanone—and several amino acids.[45,48]

Pharmacological screening of the nut-milk extract[49,50] and the chloroform extract [51,52] have shown that they exhibit anti-inflammatory activity in a number of experimental models of inflammation. In adjuvant-induced arthritis in albino rats the milk extract was effective at a dose level of 150 mg·kg^{-1}.[50] The drug may be acting by reducing lipid peroxidation,[53] its potent antioxidant activity,[54] by stabilizing disrupted lysosomal ezymes,[55] and at the same time normalizing carbohydrate metabolism, which is affected during adjuvant arthritis.[56] In addition, aqueous extract of *Semecarpus anacardium* shows moderate analgesic effect.[57]

Rheumatoid arthritis

In a trial with 140 rheumatoid arthritis patients, 20 patients on placebo were kept as control, whereas 120 patients were given the milk decoction of *Semecarpus anacardium* nuts for 27 days. Patients were evaluated on the basis of clinical and functional improvement and ESR levels. In addition, gastrointestinal function was evaluated on the basis of D-xylose absorption tests. Sixty-five percent of patients experienced very good relief in symptoms and improvement in walking time, pressing power, grip power, etc. Improvement was also seen in ESR, hemoglobin Hb, and D-xylose. More side effects were observed in female patients than in male patients.[58] In another open trial carried out on patients with rheumatoid arthritis *(amavata)*, who were on *Semecarpus anacardium* pills, or *bhallatakavati (vati:* pills in Sanskrit), the improvement was assessed as being "spectacular."[59]

Whole *bhallataka* nuts (endocarp and pericarp) prepared with condensed milk solids *(khoya)* and sugar were given twice a day in 5-10 g doses (10 g equivalent to 1 nut) to 25 patients with rheumatoid arthritis. Forty percent of patients showed complete remission, while 40 percent showed major improvement, and 20 percent were assessed as showing minor improvement based on the criteria enumerated by the American Rheumatic Association. Improvement was seen in body ache, general malaise, and debility; improvement in appetite, food consumption, and in hemoglobin values; in ESR values in various functional tests like walking time, dressing time, articular strength, grip power, etc.[60]

In another trial, the effect of *Semecarpus anacardium* nut-milk extract was evaluated on the basis of its effect on lysosomal enzymes, which are elevated in patients with rheumatoid arthritis. Treatment showed a decrease in the lysosomal enzymes leading the authors to conclude that the milk extract was a promising drug for rheumatoid arthritis. No side effects were observed and the drug was well tolerated. One patient had urticaria, which disappeared on reduction of the dose from 5 g to 2.5 g.[61]

In a placebo-controlled study, 40 patients were enrolled in the trial: 30 in the drug group and 10 in the placebo group. The drug consisted of 3-5 g of *amrit bhallataka* twice daily with milk together with

500 mg of *Boswellia serrata (sallaki)* gum in capsules taken thrice daily for 10 weeks. It was found that 60 percent of patients receiving the drug showed very good change in laboratory findings and in clinical improvement, with eight patients showing normal improvement and four patients showing no improvement. Unfortunately, no other details are available since the trial was reported as an abstract.[62]

A three-drug combination of *Semecarpus anacardium (bhallatak), Dalbergia lanceolaria (gourakh),* and *Commiphora mukul (guggulu)* has already been covered under *Commiphora mukul* earlier in this chapter. This combination has been shown to be better than the individual herbs for rheumatoid arthritis, sciatica, frozen shoulder, and osteoarthritis.

Sciatica

In an open trial, 42 patients with sciatica *(gridhrasi)* were given *Naimittika rasayana* containing purified *bhallataka* in dosages of 100 mg to 1,000 mg twice a day. The *Naimittika rasayana* regimen consists of increasing the dosage every day by 100 mg starting from 100 mg and going up to 1,000 mg after which it is again reduced to 100 mg for 2-12 weeks with milk and ghee. Twenty-five patients were completely relieved of their complaints, although 12 patients experienced partial relief. Also observed was an overall improvement in their physical condition. Side effects were observed in five patients when the dosage was increased to more than 500 mg.[63]

In a dose-searching study conducted with purified *Semecarpus anacardium (bhallataka),* good results were obtained at the 4 g·day^{-1} dosage, which was judged to be the optimum dosage for treatment of sciatica.[64]

As mentioned earlier in the opening paragraph, the drug is toxic before processing, but after suitable treatment it is considered nontoxic. There is an irritant oil in the pulp of the fruit that needs to be removed or modified.[46] Thus, a chloroform extract of the nuts of *Semecarpus anacardium* was toxic at all dose levels tested (50-400 mg·day^{-1}).[65] However, a milk extract of the nuts did not show any acute toxicity (72 hours) at the levels tested (75-2,000 mg·day^{-1}). In the subacute toxicity (30 days) no marked alteration was observed in blood and biochemical values at 50-500 mg·day^{-1} body weight.

However, at 500 mg·day[-1] there was an increase in blood glucose, serum creatinine, uric acid, and blood urea. In addition, changes in lipid profile were observed owing to the fact that clarified butter (ghee) is used as the base. Vital organs showed normal architecture.[66] The clinical toxicity of the nuts studied in 266 patients showed no toxicity or side effects.[67] In a trial on the role of *Semecarpus anacardium* on the management of rheumatoid arthritis, side effects such as urticarial rashes, mucosal irritation, and bleeding were seen. The patients in this trial were carefully monitored and the drug withdrawn, if needed.[58] In another trial, the drug prepared by boiling first in water then adding the solidified milk known as *khoya,* prepared by boiling off the water, was well tolerated, with only one patient developing urticaria, which disappeared at half dose and the drug was well tolerated.[60]

Tinospora cordifolia *(Willd.) Miers ex Hook f. & Thoms. (Family: Menispermaceae)*

Tinospora cordifolia (see Plate 4 in color gallery) is a climber found throughout India growing on trees and shrubs. The stem and the aerial roots are generally used fresh. Other aspects of the plant are covered in Chapter 4, "Hepatoprotective agents" where the herb is first described. It is one of ten plants commonly used in preparations for the treatment of joint diseases.[68,69] The stem is an official drug in the *Indian Herbal Pharmacopoeia,* 2002, as an analgesic and an antipyretic agent.[70]

Experimental studies on small animals have demonstrated the anti-inflammatory effects of the aqueous extract of *Tinospora cordifolia* in acute and chronic inflammation.[71-74] In experimental adjuvant–induced arthritis it inhibited both phase I and II.[73] The aqueous extract at 1 g·kg[-1] showed maximum anti-inflammatory effect in cotton pellet granuloma and formalin-induced arthritis.[74,75]

In an open trial, 50 patients with various joints problems diagnosed according to Ayurveda as *amavata* (usually equated as rheumatoid arthritis in modern parlance) and *sandhigatavata* (usually equated as osteoarthritis in modern parlance), degenerative arthritis, senile arthritis, and psoriatic arthritis were treated with capsules containing 480 mg of a dried aqueous extract of *Tinospora cordifolia.*

The results were assessed in 24 patients as showing complete relief, 16 with partial relief, and 10 patients with no relief at all. Good improvement was seen within 10 days of starting the treatment in 72 percent of cases with the drug being well tolerated. In addition, many patients obtained relief from constipation.[69]

Other trials with *Tinospora cordifolia* on patients with rheumatoid arthritis have been reported either as a single drug[76] or in combination with ginger,[77] which is covered under the section on ginger.

The safety of *Tinospora cordifolia* is covered in Chapter 4, "Hepatoprotective agents."

Vitex negundo *Linn. (Family: Verbenaceae)*

Sanskrit: Nirgundi, Sinduwar	Tamil: Nochi
Hindi: Sambhalu	English: Five-leaved chaste tree

Vitex negundo is a large aromatic shrub commonly found growing in many parts of India.[78] The Sanskrit name *nirgundi* implies that it works against a number of ailments (*nir:* no; *gunda/gundi:* notorious). There are two varieties available in India that differ in the color of the stems—white *(Vitex negundo* var. *negundo)*, because it is covered with white hair, and purple *(Vitex negundo* var. *purpurescens);* however, it is not clear from published literature which variety has been used in studies. Although all parts of the plant are used, the leaf and root are commonly used in medicine; however, the leaf is used widely. The leaves are used both internally and externally to treat joints swellings and pains, rheumatism, fever, cough, and sinus problems.[79]

The leaves contain approximately 0.04-0.07 percent of an essential oil containing several terpenes (with β-caryophyllene as the major constituent), flavonoids (casticin, orientin, isoorientin, luteolin, luteolin-7-O-glucoside, corymbosin, gardenins A and B, etc.), flavanones, several iridoid glycosides (aucubin, agnuside, nishindaside, negundoside, 6'-p-hydroxybenzoyl-mussaenosidic acid), alkaloids (nishindine and hydrocotylene),[78,80] betulinic acid, and ursolic acid.[81]

The leaf and leaf extracts (petroleum ether, methanol, aqueous methanol, and water) also showed significant analgesic activity.[82-86]

The leaves have been shown to have anti-inflammatory activity in a number of experimental models.[83,86-88] The leaves have also been shown to have antiarthritic activity in rats.[89]

The anti-inflammatory effect of *Vitex negundo* leaves is considered to be mediated through histamine and 5-hydroxytrytamine (5-HT) both in the initial phase and in the delayed phase.[90] In addition, it has been suggested that the anti-inflammatory and analgesic effects may be due to the inhibition of prostaglandin synthesis,[83,86] membrane stabilizing, and antioxidant activity.[86]

In an open trial, 50 cases with rheumatoid arthritis were treated with *Vitex negundo* and found to show encouraging results.[91] In another open trial on 30 patients with deranged *"vata"* described as *"vatavyadhis"* (problems with motion), which could be loosely considered to be rheumatism, 10 patients had rheumatoid arthritis *(amavata)*, whereas 10 patients had osteoarthritis *(sandhigatavata)* and were treated with 1 g *Vitex negundo* leaf powder taken orally twice a day, while an oil extract of the leaves—prepared by boiling a decoction of the leaves in sesame oil till the water evaporated—was used to massage the affected areas. Five patients in each group with rheumatoid arthritis and osteoarthritis received *Commiphora mukul* orally and served as control. Patients had the disease for periods ranging from 1 to 10 years. Of the ten patients on *Vitex* with rheumatoid arthritis, four patients showed improvement ranging from 25 to 50 percent based on clinical parameters, lowering of leukocytosis and improvement in ESR values after 3 months, whereas no improvement was seen in the remaining six cases even after 6 months, and the medication was changed to *Commiphora mukul.* In the control group all the five patients showed improvement, two cases recovering fully, one with 75 percent improvement, another with 50 percent, and the remaining patient dropping out due to loose motions as a result of *guggul* treatment. In the group with *sandigata vata* (osteoarthritis) all the ten patients using *Vitex* showed improvement based on lessening of pain, decrease in swelling, and clinical improvement. No side effects were observed. In two cases that were followed using X-ray, there was no radiological improvement. In the *gugggul* group improvement was not as good as the trial group.[92] Thus *Vitex negundo* was found more effective in noninflammatory cases, such as osteoarthritis *(sandhigata vata),* whereas *Commiphora mukul* worked better in patients with rheumatoid arthritis *(amavata).* In addition, *Vitex negundo* was considered useful in cases where *Commiphora mukul* caused gastric irritation and diarrhea.[92]

However, the numbers in both arms are small and the patient population appears to have been nonhomogenous. Further trials are warranted with larger patient numbers and standardized plant material considering the promising nature of the results.

Sciatica

In a trial of 20 patients with sciatica, 10 patients were treated with *sodhana,* which includes certain Ayurvedic "purificatory" procedures for detoxification and *samana* (drug treatment), and 10 patients were treated with *Vitex negundo* and *Commiphora mukul* (*samana* alone). In group I, 60 percent of patients had complete relief and 40 percent had marked relief; however, in group II, 40 percent had complete relief, 40 percent had marked relief, and 20 percent had mild relief.[93]

The combination of *guggul* and *Vitex negundo* has been tried out both in ankylosing spondylitis and in cervical spondylosis; see *Commiphora mukul* earlier in this chapter. Another combination *rasonadi kwath* using garlic, ginger, and *nirgundi (Vitex negundo)* in rheumatoid arthritis has been tried out.[94] Fifty patients were included in the trial based on the American Rheumatic Association 1959 guidelines. A decoction made from equal parts of dried ginger, garlic, and *Vitex negundo* was given daily at a dose of 25 ml thrice daily for 6 weeks. The daily dosage corresponded to 25 g each of the three ingredients. Initially, acute pain was controlled both by oral Ayurvedic medication and external application as required. Results were assessed based on pain relief, diminishing of swelling and tenderness, and increase in freedom of movement of joints, functional tests, and ESR. There was significant relief in swelling and pain in the joints in 2-3 weeks. Improvement in functional tests and ESR was also seen. Most patients were assessed as having "complete relief" or "partial relief." Patients having the disease for a shorter time had greater relief.[94]

The leaves are well tolerated in clinical dosages.[95] In an experimental study using fresh mature leaves of *Vitex negundo,* no acute toxicity or stress was found up to 5 g·day^{-1} body weight.[86]

Withania somnifera *Dunal. (Family: Solanaceae)*

Sanskrit: Ashwagandha	English: Winter Cherry
Hindi: Asgandh	Tamil: Ammukara

Withania somnifera is an erect shrub found growing wild through-out the hotter parts of India and cultivated for its roots, which are well known in Ayurveda for their rejuvenative or *rasayana* properties. The roots are considered to have the smell of a horse, as the Sanskrit name *ashwagandha* denotes (*ashwa:* horse; *gandha:* smell), and are said to confer upon the person consuming them the strength and vitality of a horse. The roots are thus used in debility and convalescence—by sportspeople to increase endurance; in cough and sore throat; for re-ducing glandular swellings; as a sedative—for insomnia; and in rheu-matism and gout.[96] *Ashwagandha* is commonly referred to as "Indian Ginseng" because of its beneficial properties. The root has an official status as an adaptogen in the *Indian Herbal Pharmacopoeia, 2002.*[97]

The roots contain 0.2-0.3 percent of alkaloids and withaferin A to-gether with several withanolides, which are C-28 steroidal lactones of the ergostane type.[97,98] In addition, the roots contain starch, reduc-ing sugars, hentriacontane, and a number of amino acids.[98] Also pres-ent are sitoindosides VII and VIII, which are acylsterylglucosides and sitoindosides IX and X, which are C-27 glycowithanolides that may contribute to the adaptogenic property displayed by *Withania somnifera.*[99]

Withania somnifera root powder,[100] root methanol extract,[101] and its active principles—a mixture containing equimolar concentrations of withaferin A and sitoindosides VII-X[102]—were shown to possess an-tioxidant activity, which may explain the antistress, anti-inflamma-tory, immunomodulatory, and cognition-enhancing and rejuvenative effects shown in experimental and clinical studies. Withaferin A has been shown to have anti-inflammatory and antiarthritic property in several experimental models.[103]

The roots of *Withania somnifera* have been shown to possess anti-inflammatory activity in acute, subacute, and chronic models of in-flammation. In experimental animals, the powdered root showed considerable anti-inflammatory activity, although less than phenyl butazone at 1 g·kg^{-1} body weight, while showing greater effect on acute phase reactants,[104] which are released into the blood during the acute phase of inflammation. NSAIDS have only a poor control of acute phase reactants in contrast to steroidal anti-inflammatory drugs. *Ashwagandha* in doses of 100 mg·100g^{-1} body weight of rat showed a 32 percent reduction of paw volume as against 46 percent shown by phenyl butazone. In addition, *ashwagandha* influences most of the acute phase reactants in a very short time.[104] It has, especially, a good lowering effect on alpha-2 macroglobulin, an acute phase reactant, which is considered a sensitive index of the efficacy of anti-inflammatory drugs.[105] At a dose of 1 g·kg^{-1} it produced significant anti-inflammatory effect in cotton pellet granuloma in rats.[106] When tested for its long-term effect on adjuvant-induced arthritis in rats, it was found to exert a beneficial effect on swelling, and also prevented weight loss and degenerative changes seen in the bones in long-standing arthritis.[107]

In carrageenin-induced paw edema,[108] the aqueous extract of *Withania somnifera* acts as an anti-inflammatory by blocking histamine H$_1$ and H$_2$, and 5-hydroxytryptamine receptors in the early phase and prostaglandin synthesis in the delayed phase of inflammation. However, in cotton pellet granuloma, the anti-inflammatory activity of *Withania somnifera* is mediated by blocking the H$_2$ receptors.[106]

In an open, exploratory trial with 63 patients with various arthropathies, 46 patients with rheumatoid arthritis were given 4, 6, or 9 g of *Withania somnifera* root powder orally for a period of 3-4 weeks. It was found that pain and swelling disappeared in 12 patients; there was considerable improvement in 10; mild improvement in 11; 4 patients had no relief; and there were 7 dropouts.[109]

In another open trial, 77 patients with rheumatoid arthritis *(amavata)* were treated with 3 g of *Withania somnifera* root powder thrice a day with milk for 6 weeks. The results were evaluated as "good" in 22 percent, "fair" in 53 percent, "poor" in 22 percent, whereas 3 percent did not respond. It was observed that patients who had the disease for less than a year responded better to the treatment.[110]

In a comparative randomized trial using three different treatment options, 120 patients with rheumatoid arthritis were assigned randomly to receive *Cyperus rotundus (musta)* powder, *Withania somnifera (ashwagandha)* powder, or *Panchakarma* treatment consisting of various treatment modalities (such as vomiting, two forms of enema or bloodletting and enema, purgation, and nasal application of medicine) for detoxification. All three arms gave highly significant results ($p < 0.001$); however, maximum improvement was seen in the *Panchakarma* group.[111]

In a preliminary open trial, 25 patients with radiologically confirmed cervical spondylosis were administered 4 g of *Withania somnifera* powder along with 100 ml of decoction from *Smilax china* given thrice a day for 30 days. The results were compared with brufen—an allopathic NSAID.[112]

In clinical trials for arthritis, using up to 6 g of *Withania somnifera* root powder for 3-4 weeks was well tolerated.[109] In a long-term trial on healthy volunteers in the age group of 50-59 years to study its tonic antiaging effect, 3 g of the root powder in three divided doses for 1 year showed no untoward side effects, and there was an increase in hemoglobin levels in the subjects.[113] Acute toxicity and a 4-week subacute study with aqueous extract of *Withania somnifera* in doses from 50 mg to 1 $g \cdot kg^{-1}$ showed no toxic effects. There was no hepatic or renal toxicity.[114] Also chronic feeding of *Ashwagandha* at 100 $mg \cdot kg^{-1}$ for 180 days did not show any toxicity or significant changes in the biochemical profile of blood; [115] the safety data on *Withania somnifera* has been summarized.[116]

Zingiber officinale *Roscoe (Family: Zingiberaceae)*

Ginger is a widely used traditional medicine for a variety of ailments, including its use for specific action in rheumatism and inflammation. Other aspects of the rhizome and its pungent principles have been covered in greater detail in Chapter 3, "Gastrointestinal agents," where it first appears in this book. According to Ayurveda, impaired digestion is a major cause of all diseases, and ginger is considered to act on all the three phases of digestion—digestion, absorption, and elimination, and therefore help in ameliorating various problems. In Chapter 3, the use of ginger in relieving malabsorption—a contributory factor in the causation of inflammatory disorders, such as rheumatoid arthritis—has been described. Ginger is an official drug in the *Indian Herbal Pharmacopoeia,* 2002, for its carminative, antiemetic, and anti-inflammatory properties.[117]

Ginger exhibits an anti-inflammatory effect in carrageenan-induced paw edema[118-121] and in cotton pellet–induced granuloma in rats.[120] Ginger oil has been shown to exhibit anti-inflammatory activity inhibiting chronic adjuvant arthritis in rats.[122] More specifically, the gingerols and shoagols are among the active constituents of ginger.[123] 6-Gingerol and four other compounds, namely, [6]- and [10]-dehydrogingerdione, and [6]- and [10]-gingerdiones, were found to be potent inhibitors of prostaglandin biosynthesis.[124] Ginger and its various pungent constituents behave as dual inhibitors of the arachidonic acid pathway, inhibiting both cyclooxgenase [125,126] and lipoxygenase.[125,127,128] Of special interest is the inhibition of COX-2.[126] In addition, ginger extract[129] and gingerol[130] inhibit platelet aggregation, thromboxane synthase, and the incorporation of arachidonic acid into thrombocytes. [6]- Gingerol has also been shown to be a potent inhibitor of NO-synthesis, and is effective in protecting against peroxynitrite-induced damage.[131]

One of the first studies using ginger was reported in 1977.[132] In an open study, seven patients with rheumatic disorders given ginger found relief in pain and associated symptoms.[133] In a larger group of 56 patients, 28 with rheumatoid arthritis, 18 with osteoarthritis, and 10 with muscular discomfort, were treated with powdered ginger. Of these, 75 percent of arthritis patients found relief in pain and swelling. All patients with muscular discomfort had relief from pain. No side effects were reported during ginger administration in periods ranging from 3 months to 2.5 years.[134]

A number of combinations of ginger with other drugs have been reported to study the effect of gastrointestinal stimulant drugs for the treatment of rheumatoid arthritis. Thus, four groups with three combination drugs were tried out. In group 1, ginger was combined with *Tinospora cordifolia,* in group 2 and in group 4 ginger was combined with *Commiphora mukul,* whereas in group 3 a decoction of the three plants of ginger, *Vitex negundo,* and *rasna* (Botanical name not mentioned) was tried out. In order to estimate the comparative efficacy of the drugs they were compared against standard Ayurvedic drugs that are traditional multiplant preparations commonly used in the treatment of rheumatism—*Yogaraja guggulu, Vatagajankusha Rasa/Amavatari Rasa,* and *Maharasnadi Kwatha.* Patients were selected on the basis of the 1959 criteria of the American Rheumatic Association.

In the first trial, 77 patients were enrolled and given 25-50 ml of a decoction of *Zingiber officinale (sunthi)* and *Tinospora cordifolia (guduchi)* thrice a day or given the traditional formulations—*Yogaraj guggulu, Vatagajankusa rasa,* and *Maharasanadi kwatha.* There was slow improvement in the major presenting features (pain, swelling, and restriction in movement). The results from the *sunthi-guduchi* group were assessed to be better because more patients experienced partial relief, fewer patients had no relief, and there were fewer dropouts. The ESR showed significant decrease in the *sunthi-guduchi* group coming within normal limits at the end of the treatment period.[135,136]

The second combination of ginger with *Commiphora mukul (guggul)* was tried out first in an open comparative format with 63 patients, of which 36 patients received 2 g of *sunthi-guggul* (1 g each of powdered rhizome of *Zingiber officinale* and purified resin of *Commiphora mukul*) thrice a day for 6 weeks, whereas the second group received the traditional combination of 1 g *Yogaraja guggulu,* 0.5 g *Amavatari Rasa,* and 25 ml *Maharasnadi Kwatha* thrice a day. Inclusion parameters were evolved based on the 1959 criteria of the American Rheumatic Association. These were morning stiffness, pain while passing motion, tenderness, swelling in one or more joints, and symmetrical joint involvement. Apart from clinical assessment, ESR levels were also monitored. The improvement in the *sunthi-guggulu* group was assessed as being "remarkable" and the number of patients obtaining complete relief and partial relief was more than the patients in the standard treatment group. However, the majority of patients had the disease for less than 1 year.[135,137]

Based on the good results obtained with the combination of *sunthi-guggulu,* another trial with 75 patients was carried out for 6 weeks with the drug along with external treatment. All patients who completed the trial showed definite improvement although the number of patients who obtained complete relief was small; partial relief was obtained by more than 50 percent of patients. It was observed that male patients and those with a shorter duration of the disease showed better results.[137,138]

The third group of 50 patients was treated for 6 weeks with 25 ml decoction of the combination containing *rasna* (Botanical name not mentioned), *sunthi (Zingiber officinale)*, and *nirgundi (Vitex negundo)* taken thrice daily. Complete relief was experienced by 28 percent of the patients, whereas 46 percent had partial relief. It was observed that female patients had better relief; however, the patient number is perhaps too small to make definite conclusions and this observation needs to be confirmed.[135] The drug *rasna* has not been botanically identified in the paper by the Latin name, which is unfortunate considering the fact that *rasna* is one of the so-called controversial drugs of Ayurveda where the identity of the plant is disputed and more than one plant is considered to be the genuine source of the drug.

In a recent, randomized, double-blind, placebo-controlled, multicentric, parallel group study, the efficacy and safety of *Zingiber officinale* with *Alpinia galanga* was evaluated in 261 patients with moderate-to-severe knee pain because of osteoarthritis. The drug was a standardized and highly concentrated extract containing the two species. The primary efficacy criterion was a reduction in knee pain on standing. There was statistically significant reduction in symptoms of osteoarthritis of the knee (63 percent responders in the ginger group versus 50 percent in the placebo group). Patients receiving the ginger extract experienced more gastrointestinal side effects than the placebo group (59 versus 21).[139]

The safety of ginger is covered in Chapter 3, "Gastrointestinal agents." In a trial using ginger in 56 patients for periods ranging from 3 months to 2.5 years no side effects were experienced.[134]

Further clinical trials are needed to establish the efficacy in larger patient numbers, especially for the two combination preparations of ginger with *Tinospora cordifolia* and with *Commiphora mukul,* which appear to offer advantages over monotherapy.

NOTES

1. Pachnanda VK, Kant S, Singh D, Singh GB, Gupta OP, Atal CK. Clinical evaluation of *Salai guggal* in patients of arthritis. *Indian J Pharm* 13:63 (1981).

2. Gupta VN, Yadav DS, Jain MP, Atal CK. Chemistry and pharmacology of gum resin of *Boswellia serrata (salai guggal). Indian Drugs* 24 (5):1-6 (1987) and references cited therein.

3. Ammon S. Indischer Weihrauch: Ein pflanzliches Antirheumatikum. *Deutsche Apoth Ztg* 131:972-974 (1991).

4. Weihrauch—ein neuer Weg in der Therapie von Entzündungen? An interview with Prof HPT Ammon. *Deutsche Apoth Ztg* 132:2442-2444 (1992).

5. Singh GB, Singh S, Bani S, Kaul A. Boswellic acids—A new class of anti-inflammatory drugs with a novel mode of action (pp. 81-82). Calcutta: International Seminar on Traditional Medicine, November 7-9, 1992.

6. Von Keudell C. Therapie mit Boswellinsäuren (Weihrauch)—eine Ergänzung oder sogar Alternative in der Therapie autoaggressiver Erkrankungen? *Bauchredner DCCV- Journal* (2):20-28 (1995).

7. Etzel R. Special extract of *Boswellia serrata* (H15) in the treatment of rheumatoid arthritis. *Phytomedicine* 3:91-94 (1996).

8. Sander O, Herborn G, Rau R. Is H15 (resin extract of *Boswellia serrata*, "incense") a useful supplement to established drug therapy of chronic polyarthritis? Results of a double-blind pilot study. *Z Rheumatol* 57:11-16 (1998).

9. Gujral ML, Sareen K, Tangri KK, Amma MKP, Roy AK. Anti-arthritic and anti-inflammatory activity of gum *guggul* (*Balsomodendron mukul* Hook.). *Indian J Physiol Pharmacol* 4:267-273 (1960).

10. Satyavati GV, Raghunathan K, Prasad DN, Rathor RS. *Commiphora mukul* Engl. and *Tinospora cordifolia* Willd. A study of the anti-inflammatory activity. *Rheumatism* 4:141 (1969).

11. Gulati OD, Parikh HM, Panchal DI, Karbhari SS. Anti-inflammatory activity of *guggul (Balsamodendron mukul)* in white rats. *Rheumatism* 8(3):83-89 (1973).

12. Shanthakumari G, Gujral ML, Sareen K. Further studies on the anti arthritic and anti-inflammatory activities of gum *guggul*. *Indian J Physiol Pharmacol*. 8 (2):36-37 (1964).

13. Sharma JN, Jain SC. Antiarthritic activity of a newly isolated steroidal component from fraction of *Commiphora mukul* in the adjuvant arthritis in rabbits. *Indian J Pharmacol* 10(1):87 (1978).

14. Arora RB, Taneja V, Sharma RC, Gupta SK. Anti-inflammatory studies on a crystalline steroid isolated from *Commiphora mukul*. *Indian J Med Res* 60:929-931 (1972).

15. Sharma JN, Sharma JN. Comparison of the anti-inflammatory activity of *Commiphora mukul* (an indigenous drug) with those of phenylbutazone and ibuprofen in experimental arthritis induced by mycobacterial adjuvant. *Arzneimitellforschung* 27:1455-1457 (1977).

16. Duwiejua M, Zeitlin IJ, Waterman PG, Chapman J, Mhango GJ, Provan GJ. Anti-inflammatory activity of resins from some species of the plant family Burseraceae. *Planta Med* 59:12-16 (1993).

17. Dahanukar S, Sharma S, Karandikar SM. Evaluation of anti-inflammatory potentials of *guggul*. *Indian Drugs* 20 (10):405-408 (1983).

18. Vyas SN, Shukla CP. A clinical study on the effect of *Shuddha guggulu* in rheumatoid arthritis. *Rheumatism* 23(1):15-26 (1987).

19. Pandit MM, Shukla CP. Study of *shuddha guggulu* on rheumatoid arthritis. *Rheumatism* 16(2):54-67 (1981).

20. Arora RB, Sharma JN, Sharma JN, Shastri HD. Beneficial effect of fraction A of gum *guggul* in arthritic syndrome and liver function in clinical and experimental arthritis. *Rheumatism* 18(1):9-16 (1982).

21. Chandrasekharan AN, Porkodi R, Madhavan R, Parthiban M, Bhatt NS. Study of Ayurvedic drugs in rheumatoid arthritis compared to auranofin. *Indian Practioner* 57(6):489-502 (1994).

22. Singh BB, Mishra LC, Vinjamury SP, Singh VJ, Aquilina N, Shepard N. The effectiveness of *Commiphora mukul* for osteoarthritis of the knee: An outcomes study. *Altern Ther Health Med* 9:74-79 (2003).

23. Mehra BL, Singh G. A comparative study on the effect of *nirgundi patra pinda sveda* and *suddha guggulu* (controlled temperature) on the patients of *griva hundanam* (cervical spondylosis). *Rheumatism* 21(3):88-98 (1986).

24. Singh G, Mehra BL, Hejmadi S. *Trika-pristha graha* vis-à-vis ankylosing spondylitis and role of Ayurveda in its management. *Rheumatism* 21:34-44 (1986).

25. Bhat B. Effect of *katibasti* in *gridhrasi* (sciatica). *Rheumatism* 22(3):61-70 (1987).

26. Majumdar A. Clinical studies of drugs *(bhallatak, gourakh* and *guggulu)* in osteoarthritis, frozen shoulder and sciatica. *Rheumatism* 14(4):153-161 (1979).

27. *Sushruta Samhita,* ed. and trans. Bhishagratna KL (vol. 1, pp. 360, 361, "Suthrasthanam," chapter 39, verse 6, 8). Varanasi: Chowkhamba Sanskrit Series Office, 1991.

28. *Caraka Samhita,* ed. and trans. Sharma PV (vol. 1, p. 22, "Sutrasthanam," chapter 3, verse 25). Varanasi: Chaukambha Orientalia, 1981.

29. *Indian herbal pharmacopoeia* (rev. new edn., pp. 169-180). Mumbai: Indian Drug Manufacturers' Association, 2002.

30. Srimal RC, Dhawan BN. Pharmacological and clinical studies on *Curcuma longa. Hamdard Medicus* 30(1-2):131-142(1987).

31. Ammon HPT, Wahl MA. Pharmacology of *Curcuma longa. Planta Med* 57:1-7 (1991).

32. Srimal RC. Turmeric: A brief review of medicinal properties. *Fitoterapia* LXVIII:483- 493 (1997).

33. Khanna NM. Turmeric—Nature's precious gift. *Curr Sci* 76:1351-1356 (1999).

34. Fintelmann V, Wegner T. *Curcuma longa*—eine unterschätzte Heilpflanze. *Deutsche Apoth Ztg* 141:3735-3743 (2001).

35. Luthra PM, Singh R, Chandra R. Therapeutic uses of *Curcuma longa. Indian J Clinical Biochemistry* 16:153-160 (2001).

36. Chainani-Wu N. Safety and anti-inflammatory activity of curcumin: A component of turmeric *(Curcuma longa). J Altern Complement Med* 9:161-168 (2003).

37. Shoba G, Joy D, Joseph T, Majeed M, Rajendran R, Srinivas PSSR. Influence of piperine on the pharmacokinetics of curcumin in animals and human volunteers. *Planta Med* 64:353-356 (1998).

38. Wagner H, Wierer M, Bauer R. *In-vitro* Hemmung der Prostaglandin—Biosynthese durch etherische Öle and phenolische Verbindungen. *Planta Med* 52:184-187 (1986).

39. Huang MT, Lysz T, Ferraro T, Abidi TF, Laskin JD, Conney AH. Inhibitory effects of curcumin on *in vitro* lipoxygenase and cyclooxygenase activities in mouse epidermis. *Cancer Res* 51:813-819 (1991).

40. Ammon HPT, Anazodo MI, Safayhi H, Dhawan BN, Srimal RC. Curcumin: A potent inhibitor of leukotriene B$_4$ formation in rat peritoneal polymorphonuclear neutrophils (PMNL). *Planta Med* 58:226 (1992).

41. Ramsewak RS, DeWitt DL, Nair MG. Cytotoxicity, antioxidant and anti-inflammatory activities of Curcumins I-III from *Curcuma longa*. *Phytomedicine* 7:303-308 (2000).

42. Innes JF, Fuller CJ, Kelly AL, Burn JF. Randomized, double-blind, placebo-controlled parallel group study of P54FP for the treatment of dogs with osteoarthritis. *Vet Rec* 152:457-460 (2003).

43. Deodhar SD, Sethi R, Srimal RC. Preliminary study on anti-rheumatic activity of curcumin (diferuloyl methane). *Indian J Med Res* 71:632-634 (1980).

44. Satoskar SS, Shah SJ, Shenoy SSG. Evaluation of anti-inflammatory property of curcumin (diferoyl methane) in patients with postoperative inflammation. *Int J Clin Pharmacol Ther Toxicol* 24:651-654 (1986).

45. *The wealth of India, raw materials* (vol. IX, pp. 271-274). New Delhi: Publications and Information Directorate, CSIR, 1972.

46. Sivarajan VV, Balachandran I. *Ayurvedic drugs and their plant sources* (pp. 85-86). New Delhi: Oxford and IBH Publishing Co Pvt. Ltd., 1994.

47. Gogte VM. *Ayurvedic pharmacology and therapeutic uses of medicinal plants* (pp. 444-447). Trans. SPARC, Mumbai: Bharatiya Vidya Bhavan, 2000.

48. Chatterjee A, Pakrashi SC. (eds.). *The treatise on Indian medicinal plants* (vol. 3, pp. 157-158). New Delhi: Publications and Information Directorate, CSIR, 1994.

49. Satyavati GV, Prasad DN, Das PK, Singh HD. Anti-inflammatory activity of *Semecarpus anacardium* Linn. A preliminary study. *Indian J Physiol Pharmacol* 13:37-45 (1969).

50. Vijayalakshmi T, Muthulakshmi V, Sachdanandam P. Effect of the milk extract of *Semecarpus anacardium* nut on adjuvant arthritis—A dose dependent study in Wistar albino rats. *Gen Pharmacol* 27:1223-1226 (1996).

51. Saraf MN, Ghooi RB, Patwardhan BK. Studies on the mechanism of action of *Semecarpus anacardium* in rheumatoid arthritis. *J Ethnopharmacol* 25:159-164 (1989).

52. Patwardhan BK, Saraf MN, Ghooi RB. Studies on the mechanism of action of *Semecarpus anacardium* in rheumatoid arthritis. *J Res Edu Indian Med* 9(1):47-50 (1990).

53. Vijayalakshmi T, Muthulakshmi V, Sachdanandam P. Salubrious effect of *Semecarpus anacardium* against lipid peroxidative changes in adjuvant arthritis studied in rats. *Mol Cell Biochem* 175:65-69 (1997).

54. Premalatha B, Sachadanandam P. *Semecarpus anacardium* L. nut extract administration induces the *in vivo* antioxidant defence system in aflatoxin B1 mediated hepatocellular carcinoma. *J Ethnopharmcol* 66:131-139 (1999).

55. Vijayalakshmi T, Muthulakshmi V, Sachdanandam P. Effect of the milk extract of *Semecarpus anacardium* nut on glycohydrolases and lysosomal stability in adjuvant arthritis in rats. *J Ethnopharmacol* 58:1-8 (1997).

56. Vijayalakshmi T, Narayanan PJ, Sachdanandam P. Changes in glucose metabolising enzymes in adjuvant arthritis and its treatment with a Siddha drug: *Serankottai Nei. Indian J Pharmacol* 30:89-93 (1998).

57. Jabbar S, Khan MTH, Choudhri MSK, Chowdhury MMH, Gafur MA. Analgesic and anti-inflammatory activity of *Semecarpus anacardium* Linn. *Hamdard Medicus* 41(4):73-80 (1998).

58. Tripathi SN, Tiwari CM, Jaiswal LC, Upadhyaya BN, Pandey P. Role of *Semecarpus anacardium (bhallataka)* in the management of rheumatoid arthritis. *J Res Indian Med Yoga Homeopath* 14(2):33-44 (1979).

59. Rao NH. *Bhallatakavati* in *amavata* conditions. *Rheumatism* 16(1):24-29 (1981).

60. Upadhyay BN, Singh TN, Tewari CM, Jaiswal LC, Tripathi SN. Experimental and clinical evaluation of *Semecarpus anacardium* nut *(bhallataka)* in the treatment of *amavata* (rheumatoid arthritis). *Rheumatism* 21(3):70-87 (1986).

61. Muthulakshmi V, Sachdanandam P. Curative potential of *Semecarpus anacardium* Linn nut milk extract against rheumatoid arthritis patients (p. 204). Chennai: Proc Intl Congress "Ayurveda 2000," January 28-30, 2000.

62. Singh NR. Clinical study to evaluate the synergistic effect of *bhallatak (Semecarpus anacardium)* and *shallaki (Boswellia serrata)* in rheumatoid arthritis (p. 134). Chennai: Proc Intl Congress "Ayurveda 2000," January 28-30, 2000.

63. Jha SD, Pandey VN. [Clinical trial of *suddha bhallataka* on *gridhrasi*]. *J Res Ayur Siddha* 7:158-170 (1986). Abstracted in *MAPA* 8806-2059.

64. Nair PR, Vijayan NP, Madhavikutty P. The action of *bhallataka* in *gridharasi* (p. 46, abstracted in *MAPA* 9504-2220). Delhi: *Proc Sem Res Ayurveda and Siddha,* March 20-22, 1995.

65. Rao KKV, Gothoskar SV, Chitnis MP, Ranadive KJ. Toxicological study of *Semecarpus anacardium* nut extract. *Indian J Physiol Pharmacol* 23:115-120 (1979).

66. Vijayalakshmi T, Muthulakshmi V, Sachdanandam P. Toxic studies on biochemical parameters carried out in rats with *Serankotai nei,* a Siddha drug-milk extract of *Semecarpus anacardium* nut. *J Ethnopharmacol* 69:9-15 (2000).

67. Murty GK. Clinical toxicity of *Semecarpus anacardium* Linn. f. *Indian J Exp Biol* 12:444-446 (1974).

68. Raut AA, Joshi AD, Antarkar DS, Joshi VR, Vaidya AB. Anti-rheumatic formulations from Ayurveda. *Ancient Sci Life* XI (1&2):66-69 (1991).

69. Mhaiskar VB, Pandya DC, Karmarkar KB. Clinical evaluation of *Tinospora cordifolia* in *amvata* and *sandhigatvata. Rheumatism* 16:35-39 (1980).

70. *Indian herbal pharmacopoeia* (rev. new edn., pp. 449-458). Mumbai: India Drug Manufacturers' Association, 2002.

71. Pendse VK, Dadhich AP, Mathur PN, Bal MS, Madam BR. Anti-inflammatory, immunosuppressive and some related pharmacological actions of the water actions of the water extract of *neem giloe (Tinospora cordifolia). A preliminary report. Indian J Pharmacol* 9:221-224 (1977).

72. Pendse VK, Mahawar MM, Khanna NK. An experimental study of water extract of *Tinospora cordifolia* in acute and chronic inflammation. *Indian J Pharmacol* 13(1):73 (1981).

73. Pendse VK, Mahawar MM, Khanna NK, Somani KC, Gautam SK. Anti-inflammatory and related activity of water extract of *Tinospora cordifolia* (Tc-We) "*neem giloe.*" *Indian Drugs* 19(1):14-21 (1981).

74. Shah DS, Pandya DC. A preliminary study about the anti-inflammatory activity of *Tinospora cordifolia. J Res Ind Med Yoga Homeo* 11(4):77-83 (1976).

75. Gulati OD, Pandey DC. Anti-inflammatory activity of *Tinospora cordifolia. Rheumatism* 17:76-83 (1982).

76. Gulati OD, Shah CP, Kanani RC, Pandya DC, Shah DS. Clinical trial of *Tinospora* in rheumatoid arthritis. *Rheumatism* 15(4):143-148 (1980).

77. Kishore P, Pandey PN, Ruhil SD. Role of *sunthi-guduchi* in the treatment of *amavata* (rheumatoid arthritis). *J Res Ayur Siddha* 1:417- 428 (1980).

78. *The wealth of India, raw materials* (vol. X, pp. 522-524). New Delhi: Publications and Information Directorate, 1995.

79. Sivarajan VV, Balachandran I. *Ayurvedic drugs and their plant sources* (pp. 329-331). New Delhi: Oxford and IBH Publishing Co Pvt. Ltd., 1994.

80. Das B, Das R (nee Chakrabarti). Medicinal properties and chemical constituents of *Vitex negundo* Linn. *Indian Drugs* 31:431-435 (1994).

81. Chandramu C, Manohar RD, Krupadanam DGL, Dashavantha RV. Isolation, characterization and biological activity of betulinic acid and ursolic acid from *Vitex negundo* L. *Phytother Res* 17:129-134 (2003).

82. Shrivastava SC, Sisodia CS. Analgesic studies on *Vitex negundo* and *Valeriana wallachi. Indian Vet J* 47:170-175 (1970).

83. Telang RS, Chatterjee S, Varshneya C. Studies on analgesic and anti-inflammatory activities of *Vitex negundo* Linn. *Indian J Pharmacol* 31:363-366 (1999).

84. Gupta M, Mazumder UK, Bhawal SR, Swamy SMK. CNS activity of petroleum ether extract of *Vitex negundo* Linn in mice. *Indian J Pharm Sci* 59:240-245 (1997).

85. Gupta M, Mazumder UK, Bhawal SR. CNS activity of *Vitex negundo* Linn in mice. *Indian J Exp Biol* 37:143-146 (1999).

86. Dharmasiri MG, Jayakody JRAC, Galhena G, Liyanage SSP, Ratnasooriya WD. Anti-inflammatory and analgesic activities of mature fresh leaves of *Vitex negundo. J Ethnopharmacol* 87:199-206 (2003).

87. Srivastava DN, Sahni YP, Gaidhani SN. Anti-inflammatory activity of some indigenous medicinal plants in albino rats. *J Med Arom Plant Sci* 22(4A), 23 (1A): 73-77 (2000-2001).

88. Gaidhani SN, Sahni YP, Srivastava DN. Anti-inflammatory effect of *Vitex negundo* on cotton pellet induced granuloma in rats. *Indian Vet J* 79:234-235 (2002).

89. Tamhankar CP, Saraf MN. Anti-arthritic activity of *Vitex negundo* Linn. *Indian J Pharm Sci* 56:158-159 (1994).

90. Srivastava DN, Sahni YP. Anti-inflammatory activity of some indigenous plants in albino rats. *J Med Arom Plant Sci* 22 (suppl. 1):42-43 (2000).

91. Mohiddin SG. The role of shambali *(Vitex negundo)* in rheumatoid arthritis. *Rheumatism* 14(3):97-112 (1979).

92. Bhattacharya C. Clinical experiences with *nirgundi (Vitex negundo). Rheumatism* 16(3):111-117 (1981).

93. Nair PRC, Vijayan NP, Venkataraghavan S. Effect of *nirgundi panchanga* and *guggulu* in *sodhana*-cum-*samana* and *samana* treatment in *gridhrasi* (sciatica). *J Res Indian Med Yoga Homeo* 13(3):14-19 (1978).

94. Kishore P, Banerjee SN. Clinical evaluation of *rasonadi kwatha* in the treatment of *amavata*—rheumatoid arthritis. *J Res Ayur Siddha* 9(1-2):29-37 (1988).

95. *Selected medicinal plants of India. A monograph of identity, safety and clinical usage* (pp. 346-349). Bombay: Chemexcil. Basic chemicals, pharmaceuticls and cosmetics export promotion council, 1992.

96. Sivarajan VV, Balachandran I. *Ayurvedic drugs and their plant sources* (pp. 65-66). Oxford and IBH Publishing Co Pvt. Ltd., New Delhi, 1994.

97. *Indian herbal pharmacopoeia* (rev. new edn., pp. 467-478). Mumbai: Indian Drug Manufacturers' Association, 2002.

98. *The wealth of India, raw materials* (vol. 10, pp. 581-585). New Delhi: Publications and Information Directorate, 1995.

99. Wagner H, Nörr H, Winterhoff H. Plant Adaptogens. *Phytomedicine* 1:63-76 (1994).

100. Panda S, Kar A. Evidence for free radical scavenging activity of *ashwagandha* root powder in mice. *Indian J Physiol Pharm* 41:424-426 (1997).

101. Russo A, Izzo AA, Cardile V, Borrelli F, Vanella A. Indian medicinal plants as antiradicals and DNA cleavage protectors. *Phytomedicine* 8:125-132 (2001).

102. Bhattacharya SK, Satyan KS, Ghosal S. Antioxidant activity of glycowithanolides from *Withania somnifera*. *Indian J Exp Biol* 35:236-239 (1997).

103. Sethi PD, Thiagarajan AR, Subramanian SS. Studies on the anti-inflammatory and anti-arthritic activity of withaferin A. *Indian J Pharmacol* 2:165-172 (1970).

104. Anbalagan K, Sadique J. Influence of an Indian medicine *(ashwagandha)* on acute phase reactants in inflammation. *Indian J Exp Biol* 19:245-249 (1981).

105. Anbalagan K, Sadique J. *Withania somnifera (aswagandha)*, a rejuvenating drug which controls alpha-2 macroglobulin synthesis during inflammation. *Int J Crude Drug Res* 23:177-183 (1985).

106. Sahni YP, Srivastava DN. Role of inflammatory mediators in anti-inflammatory activity of *Withania somnifera* on chronic inflammatory reaction. *Indian Vet Med J* 19:150-153 (1995).

107. Begum VH, Sadique J. Long term effect of herbal drug *Withania somnifera* on adjuvant induced arthritis in rats. *Ind J Exp Biol* 26:877-882 (1988).

108. Nashine K, Srivastava DN, Sahni YP. Role of inflammatory mediators in anti-inflammatory activity of *Withania somnifera*. *Indian Vet Med J* 19:286-288 (1995).

109. Bector NP, Puri AS, Sharma D. Role of *Withania somnifera (ashwagandha)* in various types of arthropathies. *Indian J Med Res* 56:1581-1583 (1968).

110. Bikshapathi T, Kumari K. Clinical evaluation of *ashwagandha* in the management of *amavata*. *J Res Ayur. Siddha* 20(1-2):46-53 (1999).

111. Madhavikutty P, Santhakumari K, Vijayan NP, Nair PR, Kumar S. Comparative clinical study on *musta, ashwagandha* and *panchakarma* therapy in *amavata* (rheumatoid arthritis). *J Res Ayur Siddha* 18(1-2):1-10 (1997).

112. Shareef MA. Management of cervical spondylosis through herbal drugs *Withania somnifera* and *Smilax china* Linn. A preliminary clinical study. In Govil JN,

Singh VK, Hashmi S (eds.), *Medicinal plants: New vistas of research* (vol. X, pp. 97-101). New Delhi: Today and Tomorrow's Printers and Publishers, 1993.

113. Kuppurajan K, Rajagopalan SS, Sitaraman R, Rajagopalan V, Janaki K, Revathi R, Venkataraghavan S. Effect of *aswagandha (Withania somnifera* Dunal) on the process of ageing in human volunteers. *J Res Ayur Siddha* 1:247-258 (1980).

114. Rege NN, Thatte UM, Dahanukar SA. Adaptogenic properties of six rasayana herbs used in Ayurvedic medicine. *Phytother Res* 13:275-291 (1999).

115. Dhuley JN. Adaptogenic and cardioprotective action of *ashwagandha* in rats and frogs. *J Ethnopharmacol* 70:57-63 (2000).

116. Mishra LC, Singh BB, Dagenais S. Scientific basis for the therapeutic use of *Withania somnifera (ashwagandha)*: A review. *Altern Med Rev* 5:334-346 (2000).

117. *Indian herbal pharmacopoeia* (rev. new edn., pp. 479-490). Mumbai: Indian Drug Manufacturers' Association, 2002.

118. Sharma AK, Singh RH. Screening of anti-inflammatory activity of certain indigenous drugs on carrageenin induced paw oedema in rats. *Bull Ethnobot Res* 1:262 -271 (1980).

119. Mascolo N, Jain R, Jain RC, Capasso F. Ethnopharmacologic investigation of ginger *(Zingiber officinale)* L. *J Ethnopharmacol* 27:129-140 (1989).

120. Jana U, Chattopadhyay RN, Shaw BP. Preliminary studies on anti-inflammatory activity of *Zingiber officinale* Rosc. *Vitex negundo* Linn and *Tinospora cordifolia* (Willd) Miers in albino rats. *Indian J Pharmacol* 31:232-233 (1999).

121. Penna SC, Medeiros MV, Aimbire FSC, Faria-Neto HCC, Sertié JAA, Lopes-Martins RAB. Anti-inflammatory effect of the hydroalcoholic extract of *Zingiber officinale* rhizomes on rat paw and skin edema. *Phytomedicine* 10:381-385 (2003).

122. Sharma JN, Srivastava KC, Gan EK. Suppressive effects of eugenol and ginger oil on arthritic rats. *Pharmacol* 49:314-318 (1994).

123. Suekawa M. Pharmacological actions of pungent constituents, [6]-gingerol and [6]-shoagol. *J Pharmacobio-Dyn* 7:836-848 (1984).

124. Kiuchi F, Shibuya M, Sankawa U. Inhibitors of prostaglandin biosynthesis from ginger. *Chem Pharm Bull* 30:754-757 (1982).

125. Kiuchi F, Iwakami S, Shibuya M, Hanaoka F, Sanakawa U. Inhibition of prostaglandin and leukotriene biosynthesis by gingerols and diarylheptanoids. *Chem Pharm Bull* 40:387-391 (1992).

126. Noh MS, Ha JY, Lee CH, Leu WY, Lee SH, Lee JJ. Inhibitory activities of natural products on lipopolysaccharide induced prostaglandin production in mouse macrophages. *Yakkak Hoeji* 42:558-566 (1998).

127. Iwakami S, Shibuya M, Tseng CF, Hanaoka F, Sankawa U. Inhibition of arachidonate 5-lipoxygenase by phenolic compounds. *Chem Pharm Bull* 34:3960-3963 (1986).

128. Flynn DL, Rafferty MF, Boctor AM. Inhibition of human neutrophil 5-lipoxygenase activity by gingerdione, shogaol, capsaicin and related pungent compounds. *Prostaglandins Leukot Med* 24:195-198 (1986).

129. Srivastava KC. Aqueous extracts of onion, garlic and ginger inhibit platelet aggregation and alter arachidonic acid metabolism. *Biomedica Bichimica Acta* 43:335-346 (1984).

130. Guh JH, Ko FN, Jong TT, Teng CM. Antiplatelet effect of gingerol isolated from *Zingiber officinale. J Pharm Pharmacol* 47:329-332 (1995).

131. Ippoushi K, Azuma K, Ito H, Horie H, Higashio H. [6]-gingerol inhibits nitric oxide synthesis in activated J774.1 mouse macrophages and prevents peroxynitrite-induced oxidation and nitration reactions. *Life Sci* 73: 3427-3437 (2003).

132. Rao RS. Efficacy of *sunthi (Zingiber officinale)* in *amavata. Rheumatism* 12(2):29-31 (1977).

133. Srivastava KC, Mustafa T. Ginger *(Zingiber officinale)* and rheumatic disorders. *Med Hypotheses* 29(1):25-28 (1989).

134. Srivastava KC, Mustafa T. Ginger *(Zingiber officinale)* in rheumatism and musculoskeletal disorders. *Med Hypotheses* 39:342-348 (1992).

135. Kishore P, Padhi MM. Studies on ancient Indian concept of 'Role of impaired gastro-intestinal function—enteropathy' in the pathogenesis and treatment of rheumatoid arthritis—*amavata. Ancient Sci Life* VI:203-216 (1987).

136. Kishore P, Pandey PN, Ruhil SD. Role of *sunthi-guduchi* in the treatment of *amavata*—rheumatoid arthritis. *J Res Ayur Siddha* 1:417-428 (1980).

137. Kishore P, Devi Das KV, Banarjee S. Clinical studies on the treatment of *amavata*—rheumatoid arthritis with *sunthi-guggulu. J Res Ayur Siddha* III (3&4): 133-146 (1982).

138. Kishore P, Padhi MM. Further clinical evaluation of *sunthi-guggulu* in the treatment of *amavata*—rheumatoid arthritis. *J Res Ayur Siddha* IX(3-4):89-104 (1988).

139. Altmann RD, Marcussen KC. Effects of a ginger extract on knee pain in patients with osteoarthritis. *Arthritis Rheum* 44:2531-2538 (2001).

Chapter 9

Skin and Trauma Care Agents

The skin, which covers an area of 2 m^2, is the largest organ in the body and, therefore, also subject to external influences such as heat and light; apart from numerous agents, for example bacteria, fungus, virus, etc.; physical damage due to accidents, cuts, wounds, burns; and—in the case of traumatic injuries—breaking of bones. In Ayurveda, plants have been the mainstay of treatment and the management of skin diseases, or *kustha.* In the field of traumatic injuries (methods of treatment and care of injury), there are experts who specialize in the setting of bones and the treatment of the injury. The hereditary bonesetters of Puthur, a small village in Andhra Pradesh, are well known for their bonesetting skills. Herbs are applied externally on the injured site, and are also given internally to help healing and strengthening of the bone. People come from far and wide to get their injuries treated.

A large number of plants have been found to be used in the treatment of skin disorders.[1] However, relatively few of them have been subjected to clinical trials although or perhaps because, they form part of the day-to-day practice of Ayurvedic physicians. Plants and plant products are frequently used in homes to preserve healthy skin. Common among these are turmeric and sandalwood. Others include neem leaves, the astringent barks of different *Ficus* species, and members of the Labiateae such as holy basil, *Leucas aspera,* etc.

This chapter is divided into three sections—the first section is on skin diseases and includes the different categories given by Willuhn. It covers diseases caused by external agents (Virus: *Shingles zoster;* Bacteria: Impetigo, *Pityriasis versicolor;* Fungus: ringworm; Mites:

doi:10.1300/5683_09

Scabies), and those caused without an external agent, such as psoriasis, eczema, leukoderma, neurodermatitis, and allergic skin problems.[2] The second section covers herbs used in wound healing and the third section is on herbs used for healing of bones.

NOTES

1. Vohora SB, Mishra GV. Rational basis of the use of medicinal plants in skin diseases. *Indian Drugs* 35:1-17 (1998).
2. Willuhn G. Pflanzliche Dermatika—Eine kritische Übersicht. *Deut Apoth Ztg* 132:1873-1883 (1992).

SKIN DISEASES

Since most of the trials are of a preliminary and exploratory nature covering several indications, it is not possible to group them into different categories and they are covered according to the plant. Among various skin problems, eczema, scabies, and ringworm are commonly found in India. In addition, numerous skin disorders caused by fungi, bacteria, virus, or due to allergy also abound.

Azadirachta indica *A Juss. (Family: Meliaceae)*

Latin: *Melia azadirachta* Linn.	Hindi: Neem, Nimb
Sanskrit: Nimba	Tamil: Veppan, Vembu
English: Margosa	

Azadirachta indica or the *neem* tree is considered to be a veritable pharmacy, all parts being used for a wide variety of ailments, especially for the treatment of skin disorders of varied etiology. Just sleeping under a *neem* tree is said to promote one's health. Whereas all parts of the tree are used medicinally, the leaves and seed oil are used most widely for the treatment of skin diseases. The fresh green leaves have long been used as a household remedy to relieve itch in smallpox, chicken pox, and measles. It is also customary to apply a freshly ground paste of turmeric and *neem* leaves on the body while taking the first bath after recovering from measles, chicken pox, and small pox. Other aspects of neem, its chemistry, and use in diabetes are covered in Chapter 11, "Antidiabetic agents."

There is evidence to show that *neem* is active against a wide range of bacteria, fungi, and viruses. The aqueous and alcoholic extract of the leaf and bark,[1] the chloroform extract of leaves, the seed oil, and the gum showed antibacterial activity against a variety of pathogens.[2-5] The oil obtained by steam distillation of fresh mature leaves showed antifungal activity against *Trichophyton mentagrophytes*[6] in vitro; stem bark extract[7] and the ethanolic extract of seeds had antimycotic activity against *Candida albicans.*[8] *Neem* leaf extract has also shown antiviral activity against several viruses. Water extract of tender leaves showed antiviral activity against vaccinia[9,10] and variola[9] viruses. In addition, *neem* leaf extract shows activity against fowl pox virus, chikungunya, and measles viruses, group B coxsackieviruses and dengue virus type-2.[10-13]

It has been suggested that the range of diseases on which *neem* has a favorable effect is owing to the immunomodulatory effect shown by several parts of the tree.[14,15] Thus the bark,[14,15] leaf,[15,16] and seed oil[17] have been shown to have an immunomodulatory effect. The leaf aqueous extract modulates both cell-mediated and humoral responses in mice.[16] In addition, *neem* exerts an anti-inflammatory effect. Thus, the alcoholic extract of leaves[18] and the water-soluble portion of the alcoholic extract,[19] but not the ether soluble fraction,[20] show anti-inflammatory effect. However, the ether-soluble fraction has a potent analgesic effect under acute inflammatory conditions.[20]

Eczema, ringworm, scabies

Eczema is an inflammation of the skin that is accompanied by itching, scaling, or blisters. Ringworm (tinea) is a fungal infection of the skin, hair, and nails; whereas, scabies is caused by the mite *Sarcoptes scabei* that causes itching.

In an open study, patients with common skin disorders such as eczema, ringworm, and scabies were treated with a lotion prepared by dissolving the residue of a 70-percent alcoholic extract of neem leaves in propylene glycol in the ratio of 2:3 and applying it on the affected part. The lotion was applied twice a day for 3 days to treat scabies, and 4-8 days to treat cases of ringworm. The lotion was found to be effective in all cases of acute weeping and chronic eczema, ringworm, and scabies.[21,22] Many of these patients were nonresponding to conventional treatments, such as salicylic acid, benzoyl benzoate, and sulfur.

In an open trial, the oil obtained by boiling *Strychnos nux vomica* nut in neem oil was applied externally on patients with eczema and was found to yield good results.[23] In patients with scabies, a 4:1 mixture of fresh neem leaves and turmeric powder was applied on 814 patients with scabies. More than 97 percent of the patients were cured within 3-15 days by this treatment.[24] No toxic or adverse effects were seen. In a report, the use of one to two 500 mg neem capsules made from leaves, flowers, and twig powder, taken orally with food twice a day for long periods, "dramatically" helped patients with chronic fungal infections of skin and nails, boils, and other bacterial infections. It was also reported to be useful in cases of allergic skin conditions and psoriasis.[25] Other neem products that have been reported to be useful in psoriasis are the bitter compound nimbidin[26] and neem toddy[27] taken together with a compound herbomineral preparation *Arogyavardini vati,* which is used in a number of conditions—skin problems, obesity, hepatitis, chronic constipation, anorexia, heart problems, and many others. Studies involving the use of neem preparations in wound healing are discussed later in this chapter.

It would thus be worthwhile to explore the nature of the products required and conduct further trials to establish the efficacy parameters to confirm the success that has been reported with a variety of neem preparations.

Preparations derived from the neem tree, such as from the bark and the leaf, generally have a wide margin of safety except for the seed oil for which some data exists that it may be unsafe, especially in oral consumption by infants in doses of 5-30 ml,[28] which is in any case a high dosage for any oil to be given to infants. One study has shown that the seed oil is safe for topical use in wounds;[29] however, care needs to taken in assessing the quality of the starting material, the method of processing, and the composition of oil derived from it.

Cardiospermum halicacabum *Linn. (Family: Sapindaceae)*

Sanskrit: Indravalli, karnasphota   English: Balloon Vine

Tamil: Moddakattan

Cardiospermum halicacabum is a slender climber found growing throughout India up to 1,200 m elevation. The tender shoots are used as a vegetable, whereas the whole plant is used for medicinal purposes. The plants belong to the group of ten auspicious herbs or *dasapushpa* (dasa: ten; pushpa: flowers), which are supposed to promote health and remove unhealthy tendencies, including the urge to commit sinful acts.[30] The drug appears in later Ayurvedic texts. The herb is used for rheumatism, nervous disorders, sprains, lumbago, edema, and earache. The leaves are used for wound healing, in piles, for treatment of asthma, and to relieve fever associated with cough.[30,31] The herb is very commonly used in food in Tamil Nadu to get relief from rheumatic complaints, probably because of its use in Siddha medicine. It is also used in skin disorders to treat eczema and herpes.[32]

There are two varieties of *Cardiospermum halicacabum* with differences in the size and shape of the fruit, and in the size and shape of the leaves; the fruits of *Cardiospermum halicacabum* var. *microcarpum* have smaller, winged sharply three-lobed fruits, and smaller leaves, whereas *Cardiospermum halicacabum* var. *luridum* has larger bloated three-lobed fruits, which are not winged, and larger leaves.[33] It is not certain which of these varieties has been used in the various investigations, and the impact of this on the results obtained; both varieties are probably similar in activity and used interchangeably; however, this needs to be verified. The results are cited as in literature. It is likely that the investigations from India used the more widespread var. *microcarpum;* there is also the fact that *Cardiospermum halicacabum* var. *luridum* was earlier identified as *Cardiospermum canescens* in India. Investigations from Germany probably used the var. *luridum* from the picture of the plant published along with the review article summarizing German investigations.[34]

A large number of constituents have been isolated from the aerial parts—flavonoids (apigenin, luteolin, kaempferol-3-rhamnoside and quercetin-3-rhamnoside), several pentacyclic tritepenoids, hydrolysable tannins, sterols (campesterol, β-sitosterol, stigmasterol, β-amyrin), and quebrachitol.[34]

The anti-inflammatory activity has been studied in several experimental models—granuloma pouch,[35] cotton pellet implantation,[35,36] carrageenan-induced paw edema,[36] and in vitro studies.[37] The topical anti-inflammatory activity of a 95-percent ethanolic extract has also been studied in mice and the heptane fraction of this extract at 232 μg per ear was found to exhibit potent activity, probably through inhibition of the enzyme phospholipase A2.[38]

Studies conducted using an alcoholic extract of the fresh flowering plant of *Cardiospermum halicacabum* in the form of a cream has been included here since it is used in the form of a homeopathic mother tincture, and hence is comparable to that used in herbal medicine.

Neurodermatitis, atopic dermatitis, and eczema

Neurodermatitis is an itchy, eczema-like skin condition caused by repeated scratching, whereas atopic dermatitis is inflammation of the skin caused by allergy. In an open observational study, 512 patients with neurodermatitis were treated with *Cardiospermum* cream; 42 patients served as control and used both the base cream without the active drug and the *Cardiospermum* cream. It was found that there was reduction in the erythema when using the active cream as judged by reduction in redness. In addition, patients could reduce their other medications— corticosteroids and antihistamines.[39] In another open observational study, similar results were obtained from patients with eczema.[40] In another controlled double-blind study in patients with atopic dermatitis, the superior efficacy of the *Cardiospermum* cream against the base cream[41] and of comparable efficacy to bufexamac has been observed.[42] These results have led to the cream being allowed to be used in Germany in 1995 for inflammatory skin disorders accompanied by itching, such as eczema and neurodermatitis.[34]

Aerial parts of *Cardiospermum halicacabum* var. *microcarpum* are sold as fresh herbs in the market in Chennai (earlier Madras) especially after the rains. The leaves are often eaten both raw and cooked as food in Chennai to relieve joint pain. The LD_{50} of the alcoholic extract when injected intraperitoneally in mice is 20 mg·25 g^{-1} body weight.[35] In the open study, the tolerability of the *Cardiospermum* cream was evaluated as good to very good by 82 percent of the patients.[39] The *Cardiospermum halicacabum* ointment was well tolerated, and in efficacy distinctly superior to the ointment base in a double-blind study.[41] The tolerability of the bases used for the ointment and the tincture of *Cardiospermum halicacabum* did not show any irritation or allergic reaction.[34]

Pongamia pinnata *Pierre (Family: Fabaceae)*

Latin syn: *Pongamia glabra* Vent.	Hindi: Karanj
Sanskrit: Karanj	Tamil: Poongam
English: Indian Beech, Pongam oil tree	

Pongamia pinnata is a medium-sized tree with shiny leaves found almost throughout India up to an elevation of 1,200 m. All plant parts are used medicinally and the plant is a reputed drug for skin problems. The leaves, seed, and bark are considered to be useful in skin problems because of their anti-inflammatory, analgesic, and antiseptic properties.[43] The seed paste and seed oil especially are highly regarded for the treatment of scabies, herpes, leukoderma, and other skin diseases.[44]

The tree has been extensively investigated for its chemical constituents and a large number of different classes of compounds have been isolated—flavones, flavone glycosides, furanoflavones, and chromenoflavones, sterols, triterpenes, phenylpropanoid compounds, fatty acids, aminoacids, etc. The seeds contain furanoflavones— karanjin, pongapin, kanjone, and pongaglabrone, the diketone— pongamol. The oil has been clinically shown to be nonirritating. Karanjin, one of the major flavones of the seeds, is said to be the active principle, which is responsible for the curative effect of the oil in skin diseases.[44]

The few studies carried out so far support the use of *Pongamia pinnata* in skin problems. Thus *Pongamia pinnata* seed extracts at 50 mg·kg^{-1} to 100 mg·kg^{-1} given intraperitoneally showed anti-inflammatory, analgesic, and antiulcerogenic effect in rats.[45,46] It has been suggested that the anti-inflammatory effect may be owing to the modulation of eicosanoid formation in inflammation.[45] In addition, the seed oil has been shown to possess antibacterial activity against 14 strains of pathogenic bacteria mainly because of inhibition of cell membrane synthesis in the bacteria.[47] In vitro experiments have shown that the aqueous seed extract inhibits growth of the herpes - virus—HSV-1 at 1 mg·ml^{-1} and HSV-2 at 20 mg·ml^{-1}—in Vero cells.[48]

The only clinical evidence comes from a study that has been published as an abstract.[49] Thus, in an open, exploratory study, patients with a wide variety of skin complaints—herpetic lesions due to *Shingles zoster* (infection of the nerves characterized by painful rash) and *Herpes genitalis* (painful blisters caused by the herpes simplex virus 2 producing soreness, itching, and painful blisters in the genital area), impetigo (blisters around the mouth due to skin infection caused by bacteria, especially *Staphylococci*), ringworm, *Pityriasis versicolor* (a skin problem caused by fungus and characterized by white, brown, or colored flaking skin on the neck and trunk), and eczema were treated with *Pongamia* seed oil, a 1:1 sterile aqueous extract of *Pongamia* seed, or *Pongamia* root. The control group received only paraffin oil for application. "Remarkable" healing effects were seen with *Pongamia* seed oil for herpetic lesions due to *Shingle zoster* and *Herpes genitalis,* whereas the seed extract helped in treating *Shingles zoster.* Impetigo was helped by both the oil and seed extract, whereas oil, seed extract, and root extract were all active in the case of ringworm. There is no mention of its effect on eczema and *Pityriasis versicolor.*

Further clinical studies are warranted since the preliminary results are promising. Although a lot of work has been done on the chemical constituents of the seed oil, it would be useful to establish the composition of the material being used for the trials. This would be important since it has been mentioned in earlier work, that seed[50] and seed oil[51] are toxic. However, seeds were nontoxic after solvent extraction[51] and the purified oil is safe for use.[52] Safety studies have been carried out on the seed aqueous extract.[53]

NOTES

1. Ahmad I, Ahmed F, Hussain S. *In vitro* antimicrobial activity of leaf and bark extracts of *Azadirachta indica* A Juss. *Indian Vet Med J* 19:204–206 (1995).

2. Thaker AM, Anjaria JV. Antimicrobial and infected wound healing response of some traditional drugs. *Indian J Pharmacol* 18:171-174 (1986).

3. Chaurasia SC, Jain PC. Antibacterial activity of essential oils of four medicinal plants. *Indian J Hosp Pharmacy* 15(6):166-168 (1978).

4. Baswa M, Rath CC, Dash SK, Mishra RK. Antibacterial activity of *karanj (Pongamia pinnata)* and *neem (Azadirachta indica)* seed oil: A preliminary report. *Microbios* 105:183-189 (2001).

5. Banerjee G, Nagar PA. Antimicrobial activity of the gum obtained from *Roystonia regia* and *Melia azadirachta* (p. 86, Abstract no: EP 09). Manipal: *Proc 42nd Indian Pharmaceutical Cong,* December 28-30, 1990.

6. Pant N, Garg HS, Madhusudanan KP, Bhakuni DS. Sulfurous compounds from *Azadirachta indica* leaves. *Fitoterapia* 57:302-304 (1986).

7. Fabry W, Okemo P, Ansorg R. Fungistatic and fungicidal activity of East African medicinal plants. *Mycoses* 39:67-70 (1996).

8. Khan M, Zubairy HN. Mycoses Part I: Antimycotic effect of *Azadirachta indica* on *Candida albicans*. *Hamdard Medicus* 41(4):33-34 (1998).

9. Rao AR, Sukumar S, Paramasivam TV, Kamalakshi S, Parashuraman AR, Shantha M. Study of antiviral activity of tender leaves of margosa tree *(Melia azadericta)* on vaccinia and variola virus. *Indian J Med Res* 57:495—502 (1969).

10. Rai A, Sethi MS. Screening of some plants for their activity against vaccinia and fowl-pox viruses. *Indian J Animal Sci* 42:1066-1070 (1972).

11. Gogate SS, Marathe AD. Antiviral effect of *neem* leaf (*Azadirachta indica* Juss.) extract on chikungunya and measles viruses. *J Res Edu Indian Med* 8(1):1-5 (1989).

12. Badam L, Joshi SP, Bedekar SS. *In vitro* antiviral activity of *neem* (*Azadirachta indica* A. Juss.) leaf extract against group B Coxsackie viruses. *J Commun Dis* 31(2):79-90 (1999).

13. Parida MM, Upadhyay C, Pandya G, Jana AM. Inhibitory potential of *neem* (*Azadirachta indica* A. Juss.) leaves on dengue virus type-2 replication. *J Ethnopharmacol* 79:273-278 (2002).

14. van der Nat JM, t'Hart LA, van der Sluis WG, van Dijk H, van den Berg AJJ, de Silva KTD, Labadie RP. Characterization of anti-complement compounds from *Azadirachta indica*. *J Ethnopharmacol* 27:15-24 (1989).

15. Upadhyaya S, Dhawan S. *Neem (Azadirachta indica):* Immunomodulatory properties and therapeutic potential (p. 34). Bombay: Update Ayurveda-94, February 24-26, 1994.

16. Ray A, Banerjee BD, Sen P. Modulation of humoral and cell-mediated immune responses by *Azadirachta indica (Neem)* in mice. *Indian J Exp Biol* 34: 698-701 (1996).

17. Upadhyay SN, Dhawan S, Garg S, Talwar GP. Immunomodulatory effects of *neem (Azadirachta indica) oil. Int J Immunopharmacol* 14:1187-1193 (1992).

18. Koley KM, Lal J, Tandan SK. Anti-inflammatory activity of *Azadirachta indica (neem)* leaves. *Fitoterapia* 65:524-528 (1994).

19. Chattopadhyay RR. Possible biochemical mode of anti-inflammatory action of *Azadirachta indica* A. Juss in rats. *Indian J Exp Biol* 36:418-420 (1998).

20. Tandan SK, Chandra S, Gupta S, Tripathi HC, Lal J. Pharmacological effects of *Azadirachta indica* leaves. *Fitoterapia* 61:75-80 (1990).

21. Singh N, Mishra N, Singh SP, Kohli RP. *Melia azadirachta* in some common skin disorders—A clinical evaluation. *The Antiseptic* 76:677-680 (1979).

22. Singh N. Role of *Azadirachta indica (neem)* in some common skin disorders of man (p. 16). Lucknow: Proc Natl Sem Use of Traditional Medicinal Plants in Skin Care, CIMAP, November 25-26, 1994.

23. Masilamani G, Bharadwaj TPR, Purushothaman KK. Role of *Etti Ennei* and *Naguneri Ennei* in the treatment of "*Karappan*" (eczema)—A pilot study. *J Res Indian Med Yoga Homeo* 14:74-80 (1979).

24. Charles V, Charles SX. The use and efficacy of *Azadirachta indica* ADR ("*neem*") and *Curcuma longa* ("turmeric") in scabies. A pilot study. *Trop Geogr Med* 44:178-181 (1992).

25. Dhasmana KM, Singh V, Abbas SS, Singh N. An herbal antibiotic in the treatment of skin and upper respiratory tract disorders (p. 149). Lucknow, UP: Second World Congress on "Biotechnological Developments of Herbal Medicine" NBRI, February 20-22, 2003.

26. Rajasekharan S, Pillai NGKP, Kurup PB, Pillai KGB, Nair CPR. Effect of nimbidin in psoriasis-a case report. *J Res Ayur Siddha* 1:52-58 (1980).

27. Sharma UD. *Neem*—An important medicine for psoriasis. *Sachitra Ayurved* 47:281-282 (1994). Abstracted in *MAPA* 9503-2036.

28. van der Nat JM, van der Sluis, de Silva KTD, Labadie RP. Ethnopharmacognostical survey of *Azadirachta indica* A. Juss. (Meliaceae). *J Ethnopharmacol* 35:1-24 (1991).

29. Tandan SK, Gupta S, Chandra S, Lal J, Singh R. Safety evaluation of *Azadirachta indica* seed oil, an herbal wound dressing agent. *Fitoterapia* 66:69-72 (1995).

30. Sivarajan VV, Balachandran I. *Ayurvedic drugs and their plant sources* (pp. 178-179). New Delhi: Oxford and IBH Publishing Co Ltd, 1994.

31. *The wealth of India, raw materials* (vol. 3, pp. 269-271). New Delhi: Publications and Information Directorate, CSIR, 1992.

32. Shanmugam NK. *Dictionary of medicinal plants* (pp. 686-687). Madras: Nakkeeran Paddipakkam Vellitu, 1989.

33. Matthew KM. *An excursion flora of central Tamilnadu* (p. 97). New Delhi: Oxford and IBH Publishing Co Ltd., 1991.

34. Niederle S. *Cardiospermum halicacabum* (L)—Die Ballonrebe. *Z Phytotherapie* 17:61-66 (1996).

35. Gopalakrishnan C, Dhananjayan R, Kameswaran L. Studies on the pharmacological actions of *Cardiospermum halicacabum. Ind J Physiol Pharmacol* 20:203-208 (1976).

36. Sadique J, Chandra T, Thenmozhi V, Elango V. Biochemical modes of action of *Cassia occidentalis* and *Cardiospermumn halicacabum* in inflammation. *J Ethnopharmacol* 19:201-212 (1987).

37. Chandra T, Sadique J. Anti-inflammatory effect of the medicinal plant *Cardiospermumn halicacabum* L. *In vitro* study. *Arogya J Health Sci* X:57-60 (1984).

38. Koch E, Chatterjee SS, Jaggy H. Topical anti-inflammatory activity of lipophilic extracts from *Cardiospermum halicacabum. Phytomedicine* 3 (suppl.1): 229 (1996).

39. Rudolph R, Benthien H, Jappe U, Kunz B. Lokaltherapie der atopischen Dermatitis mit *Cardiospermum halicacabum. Haut* 1:63-66 (1994).

40. Rudolph R. Brüggemann B, Schenk WH, Wandel G. Klinische Erfahrungen in der Therapie berufsbedingter Abnutzungseczeme mit *Cardiospermum-halicacabum-*Salbe. *Allergologie* 18:216-217 (1995).

41. Merklinger S, Messemer C, Niederle S. *Cardiospermum-*Salbe und Salbengrundlage im Halbseitenvergleich-eine kontrollierte Studie. *Z Phytotherapie* 16:263-266 (1995).

42. Brüggemann B, Rudolph R. Lokale Therapie der atopischen dermatitis: *Cardiospermum halicacabum* und Bufexamac im Vergleich. *Haut* 6:2818-2822 (1995).

43. Gogte VM. *Ayurvedic pharmacology and therapeutic uses of medicinal plants* (pp. 336-337). Trans. SPARC, Mumbai: Bharatiya Vidya Bhavan, 2000.

44. *The wealth of India, raw materials* (vol. VIII, pp. 206-211). New Delhi: Publications and Information Directorate, CSIR, 1969.

45. Singh RK, Pandey BL. Anti-inflammatory activity of seed extracts of *Pongamia pinnata* in rat. *Indian J Physiol Pharmacol* 40:355-358 (1996).

46. Singh RK, Joshi VK, Goel RK, Gambhir SS, Acharya SB. Pharmacological actions of *Pongamia pinnata* seeds—A preliminary study. *Indian J Exp Biol* 34:1204-1207 (1996).

47. Baswa M, Rath CC, Dash SK, Mishra RK. Antibacterial activity of *karanj (Pongamia pinnata)* and *neem (Azadirachta indica)* seed oil: A preliminary report. *Microbios* 105:183-189 (2001).

48. Elanchezhiyan M, Rajarajan S, Rajendran P, Subramanian S, Thyagarajan SP. Antiviral properties of the seed extract of an Indian medicinal plant, *Pongamia pinnata* Linn. against herpes simplex viruses: *In-vitro* studies on Vero cells. *J Med Microbiol* 38:262-264 (1993).

49. Rajarajan S, Subramanian S, Thygarajan SP, Sundaram M, Venkatraman TK. A study on the clinical efficacy of two medicinal plants *Pongamia pinnata* (Linn) Merr. [(*Pongamia glabra* Vent.)] *Thespesia populnea* (L.) Sol against certain skin disorders of viral, bacterial and fungal origin. Jaipur: 13th Natl Cong Indian Medical Assoc Medical Micribiol, November 10-12, 1989.

50. Chakaraborty N, Mandal L. Effect of toxic factor(s) of *karanja (Pongamia glabra* Vent.) oil and its different fractions on mice. *Indian Vet J* 60:138-142 (1983).

51. Samanta G, Adityachowdhury N, Banerjee GC. Nature of deleterious factors occurring in *karanja* (*Pongamia glabra* Vent.) seed. *Indian J Animal Sci* 57(1):37-41 (1987).

52. Sasmal D, Makli SS, Basu SP. Preliminary study on the effect of purified *Pongamia* oil on liver and kidney functions in rats. *Fitoterapia* 68:35-38 (1997).

53. Elanchezhian M, Udaysankar K, Rajarajan S, et al. *In vitro* and *in vivo* study on the toxicity studies of an Indian medicinal plant *Pongamia pinnata* (Linn). *Biomedicine* 12 (2):47-52 (1992).

LEUKODERMA/FOLLICULAR ECZEMA

Leukoderma is a skin condition caused by the inability of melanoblasts to synthesize melanin. White patches appear on the skin wherever melanin is lost. Many plants have been described for its treatment in Ayurveda. The incidence of the disease is estimated to be 3 percent higher in India than the world incidence of 1 percent.[1]

Psoralea corylifolia *Linn. (Family: Fabaceae)*

Sanskrit: Bakuchi	Tamil: Karporgam
Hindi: Bavchi	English: Scurfy pea

Psoralea corylifolia is an erect annual herb with bluish purple flowers found growing wild throughout India. The seeds are a reputed drug for the skin in Ayurveda, especially for leprosy, leukoderma, and psoriasis, and also for inflammatory skin disorders, both in the form of topical application as well as oral administration.[2]

The seeds have been extensively investigated for their chemical constituents. They contain 0.05 percent essential oil, 10 percent of a brown fixed oil, a nonvolatile oil containing terpenoids, approximately 9 percent resin, furanocoumarins—psoralen, isopsoralen identical with angelicin, coumesterol derivatives—psoralidin and isopsoralidin, flavonoids—bavachalkone, bavachinin, isobavachalkone, bavachin, and isobavachin—a monoterpenoid phenol bakuchiol, chalcones, isoflavones—corylin, neobavaisoflavone, corylinal, psoralenal—triacontane, sitosterol, and stigmasterol.[2,3]

Psoralen and isopsoralen are considered to be the active principles useful in leukoderma of nonsyphilitic origin.[2] Psoralen has been shown to stimulate melanin production by accumulation in the melanocytes and photooxidation of the dihydroxyphenylalanine present there to melanin.[4-6] The aqueous[7] and alcoholic[7,8] extracts of *Psoralea corylifolia* seeds have shown inhibitory activity against *Staphylococcus aureus*. The petroleum ether extract of the seeds inhibited the growth of *Staphylococci* at a concentration of 2-4 $\mu g \cdot ml^{-1}$, especially those of *Staphylococcus aureus* that are resistant to several antibiotics such as penicillin, streptomycin, chloramphenicol, erythromycin, and tetracycline.[9] Later on, an oily compound was isolated that inhibited *Staphylococcus aureus* at 0.5 $\mu g \cdot ml^{-1}$ with an activity comparable to that of chloramphenicol.[10,11] Bakuchiol has been studied for its anti-staphylococcal activity.[12] In addition, the seeds have also been shown to have immunomodulatory activity,[13] whereas bakuchiol and the flavonoids—isobavachin and isobavachalcone—have been shown to have potent antioxidant activity.[14] The flavonoid, bavachinin, has been shown to exert marked anti-inflammatory, antipyretic, and mild analgesic activity.[15]

Leukoderma

The preliminary exploratory studies were carried out with different preparations, derived from the seeds of *Psoralea corylifolia,* applied topically on the affected areas for a variety of skin disorders. From these exploratory studies it was found that the oleoresin of the seeds, which contained most of the essential oil, was most useful in leukoderma patches.[16]

The oral clinical use of the powdered seeds of *Psoralea corylifolia* for the treatment of leukoderma is dose dependently attended by severe side effects such as nausea, vomiting headache, and severe purging, so that in all further clinical studies, a mixture of psoralen and isopsoralen was used in doses of 10-30 mg·day^{-1} for 4 months with good results. However, the drug can no longer be considered an herbal preparation; the results of such studies have been summarized.[3]

Follicular eczema

Follicular eczema is an infection of the hair follicle caused by *Staphylococcus aureus.* The seeds of *Psoralea corylifolia,* which have exhibited good antibacterial activity, may be of use in this condition, which is characterized by chronicity. In addition, antibiotics give only temporary relief. The alcoholic extract of the seeds was dissolved in coconut oil and 5-30 ml of the oil was applied twice a day for periods ranging from 2 to 4 weeks in 21 patients. A total of 17 out of the 21 patients had significant relief and when followed up for 2 years there was no relapse. There were four dropouts after 2 weeks. At the end of 2-4 weeks of treatment 12 patients had complete relief, 2 had marked relief, and 3 patients had moderate relief. Continuation of the treatment for a few more days resulted in all patients obtaining complete relief.[17]

Topical use of the seed oil can cause irritation, blistering, and also act as a vesicant. The oleoresin extract of the seeds had the official status in the *Indian Pharmacopoeia,* 1960, as "Babchi ointment" or "Application of Psoralea." The strength of the oil or its preparation has to be adjusted to prevent redness beyond that already present in the leukoderma patch.[2,18]

It appears that the external application is useful in certain cases, but is attended by side effects such as irritation of the skin; therefore, until it is possible to standardize the product it is likely to be of use only in the form of the pure compounds and derivatives and not as a whole drug.

NOTES

1. Publications and Information Directorate. Herbal drugs for leucoderma. *Indian Drugs* 26(1):1-7 (1988).

2. *The wealth of India, raw materials* (vol. VIII, pp. 296-298). New Delhi: Publications and Information Directorate, CSIR, 1969.

3. Satyavati GV, Gupta AK, Tandon N (eds.), *Medicinal plants of India* (vol. II, pp. 518-530). New Delhi: Indian Council for Medical Research, 1987.

4. Misra AL, Agarwala SC, Mukherji B. Mode of action of psoralen in pigment production: Part I. Action of ultraviolet radiation on psoralen. *J Sci Ind Res* 20C:339-341 (1961).

5. Rashid Ali, Agarwala SC. Mode of action of psoralen in pigment production: Part II. Inactivation of –SH groups by irradiated psoralen. *J Sci Ind Res* 21C:321-323 (1962).

6. Rashid Ali, Agarwala SC. Mode of action of psoralen in pigment production: Part III. Photooxidation of dihydroxyphenylalanine in the presence of psoralen. Indian J Biochem 2:271-274 (1965).

7. George M, Pandalai KM. Investigations of plant antibiotics. Part IV. Further research for antibiotic substances in Indian medicinal plants. *Indian J Med Res.* 37:169-181 (1949).

8. Kurup PA. Studies on plant antibiotics: Screening of some Indian medicinal plants. *J Sci Ind Res* 15C:153-154 (1956).

9. Gupta KC, Bhatia MC, Chopra CL, Nath A, Chopra IC. Anti-staphylococcal activity of *Psoralea corylifolia* seed extracts, *Bull Reg Res Lab Jammu* 1:59-60 (1962).

10. Gaind KN, Dar RN, Kaul RN. Anti-staphylococcal activity of seeds of *Psoralea corylifolia* Linn. *J Pharmaceut Sci* 53:1428 (1964).

11. Gaind KN, Dar RN, Kaul RN. Isolation of an anti-staphylococcal fraction from the seeds of *Psoralea corylifolia* Linn. *Indian J Pharm* 26:141-142 (1964).

12. Kaul R. [Kinetics of the anti-staphylococcal activity of bakuchiol *in vitro*]. Arzneimittel Forsch 26:486-489 (1976).

13. Latha PG, Evans DA, Panikkar KR. Jayavardhanan KK. Immunomodulatory and antitumor properties of *Psoralea corylifolia* seeds. *Fitoterapia* 71:223-231 (2000).

14. Haraguchi H, Inoue J, Tamura Y, Mizutani K. Antioxidative components of *Psoralea corylifolia* (Leguminosae). *Phytother Res* 16:539-544 (2002).

15. Anand KK, Sharma ML, Singh B. Ghatak BJR. Anti-inflammatory, antipyretic and analgesic properties of bavachinin—A flavanone isolated from the seeds of *Psoralea corylifolia* Linn. *(Babchi). Indian J Exp Biol* 16:1216-1217 (1978).

16. Mukerjee B. *Psoralea* and other indigenous drugs used in leucoderma. *J Sci Ind Res* 15A (5) (suppl.):1-12 (1956).

17. Pillai BKR, Pillai NGK, Nair CPR. The effect of *Psoralia-*5 on follicular eczema. *J Res Ayur Siddha* XXIII(1-2):56-63 (2002).

18. *Selected medicinal plants of India. A monograph on identity, safety and clinical usage* (pp. 255-257). Bombay: Chemexcil, Basic Chemicals, Pharmaceuticals and Cosmetics Export Promotion Council, 1992.

PSORIASIS

Psoriasis is a skin condition characterized by itching, scaling, and hyperproliferation of skin, and is estimated to be afflicting 1-3 percent of populations. Although a number of plants have been used in Ayurveda for the treatment of psoriasis, only a few of them have been evaluated to some degree. The best known of these are *Aloe vera, Azadirachta indicia, Centella asiatica,* and *Wrightia tinctoria.* In the case of *Azadirachta indica,* its bitter principle, nimbidin, has been used and is therefore not covered here since nimbidin cannot be considered an herbal drug.

Aloe vera Tourn. *ex Linn (Family: Liliaceae)*

In a double-blind, placebo-controlled study, the efficacy and tolerability of a 0.5 percent of *Aloe vera* cream was studied on 60 patients with mild-to-moderate psoriasis. Patients had the disease for an average of 8.5 years before entry to the trial. Patients were given either *Aloe vera* cream or placebo and asked to apply the cream thrice a day for 5 consecutive days for a total of 4 weeks. The progress of patients was evaluated every week. By the end of the trial, the *Aloe vera* extract cream had cured 25 out of 30 patients as compared to 2 out of 30 in the placebo group, resulting in considerable clearing of psoriatic plaques. No side effects were observed.[1]

Centella asiatica *(Linn.) Urban (Family: Apiaceae)*

In a small clinical study, seven patients with psoriasis were treated with a cream containing an oil and water extract of *Centella asiatica* (see Plate 8 in color gallery) for periods ranging from 3 to 8 weeks. It was found that five out of seven patients showed complete clearance of the lesions. None of the patients experienced any side effects. One of the patients, who had frequently been using steroids in the past, showed only partial recovery.[2] Except for one patient, the remaining six patients were routinely asked to apply salicylic acid ointment 12 hours after the application of *Centella.* In vitro studies have shown that *Centella asiatica* extract has a keratinocyte antiproliferant activity.[3] Further studies are needed with larger patient numbers.

Wrightia tinctoria *R. Br. (Family: Apocyanaceae)*

Sanskrit: Sweta kutaja, Madhura kutaja	Tamil: Vetpalai
Hindi: Indrajau	English: Pala Indigo Plant

Wrightia tinctoria is a small deciduous tree found almost through-out India. The bark is sometimes used to adulterate the bark of *Holarrhena antidysentrica,* which is covered in Chapter 3, "Gastro-intestinal agents," for the treatment of amebiasis. The leaves contain indigotin, which yields 0.3-0.5 percent of the dye indigo, known as Mysore Pala Indigo, used for dyeing fabric.[4] The tree is useful medic-inally. The leaves are used in Ayurveda for toothache and hyperten-sion; the bark and seeds for dyspepsia, flatulence, leprosy, psoriasis, and fever.[5] The leaves are especially useful in skin problems, and in Siddha medicine forms part of many combination drugs used for the treatment of psoriasis.

Indigotin, indirubin, tryptanthrin, isatin, anthranilate, and rutin are the major constituents isolated from *Wrightia tinctoria.*[6] The leaves also contain β-amyrin, lupeol, β-sitosterol, and ursolic acid.[7]

Coconut oil containing the leaf extract of *Wrightia tinctoria* showed significant analgesic and anti-inflammatory activity.[8] In mice, *Wrightia tinctoria* in emulsion showed reversal of parake-ratosis, which is a feature of psoriasis.[9]

In an open running trial, 281 patients with psoriasis were treated between 1980 and 1987. The trial drug coded "777" oil was obtained by exposing fresh leaves of *Wrightia tinctoria* in coconut oil to sun-light for 3 days, followed by filtering off the oil. Patients were given 5 ml of the oil twice a day and patients were also asked to apply the oil over the affected regions and expose these areas to sunlight for 5-10 minutes.[10,11] There were 67 dropouts. Of the remaining 214 pa-tients who completed the course of treatment, 108 patients had com-plete relief, 49 patients had marked relief, 39 had moderate relief, 17 had mild relief, and 1 patient had no relief. Disappearance of scaling was taken as mild relief. Disappearance of scales and eyrthematous changes were considered as moderate relief, transformation of papu-lar to macular lesions as marked relief, whereas total disappearance of all clinical symptoms was considered as complete relief. A total of 30 patients were taken to undertake a detailed study for biopsy and also followed up for 4 years. There was no recurrence in 50 percent of the cases, although in 30 percent recurrence was postponed to more than 3 years. Recurrence was accompanied by great reduction in intensity, and there was no occurrence of any of the complications such as arthritis and carona psoriatica.[10]

Nonspecific dermatitis

In an open trial, 20 patients with histologically confirmed nonspecific dermatitis, who presented extensive skin lesions, burning, and intense itching, were treated with oil of *Wrightia tinctoria* taken orally twice a day, as well as the oil being applied topically, followed by short exposure to sunlight for a period of 6 weeks. Of these, 14 patients showed complete relief and no relapse was observed for more than 3 years.[10]

The acute toxicity (72 hours) of 777 oil prepared from *Wrightia tinctoria* leaves was studied in mice and rats and the LD_{50} was found to be 45 ml·kg^{-1} in mice and 30 ml·kg^{-1} in rats. A 30-day subacute toxicity carried out at three dosage levels—1, 5, and 10 ml of the oil extract with controls—was found to be nontoxic. Major organs such as liver, kidney, spleen, heart, and lung showed no toxicity or histopathological changes.[10]

NOTES

1. Syed TA, Ahmad SA, Holt AH, Ahmad SA, Ahmad SH, Afzal M. Management of psoriasis with *Aloe vera* extract in a hydrophilic cream: A placebo-controlled, double-blind study. *Trop Med Int Health* 1:505-509 (1996).

2. Natarajan S, Paily PP. Effect of topical *Hydrocotyle asiatica* in psoriasis. *Indian J Dermatol* 18:82-85 (1973).

3. Sampson JH, Raman A, Karlsen G, Navsaria H, Leigh IM. *In vitro* keratinocyte antiproliferant effect of *Centella asiatica* extract and triterpenoid saponins. *Phytomedicine* 8:230-235 (2001).

4. *The wealth of India, raw materials* (vol. X, pp. 588-590). New Delhi: Publications and Information Directorate, CSIR, 1976. ·

5. Warrier PK, Nambiar VPK, Ramankutty C (eds.), *Indian medicinal plants* (vol. 5, pp. 417-419). Madras: Orient Longmans Ltd. 1996.

6. Muruganandam AV, Bhattacharya SK, Ghosal S. Indole and flavonoid constituents of *Wrightia tinctoria, W. tomentosa* and *W. coccinea. Indian J Chem* 39B(2):125-131 (2000).

7. Rao MN, Rao EV, Rao VS. Triterpenoid components of the leaves and pods of *Wrightia tinctoria. Curr Sci* 35:518-519 (1966).

8. Ghosh D, Thejomoorthy P, Veluchamy G. Anti-inflammatory, analgesic and antipyretic activities of 777 oil—A Siddha medicine. *Bull Med Ethnobot Res* 6(2-4):141-154 (1985).

9. Mitra SK, Seshadri SJ, Venkatranganna MV, Gopumadhavan S. Reversal of parakeratosis, a feature of psoriasis by *Wrightia tinctoria* (in emulsion)—Histological evaluation based on mouse tail test. *Indian J Dermatol* 43(3):102-104 (1998).

10. Krishnamurthy JR, Kalaimani S, Veluchamy G. Clinical study of *vetpalai* (*Wrightia tinctoria* Linn.) oil in the treatment of *kalanjaga padai* (psoriasis). *J Res Ayur Siddha* 1:247-258 (1980).

11. Clinical and experimental studies on the efficacy of 777 oil—A Siddha preparation in the treatment of kalanjagapadai (psoriasis). Monograph published by Central Council for Research in Ayurveda and Siddha. New Delhi: Ministry of Health and Family Welfare, Government of India, 1987.

WOUND HEALING PLANTS

Plants have served as healing agents for wounds since time immemorial. The healing of wounds has been dealt with as separate topics in the major Ayurvedic texts of Sushruta, Jivika, and Vagbhata, because of the importance attached to this topic as a matter of immediate concern in those days owing to the living environment, and the frequent battles and wars. The *Sushruta Samhita* has two separate chapters dealing with the treatment of the injuries and the handling of patients, describing the use of more than one hundred plants for the treatment of wounds, both as single drugs and in combination.[1] Sushruta has mentioned not only procedures and drugs to obtain a clean wound *(vrana shodan)* followed by healing *(vrana ropan)* but also medicines to help prevent the formation of keloid scars.[2]

Aloe barbadensis *Mill. (Family: Liliaceae)*

Latin: *Aloe vera* Tourn. ex Linn.	Hindi: Ghi-kuvar
Sanskrit: Ghrita kumari, kumari	Tamil: Kattalai
English: Barbados Aloe, Indian Aloe	

Aloe barabadensis is a perennial plant with succulent leaves originally introduced from Africa into India, now found in a semiwild state in many parts of the country. The leaves are widely used in Ayurvedic medicine. Its usage varies corresponding to the part of the leaf being used—the outer thick covering of the leaf, in which the steamed leaf without pulp is applied to abscesses; the inner yellow juice or exudate, which flows out from the leaf after cutting, darkens and solidifies after a while to a dark mass called aloes containing anthraquinones, is a drastic purgative; and the inner mucilaginous leaf pulp or gel, composed mainly of carbohydrates, is considered a tonic for the liver, in female complaints such as amenorrhea and dysmenorrhea, and during menopause, good for the eyes, and for the treatment of burns, wounds, and skin diseases.[3,4]

Aloe barbadensis gel contains about 98.5 percent of water with polysaccharides as the major constituents—pectins, hemicelluloses, glucomannan, acemannan, the major carbohydrate component and mannose derivatives where mannose-6-phosphate is the major sugar component. Also present are amino acids; lipids; sterols such as campesterol, lupeol, and β-sitosterol; tannins; and enzymes.[5] In addition, glycoproteins with wound healing activity[6] and aloeride, a potent immunostimulatory polysaccharide component,[7] have been isolated.

The topical[8,9] and oral[8] wound healing activity of *Aloe vera* has been extensively studied. Studies on the healing of dermal wounds observed that there were increased levels of collagen in the granulation tissue[10] and improved synthesis of glycosaminoglycan component[11] of the extracellular matrix in a healing wound, thereby contributing to improved wound healing. *Aloe vera* also improved healing of full thickness wounds in diabetic rats, where both healing and anti-inflammatory processes are retarded because of diabetes.[12] In addition, *Aloe vera* helped faster healing of burn wounds in guinea pigs by exhibiting an antibacterial effect,[13] and in rats by its anti-inflammatory and aiding the wound healing activity.[14] The inflammatory process was inhibited by reduction of leukocyte adhesion and of inflammation-causing cytokines.[15] *Aloe vera* was also found to reverse retardation of wound healing caused by silver sulfadiazine[16] and steroids.[17] Other useful activities of *Aloe vera* gel, when applied externally, include a beneficial effect on skin regeneration[18] and its antioxidant activity.[19] The antioxidant activity is dependent on the age of the plant—3-year old plants showing greater antioxidant activity than butylated hydroxy toluene (BHT), α-tocopherol—2- and 4-year old plants, and also higher levels of polysaccharides and flavonoids.[19]

Among the constituents contributing to the observed activity, two immunomodulatory compounds were isolated from the gel of *Aloe vera*.[20] Subsequently, acemannan has been shown to accelerate wound healing.[21] Mannose-6-phosphate, a major sugar in *Aloe vera* gel, improved wound healing in mice over saline controls.[22] A glyco-protein fraction has been shown to improve wound healing via cell proliferation and migration.[6] In addition, an active glycoprotein frac-tion has been shown to exhibit radical scavenging effect apart from inhibition of cyclooxygenase-2 and thromboxane A 2 synthase inhi-bition in vitro.[23] Aloeride, a new potent immunostimulatory poly-saccharide present up to 0.015 percent of the dry weight of aloe juice, has been isolated.[7] Thus, many components of *Aloe* gel have been shown to play a useful role in wound healing.

The therapeutic effects of *Aloe vera* were examined in a number of indications in dermal ischemia due to burns, frostbite, electrical in-jury, distal dying flap, and intra-arterial drug abuse. In burn patients and those suffering from frostbite, patients healed without tissue loss. Tissue necrosis was reversed in intra-arterial drug-abuse patients. The results suggest that *Aloe* acts by inhibition of thromboxane A2 production and by maintenance of homeostasis both in the wound and also in the surrounding tissue.[24]

In a placebo-controlled study involving 27 patients with partial thickness burns were treated with *Aloe vera* gel. Patients treated with *Aloe vera* gel showed faster recovery in 11.8 days as compared to those treated with petroleum jelly gauze (18.2 days), which was con-sidered statistically significant.[25]

In a randomized double-blind study, 100 patients with 10-40 per-cent burns had wounds dressed either with *Aloe vera* extract or rou-tine dressing done every 3 days. The main wound healing time was significantly lower ($p < 0.001$) in the case of those treated with *Aloe vera* as was bacteriological control ($p < 0.012$).[26]

There are a number of factors involved in the use of *Aloe vera* gel. The gel itself is preferably used fresh due to possible decomposition[5] and also the probable negative effect on the clinical outcome of added stabilizers[27] and the further processing that the gel undergoes.[28] Experimental studies have shown that *Aloe vera* gel may delay wound healing in the later stages.[29] In first- and second-degree burns in mice, *Aloe vera* gel increased the rate of healing, improved epithelialization, and reduced inflammation, but proved to be not very effective for third-degree burns.[30] As information becomes available on the contribution of the various components of the gel and the time of application to wound healing, it should be possible to obtain more consistent results, since negative trials have also been reported with *Aloe* gel. More clinical trials are required to further validate the use of *Aloe vera* gel. The topical use of the gel is generally considered safe. Cases of irritation may be attributed to the presence of traces of anthraquinones. However, the possibility of allergic reactions needs to be borne in mind.[5]

Centella asiatica *(Linn.) Urban (Family: Apiaceae)*

The use of *Centella asiatica* (see Plate 8 in color gallery) in chronic venous insufficiency has been covered in Chapter 6, "Cardiovascular drugs," and its use as a mental rejuvenator in Chapter 12. *Centella asiatica* is well known in Ayurveda[31,32] as a local stimulant of the skin, and is used therefore in skin diseases, such as herpes, eczema, and psoriasis and in wound healing.

Extracts of *Centella asiatica* have been evaluated in experimental animals. Thus both alcoholic[33] and aqueous extract[34] of *Centella asiatica* when applied to open wounds in rats showed an increased cell proliferation and protein synthesis. Treated wounds healed faster as compared to untreated controls showing faster epithelialization and rate of wound contraction[33,34] in experimental wounds. The extract as well as the total triterpenes—asiaticoside, asiatic acid, and madecassic acid reconstituted from the plant in the ratio 4:3:3 have been shown to increase the percentage of collagen in human skin fibroblast cultures[35] and also to stimulate glycosaminoglycan synthesis in experimental wounds in rats.[36] These three triterpenes have been shown to hasten wound healing by increasing human collagen I synthesis.[37] In addition, it was shown that the presence of the glucose moiety was not necessary for collagen synthesis.[37] Asiaticoside improved wound healing in both normal and delayed healing models owing to increased collagen synthesis and angiogenesis,[38] and was also shown to enhance induction of antioxidant levels at initial levels of healing in excision type cutaneous wounds in rats.[39]

In a study with 27 patients with slow healing wounds of varied etiology, patients were treated topically with an ointment containing 1 percent *Centella asiatica* extract or with a 2 percent powder in addition to three intramuscular injections of asiaticoside per week. Accelerated healing of wounds was seen in 55 percent of patients, with improvement in 15 percent. The remaining 30 percent of patients showed no perceptible effect of treatment.[40] In another study, 64 percent healing was observed when a preparation in which asiaticoside was the major ingredient was used in patients with intractable and soiled wounds.[41] In another open study, a formulation containing 89.5 percent of *Centella asiatica* produced healing in 64 percent patients, whereas 16 percent showed improvement in wounds.[42] In second- and third-degree burns, topical application of a preparation of *Centella asiatica* hastened healing, averted infection, and prevented the formation of hypertrophic scars.[43]

In some individuals, hypersensitivity reactions can occur when *Centella asiatica* is applied topically;[44] however, it has been suggested that this could be due to other ingredients.[45]

NOTES

1. Idris M, Singh B, Singh G. The use of medicinal plants in wound healing (pp. 37-41). Lucknow: Proc Natl Sem Use of Traditional Medicinal Plants in Skin Care, CIMAP, November 25-26, 1994.

2. Deshpande PJ, Pathak SN, Gode JD. Wound healing under the influence of certain indigenous drugs. In Udupa KN, Chaturvedi GN, Tripathi SN (eds.), *Advances in research in Indian medicine* (pp. 269-303). Varanasi: Banaras Hindu University, 1970.

3. Pandey G. *Dravyaguna vijnana (materia medica—vegetable drugs)* (1st edn., vol. II, pp. 312-320). Varanasi: Krishnadas Academy, 2001.

4. Lad V, Frawley D. *The yoga of herbs* (pp. 100-101). Santa Fe: Lotus Press, 1986.

5. *WHO monographs on selected medicinal plants* (vol. 1, pp. 43-49). Geneva: World Health Organization, 1999.

6. Choi SW, Son BW, Son YS, Park YI, Lee SK, Chung MH. The wound-healing effect of glycoprotein fraction isolated from *Aloe vera*. *Br J Dermatol* 145:535-545 (2001).

7. Pugh N, Ross SA, ElSohly MA, Pasco DS. Characterization of Aloeride, a new high molecular-weight polysaccharide from *Aloe vera* with potent immunostimulatory activity. *J Agric Food Chem* 49:1030-1034 (2001).

8. Davis RH, Leitner MG, Russo JM, Byrne ME. Wound healing. Oral and topical activity of *Aloe vera. J Am Podiatr Med Assoc* 79:559-562 (1989).

9. Heggers JP, Kucukcelebi A, Stabenau CJ, Ko F, Broemling JD, Winters WD. Wound healing effects of Aloe gel and other topical antibacterial agents in rat skin. *Phytother Res* 9:455-457 (1995).

10. Chithra P, Sajithlal GB, Chandrakasan G. Influence of *Aloe vera* on collagen characteristics in healing dermal wounds in rats. *Mol Cell Biochem* 181:71-76 (1998).

11. Chithra P, Sajithlal GB, Chandrakasan G. Influence of *Aloe vera* on the glycosaminoglycans in the matrix of healing dermal wounds in rats. *J Ethnopharmacol* 59:179-186 (1998).

12. Chithra P, Sajithlal GB, Chandrakasan G. Influence of *Aloe vera* on the healing of dermal wounds in diabetic rats. *J Ethnopharmacol* 59:195-201 (1998).

13. Rodríguez-Bigas M, Cruz NI, Suárez A. Comparative evaluation of *Aloe vera* in the management of burn wounds in guinea pigs. *Plast Reconstr Surg* 81:386-389 (1988).

14. Somboonwong J, Thanamittramanee S, Jariyapongskul A, Patumraj S. Therapeutic effects of *Aloe vera* on cutaneous microcirculation and wound healing in second degree burn model in rats. *J Med Assoc Thai* 83:417-425 (2000).

15. Duansak D, Somboonwong J, Patumraj S. Effects of *Aloe vera* on leukocyte adhesion and TNF-alpha and IL-6 levels in burn wounded rats. *Clin Hemorheol Microcirc* 29:239-246 (2003).

16. Muller MJ, Hollyoak MA, Moaveni Z, Brown TL, Herndon DN, Heggers JP. Retardation of wound healing by silver sulfadiazine is reversed by *Aloe vera* and nystatin. *Burns* 29:834-836 (2003).

17. Udupa SL, Udupa AL, Kulkarni DR. A comparative study of the effect of some indigenous drugs on normal and steroid-depressed healing. *Fitoterapia* LXIX:507-510 (1998).

18. Verma SBS, Schulze HJ, Steigleder GK. The effect of externally applied remedies containing *Aloe vera* gel on the proliferation of the epidermis. *Parfumerie und Kosmetik* 70:452-459 (1989).

19. Hu Y, Xu J, Hu Q. Evaluation of antioxidant potential of *Aloe vera* (*Aloe barbadensis* Miller) extracts. *J Agri Food Chem* 51:7788-7791 (2003).

20. t'Hart LA, van Enckevort PH, van Djik H, Zaat R, de Silva KT, Labadie RP. Two functionally and chemically distinct immunomodulatory compounds in the gel of *Aloe vera. J Ethnopharmacol* 23:61-71 (1988).

21. Tizard AU et al. Effects of acemannan, a complex carbohydrate on wound healing in young and aged rats. *Wounds, a compendium of clinical research and practice* 6:201-209 (1995).

22. Davis RH, Donato JJ, Hartmann GM, Haas RC. Anti-inflammatory and wound healing activity of a growth substance in *Aloe vera. J Am Podiatr Med Assoc* 84:77-81 (1994).

23. Yagi A, Kabash A, Mizuno K, Moustafa SM, Khalifa TI, Tsuji H. Radical scavenging glycoprotein inhibiting cyclooxgenase-2 and thromboxane A2 synthase from *Aloe vera* gel. *Planta Med* 69:269-271 (2003).

24. Heggers JP, Pelley RP, Robson MC. Beneficial effects of *Aloe* in wound healing. *Phytother Res* 7 (suppl.):S48-S52 (1993).

25. Visuthikosol V, Chowchuen B, Sukwanarat Y, Sriuriratana S, Boonpucknavig V. Effect of *Aloe vera* gel on healing of burn wounds: A clinical and histologicial study. *J Med Assoc Thai* 78:403-409 (1995).

26. Murtaza A, Hatwar SK. *Aloe* extract in management of burn wounds. *Curr Med Trends* 6(1):1071-1077 (2002).

27. Tyler VE. *Herbs of choice, the therapeutic use of phytomedicinals* (pp. 155-157). New York: Pharmaceuticals Products Press, 1994.

28. Reynolds T, Dweck AC. *Aloe vera* leaf gel: A review update. *J Ethnopharmacol* 68:3-37 (1999).

29. Roberts DB, Travis EL. Acemannan containing wound-dressing gel reduces radiation induced skin reactions in C3H mice. *International J Radiation Oncology, Biology, Physics* 32:1047-1052 (1995).

30. Bunyapraphatsara N, Jirakulcaiwong S, Thiruwarapan S, Manokul. The efficacy of *Aloe vera* cream in the treatment of first, second and third degree burns in mice. *Phytomedicine* 2:247-251 (1996).

31. Nadkarni AK. *Dr KM Nadkarni's Indian materia medica* (vol. 1, pp. 662-666). Bombay: Popular Prakashan, 1976.

32. Gogte VM. *Ayurvedic pharmacology and therapeutic uses of medicinal plants* (pp. 466-468). Trans. SPARC, Mumbai: Bharatiya Vidhya Bhavan, 2000.

33. Suguna L, Sivakumar P, Chandrakasan G. Effects of *Centella asiatica* extract on dermal wound healing in rats. *Indian J Exp Biol* 34:1208-1211 (1996).

34. Sunilkumar, Parameshwaraiah S, Shivakumar HG. Evaluation of topical formulations of aqueous extract of *Centella asiatica* on open wounds in rats. *Indian J Exp Biol* 36:569-572 (1998).

35. Tenni R, Zanaboni G, De Agostini MP, Rossi A, Bendotti C, Cetta G. Effect of the triterpenoid fraction of *Centella asiatica* on macromolecules of the connective matrix in human skin fibroblasts cultures. *Italian J Biochem* 37:69-77 (1988).

36. Maquart FX, Chastang F, Simeon A, Birembaut P, Gillery P, Wegrowski Y. Triterpenes from *Centella asiatica* stimulate extracellular matrix accumulation in rat experimental wounds. *Eur J Dermatol* 9:289-296 (1999).

37. Bonte F, Dumas M, Chaudagne C, Meybeck A. The influence of asiatic acid, madecassic acid and asiatocoside in human collagen I synthesis. *Planta Med* 60:133-135 (1994).

38. Shukla A, Rasik AM, Jain GK, Shankar R, Kulshrestha DK, Dhawan BN. *In vitro* and *in vivo* wound healing activity of asiaticoside isolated from *Centella asiatica. J Ethnopharmacol* 65:1-11 (1999).

39. Shukla A, Rasik AM, Dhawan BN. Asiaticoside-induced elevation of antioxidant levels in healing wounds. *Phytother Res* 13:50-54 (1999).

40. Kieswetter H. Erfahrungsbericht über Behandlung von Wunden mit Asiaticosid (Madecassol). *Wien Med Wochensch* 114:124-126 (1964).

41. Morisset R, Côte NG, Panisset JC, Jemni L, Camirand P, Brodeur A. Evaluation of the healing activity of Hydrocotyle tincture in the treatment of wounds. *Phytother Res* 1:117-121 (1987).

42. Bosse J, Papillon J, Frenette G, Dansereau J, Cadotte M, Le Lorier J. Clinical study of a new antikeloid agent. *Annals of Plastic Surgery* 3:13-21 (1979).

43. Farnswoth NR, Bunyapraphatsara N (eds.), *Thai medicinal plants.* Bangkok: Prachachon, 1992, quoted in *WHO monographs on selected medicinal plants* (vol. 1, pp. 77-85). Geneva: World Health Organization, 1999.

44. Izu R, Aguirre A, Gil N, Diaz-Perez JL. Allergic contact dermatitis from a cream containing *Centella asiatica* extract. *Contact Dermatitis* 26:192-193 (1992).

45. Hausen BM. *Centella asiatica* (Indian pennywort), an effective therapeutic but weak sensitizer. *Contact Dermatitis* 29:175-179 (1993).

OTHER WOUND HEALING PLANTS

Azadirachta indica A Juss. (Family: Meliaceae)

Azadirachta indica is among other plants that have been investigated for burn wounds. The tolerability of a preparation of *Azadirachta indica* was studied in seven patients with second-degree burns and was found to be good, with an initial stinging, which passed off on continued application, and no other adverse effects reported. Healing took place in 4 weeks with burns epithelialized and scars being soft, supple, and well pigmented. A randomized comparative trial was then conducted with 17 patients who received either *Azadirachta* cream or silver sulfadiazine. Ulcer scores at the end of 2 weeks were found significantly less in the *neem* group; epithelialization was better at 88.89 percent in the *neem* group as compared to 62.5 percent in the silver sulfadiazine group. In addition, in the *neem* group, the healing of cartilaginous areas was without deformity. Only in the silver sulfadiazine group were complications such as sepsis, contractures, and hypertrophy of scars noticed, leading the authors to conclude that *neem* appeared to be a safe and effective prohealer.[1]

NOTE

1. Rege NN, Dahanukar SA, Ginde VK, Thatte UM, Bapat RD. Safety and efficacy of *Azadirachta indica* in patients with second degree burns. *Indian Practioner* 52(4):240-248 (1999).

FRACTURE HEALING PLANTS

The subject of fractures, their etiology, pathology, specific signs and symptoms, treatment, and possible complications have been dealt with in detail in the *Sushruta Samhita* dated 600 BC.[1,2] In fact, there are certain families that specialize in the setting of bones and their treatment using herbs in South India. Several plants have been used in India for hastening the healing of fractures and for strengthening the bones. Of these *Cissus quadrangularis* has been studied scientifically. There is increased interest in such plants, not only for help in bone healing when injured but also because of their possible use in osteoporosis.

Cissus quadrangularis *Linn. (Family: Vitaceae)*

Latin: *Vitis quadrangularis* Wall	Hindi: Hadjod
Sanskrit: Asthisamharaka, Vajravalli	Tamil: Perandai
English: Bonesetter, The edible-stemmed vine	

Cissus quadrangularis (see Plate 10 in color gallery) is a slender perennial climber with quadrangular stems, found leafless when old, growing throughout the hotter parts of India. The leaves and stems are commonly used as a vegetable in South India: as a paste with lentils known as chutney; or sometimes the stem juice is added to dried preparations such as *papad* that are later fried and eaten. The stem is considered to improve digestion and to be useful in piles, and is used widely in healing of fractures. The stems are administered orally and also applied topically to help heal fractures in dislocation and traumatic injury.[2,3] The Sanskrit, Hindi, and English names refer to this bone-knitting property of the plant.

The plant contains unsymmetric tetracyclic triterpenes apart from δ-amyrin and δ-amyrone in the hexane extract. In addition, several alicyclic lipid constituents have been isolated. From the methanol fraction 3, 3′, 4, 4′-tetrahydroxybiphenyl was also isolated.[4] The plant also contains calcium oxalate, vitamin C (398 mg per 100g fresh, tender stem), and β-carotene.[5]

Experimental studies using S^{35} were carried out to study the normal healing pattern of fracture in rats.[6] Weekly intramuscular injection of the alcoholic extract of *Cissus quadrangularis* (0.5 ml equivalent to 0.5 g of fresh drug) was found to accelerate fracture healing in small animals.[7,8] Histochemical and biochemical studies showed a beneficial effect of the herb.[9] Isotopic studies using S^{35}, P^{32}, and Sr^{85} showed that systemic use of the herb reduced healing time[7,8,10] by one-third.[12] Topical application of a paste of *Cissus quadrangularis* increased the healing rate of treated animals by 10-14 days.[11] The total extract has a definite influence on both the organic and mineral phase of fracture healing in experimental animals. Ca^{45} uptake studies showed that there was earlier calcification and remodeling owing to the drug. In addition, there was a 90 percent increase in tensile strength in treated animals as compared to 60 percent in untreated controls.[12] Intramuscular administration of the drug showed a stimulatory effect neutralizing the effect on cortisone-treated fractures.[13] In ovariectomized rats, feeding for 3 months with 500-750 mg·kg^{-1} of an ethanolic extract of *Cissus quadrangularis* showed significant increase in biomechanical strength comparable to raloxifene, a selective estrogen receptor modulator currently used to treat osteoporosis.[14]

In an open trial with controls, 78 patients were enrolled of which in 60 patients a paste of *Cissus quadrangularis* was applied after the fractured fragments were reduced, and the bone was immobilized in the usual fashion with a cast. Of the patients who served as controls, 18 were reduced and immobilized with a cast with no additional treatment. Patients were monitored every week and also checked using X-ray. The patients were assessed based on callus formation, improvement in the clinical picture, time of immobilization, and time required to return to normalcy. Patients using *Cissus quadrangularis* were found to experience some degree of itching, which has been attributed variously to the content of carnosine[2] and calcium oxalate.[5] Decreased swelling, greater freedom of movement; smaller callus formation, and 30-40 percent reduction in period of immobilization were some of the benefits of treatment with *Cissus quadrangularis*.[2,15,16]

In clinical practice in patients of jaw-bone fractures, it was found that addition of *Ocimum sanctum* and *Cissus quadrangularis* along with the usual management of such fractures was found to reduce significantly the time of immobilization.[17]

Cissus quadrangularis is often used in food in South India to aid digestion. It is usually well tolerated in the usual doses.[18] When the paste of the plant is applied topically, patients were found to experience some degree of itching, due to the content of carnosine[2] and calcium oxalate[5] that subsided without any treatment in a few days. This itching sensation can also occur when taken orally because of the calcium oxalate content. In experiments with *Salmonella typhimurium* tester strains *Cissus quadrangularis* was found to be mutagenic,[19] although the relevance of such experiments for human beings is not clear.

NOTES

1. *Sushrutha samhita,* trans. Bhishagratna KL (vol. II, pp. 97-100, "Nidanasthanam," chapter XV; pp. 279-288, "Chikitsasthanam," chapter III). Varanasi: Chowkhamba Sanskrit Series Office, 1991.

2. Prasad GC, Udupa KN. Role of *Cissus quadrangularis* on fracture healing. In Udupa KN, Chaturvedi GN, Tripathi SN (eds.). *Advances in research in Indian medicine* (pp. 163-196). Varanasi: Banaras Hindu University, 1970.

3. Pandey G. *Dravyaguna vijnana (materia medica—vegetable drugs)* (1st edn., vol. I, pp. 239-243). Varanasi: Krishnadas Academy, 1998.

4. Mehta M, Kaur N, Bhutani KK. Determination of marker constituents from *Cissus quadrangularis* Linn. and their quantitation by HPTLC and HPLC. *Phytochem Anal* 12:91-95 (2001).

5. Murty PBR, Seshadri TR. Chemical composition of *Vitis quadrangularis* (Wall.). *Proc Indian Acad Sci* 9:121-127 (1939).

6. Singh LM, Arnikar HJ, Udupa KN. Studies on the healing of fractures using S^{35} (Part I). *Indian J Med Sci* 15:545-550 (1961).

7. Udupa KN, Arnikar HJ, Singh LM. Experimental studies of the use of *Cissus quadrangularis* in healing of fractures (Part II). *Indian J Med Sci* 15:551-557(1961).

8. Singh LM, Udupa KN. Studies on *Cissus quadrangularis* in fracture using phosphorus[32]. Part III. *Indian J Med Sci* 16:926-931 (1962).

9. Udupa KN, Prasad GC. Chemical and histochemical studies on the organic constituents in fracture repair in rats. *J Bone and Joint Surg* 45(4):770-779 (1963).

10. Guha A, Prasad GC, Udupa KN. Studies on fracture healing *in vivo* using radioactive strontium. *Indian J Med Res* 51:298-303 (1963).

11. Udupa KN, Prasad GC. Further studies on the effect of *Cissus quadrangularis* in accelerating fracture healing. *Indian J Med Res* 52:26-35 (1964).

12. Udupa KN, Prasad GC. Biomechanical and calcium[45] studies on the effect of *Cissus quadrangularis* in fracture repair. *Indian J Med Res.* 52:480-487 (1964).

13. Prasad GC, Udupa KN. Effect of *Cissus quadrangularis* on the healing of cortisone treated fractures. *Indian J Med Res* 51:667-676 (1963).

14. Shirwaikar A, Khan S, Malini S. Antiosteoporotic effect of ethanol extract of *Cissus quadrangularis* on ovariectomized rat. *J Ethnopharmacol* 89:245-250 (2003).

15. Prasad GC, Srivastava TP, Udupa KN. A study of fracture healing with local application of *Cissus quadrangularis. J Med Surg* (June 1965) cited in note 2 above.

16. Udupa KN, Prasad GC, Sen SP. The effect of phytogenic anabolic steroid in the acceleration of fracture repair. *Life Sci* 4:317 -327 (1965).

17. Pradhan R. Herbal remedies in dental practice (p. 21). Lucknow: Proc Natl Sem Use of Traditional Medicinal Plants in Skin Care, CIMAP, November 25-26, 1994.

18. *Selected medicinal plants of India. A monograph on identity, safety and clinical usage* (pp. 93-95). Bombay: Chemexcil, Basic Chemicals, Pharmaceuticals and Cosmetics Export Promotion Council, 1992.

19. Sivaswamy SN, Balachandran B, Balanehru S, Sivaramakrishnan VM. Mutagenic activity of South Indian food items. *Indian J Exp Biol* 29:730-737 (1991).

Chapter 10

Gynecological Agents

Plants have been extensively used in Ayurveda to maintain the health of the female reproductive organs. These have been used mostly as combination drugs, and single plants have not been the subject of much scientific investigation. Much of the scientific interest has been directed toward control of fertility, which is not covered in this book. The herbs often used for the treatment of common problems of women are *Asparagus racemosus, Boerhaavia diffusa, Glycyrrhiza glabra, Saraca asoca, Symplocos racemosa, Withania somnifera, Mesua ferrea,* and others.

GALACTAGOGUE

Lactation is initiated by an increase in levels of prolactin, a hormone produced by the pituitary glands. A number of plants have been used in Ayurveda to stimulate milk production, in case of lactational inadequacy, both taken internally and also applied externally. However, there is a dearth of scientific information on such plants.

Asparagus racemosus *Willd.*
(Family: Liliaceae, Asparagaceae)

The use of roots of *Asparagus racemosus* for the treatment of duodenal ulcers has been covered in Chapter 3. The roots are used in Ayurveda for stimulating milk flow and protecting pregnant women against threatened abortion. In postpartum and estrogen-primed rats intramuscular injection of the alcoholic extract of the roots was

doi:10.1300/5683_10

shown to exert a lactogenic effect, increasing milk yield, and breast lobular-alveolar tissue, which has been attributed to an increase of prolactin levels or to a release of corticosteroids.[1] A galactagogue action was also seen in buffaloes[2] and goats.[3] The saponin fraction, especially shatavarin I, has been shown to have an antioxytocic action on uterine tissue and an anti-ADH[4,5] activity supporting its use in threatened abortions. In an open exploratory study, 15 women with deficient milk during lactation were given 2 tablets of a preparation containing *Asparagus racemosus* twice a day after meals. The trial drug contained 40 mg *Asparagus racemosus* extract, 10 mg processed iron pyrites, and 400 mg dicalcium phosphate. Out of the 15 women, 11 reported an increase in milk yield together with improved appetite. Four patients independently tried stopping the intake of the drug and the milk yield was found to decrease, which improved once again with the resumption of the intake of the drug.[6]

In a randomized controlled trial of *Asparagus racemosus,* increase in milk yield was not found different from placebo.[7] The preparation contained other herbs although *Asparagus racemosus* was the major herb in the trial preparation. The results are not necessarily attributable to *Asparagus racemosus* because of the addition of other herbs. The trial preparation also led to a decrease in prolactin levels. However, considering the reputation of *Asparagus racemosus* in increasing milk yield, studies to clarify possible reasons for this lack of response are required, preferably after standardization of the product.

NOTES

1. Sabnis PB, Gaitonde BB, Jetmalani M. Effects of alcoholic extract of *Asparagus racemosus* on mammary glands of rats. *Indian J Exp Biol* 6:55-57 (1968).

2. Patel AB, Kanitkar UK. *Asparagus racemosus* Willd-form Bordi, as a galactogogue in buffaloes. *Indian Vet J* 46:718-721 (1969).

3. Vihan VS, Panwar HS. A note on the galactogogue activity of *Asparagus racemosus* in lactating goats. *Indian J Animal Health* 27:177-178 (1988).

4. Gaitonde BB, Jetmalani M. Anti-oxytocic action of saponin isolated from *Asparagus racemosus* Willd. *(shatavari)* on uterine muscle. *Arch Int Pharmacodyn Ther* 179(1):121-129 (1969).

5. Gaitonde BB, Jetmalani M. Anti-oxytocic and anti-ADH activity of saponin fraction isolated from *Asparagus racemosus* Willd. *Indian J Pharmacy* 31:175-176 (1969).

6. Joglekar GV, Ahuja RH, Balwani JH. Galactogogue effect of *Asparagus racemosus*. A preliminary communication. *Indian Med J* 61(7):165 (1967).

7. Sharma S, Ramji S, Kumari S, Bapna JS. Randomized, controlled trial of *Asparagus racemosus (shatavari)* as a lactogogue in lactational inadequacy. *Indian Paediatr* 33:675-677 (1996).

ANTILEUKORRHEAL PLANTS

Leukorrhea or the white discharge from the vagina is commonly seen in women and termed *sweta pradara* in Sanskrit (*sweta:* white; *pradara:* discharge or flow). Clinical trial data with single herbs is scanty. A single herb for which an exploratory trial was conducted is *Boerhaavia repanda*.

Boerhaavia repanda *Willd. (Family: Nyctaginaceae)*

Boerhaavia repanda is a straggly herb found growing throughout India. The leaves and tender shoots are used as a vegetable. The root has anthelmintic activity and the root powder showed a significant therapeutic effect in the treatment of leukorrhea.[1] Fresh roots of *Boerhaavia repanda* were collected, shade-dried, powdered, and used in doses of 500 mg.

In an open clinical study, 32 patients in the age group of 20-38 years with leukorrhea were asked to take 500 mg (1 tablespoon) of *Boerhaavia repanda* root powder twice a day for 30 days. All patients reported marked improvement within a few days of treatment; white discharge stopped after 15 days but patients were asked to continue treatment for a further 2 weeks. No side effects were noticed, except for a little nausea.[2]

In an open study with controls, 20 female patients aged between 20 and 38 years with leukorrhea were asked to take 500 mg of the powder twice a day with milk or water for 15 days. A control group of 5 patients were maintained as control. At the end of the treatment period all 20 patients were found cured.[3]

NOTES

1. *The wealth of India, raw materials* (vol. 2, p. 176). New Delhi: Publications and Information Directorate, CSIR, 1988.
2. Singh SP, Grover SP. Some preliminary observations on the antileucorrheal effect of *Boerhaavia repanda* roots. *Indian J Forest* 2(4):370-371 (1979).
3. Singh SP. Therapeutic efficacy of *punarnava* (*Boerhaavia repanda* Willd.) root powder. *J Res Edu Indian Med* X(1):23-25 (1991).

ANTIMENORRHAGIAL PLANTS

Excessive loss of blood during menstruation is termed menorrhagia. It has been suggested as due to hormonal imbalance in estrogen and progesterone. Bleeding between periods is termed metrorrhagia. Excessive bleeding is termed *raktapradara* (rakta: blood; *pradara:* flow) in Ayurveda. A number of plants, especially those containing tannins, have been used to control menorrhagia; however, very few plants have been subjected to clinical trials especially as a single drug.

Saraca asoca *(Roxb.) de Wilde (Family: Caesalpiniaceae)*

Sanskrit: Ashoka	Hindi: Asok
Tamil: Asogam	

Saraca asoca is a small evergreen tree found almost everywhere in India. The stem bark is extensively used in Ayurveda for the treatment of menorrhagia especially due to uterine fibroids, uterine disorders, and leukorrhea, and to treat depression in women.[1] The bark is used in numerous multiplant preparations in the market. It has, however, been little investigated as a single drug. The bark has numerous polyphenolic compounds—procyanidin B2, leucopelargonidin, leucopelargonidin-3-O-β-D-glucoside, leucocyanidin, (-)-epicatechin, (+)-catechin, flavonoids, and sterols.[1] Experimental studies have shown that the bark has oxytocic activity in rats, guinea pigs, and isolated human uterine preparations. The uterine response to the extract was dependent on hormonal environment and the state of gestation. Estrogen-primed rats were more sensitive to the alcoholic extract.[2] A pure phenolic glycoside (P_2) showed in vitro and in vivo oxytocic activity at very low concentrations on uteri of several species.[3,4]

Considering the importance of the drug in Ayurveda it has been clinically little investigated as a single drug. Only one small trial with 10 patients has been reported in which the drug was given parentally. Commercially available "Injection *Ashoka*" 2 ml of was given intramuscularly in 10 cases of metromenorrhagia. All patients responded to the treatment with good results and menstrual flow was normalized.[5] Much more work is required experimentally to determine the mode of action in addition to holding clinical trials using the oral route.

Mimosa pudica *Linn. (Family: Mimosaceae)*

Sanskrit: Lajjalu	Tamil: Thottalsulungi
Hindi: Lajwanti	English: Sensitive plant

Mimosa pudica is a common weed found throughout the warmer parts of India. The roots contain tannin (10 percent), mimosine, and calcium oxalate. In an exploratory clinical study in patients with dysfunctional uterine bleeding, the aqueous extract of the root was given in a dose of two to three 500 mg capsules thrice a day. The period of treatment was variable from a few months to 4 years. The response was considered promising enough to warrant further studies.[6]

NOTES

1. Sharma PC, Yelne MB, Dennis TJ (eds.). *Database on medicinal plants used in Ayurveda* (vol. 3, pp. 76-87). New Delhi: Central Council for Research in Ayurveda and Siddha, 2001.

2. Satyavati GV, Prasad DN, Sen SP, Das PK. Investigations into the uterine activity of *Saraca indica* Linn. *(Ashoka). J Res Indian Med* 4(1):37-45 (1969).

3. Satyavati GV, Prasad DN, Sen SP, Das PK. Further studies on the uterine activity of *Saraca indica* Linn. *(Ashoka). Ind J Med Res* 58:947-960 (1970).

4. Satyavati GV, Prasad DN, Sen SP, Das PK. Oxytocic activity of a pure phenolic glycoside (P$_2$) from *Saraca indica* Linn. *(Ashoka)*. A short communication. *Indian J Med Res* 58:660-663 (1970).

5. Sedani MM. Role of Ayurvedic injection "*Ashoka*" in the management of metro-menorrhagia. *J Nat Integ Med Assoc* 32(9):13 (1990).

6. Vaidya GH, Sheth UK. *Mimosa pudica* (Linn.), its medicinal value and pilot clinical use in patients with menorrhagia. *Ancient Sci Life* V(3):156-160 (1986).

Chapter 11

Antidiabetic Agents

With over 100 million people affected worldwide, diabetes mellitus is the most common, chronic endocrine disorder of carbohydrate, fat, and protein metabolism. Characteristics of the disease are symptoms such as excessive thirst, hunger, weight loss, fatigue, blurred vision, etc. Diabetes has been described in Ayurveda in both the *Caraka* and *Sushruta Samhita*s under the name *madhumeha* (*madhu:* honey; *meha:* urine) or *prameha* meaning excessive urine (*pra:* excessive).

There is also a remarkable correspondence between the descriptions of the etiology and management of the disease in Ayurvedic texts and its allopathic correlates. The two types of diabetes described today are insulin-dependent diabetes mellitus (IDDM), because of nonfunctional or damaged beta cells in the pancreas, and noninsulin-dependent diabetes mellitus (NIDDM). A similar classification exists in Ayurveda with *sahaja prameha* caused due to congenital reasons and *apathyaanimittaja prameha* considered to occur due to unsuitable choice of food or consuming excessive food.[1]

A large number of plants have been used in Ayurveda for the management of diabetes mellitus, and 148 plants of 50 families have been reviewed. As, elsewhere in Ayurveda, combination drugs are the preferred mode of therapy. Some 40 plants have been used that have been reviewed by several authors.[2-4]

Scientific work has focused on phytochemical examination, and in experimentally demonstrating hypoglycemic activity in small animals made diabetic by alloxan, streptozotocin, and sometimes by adrenaline. Therefore, most studies have concentrated on the control of hyperglycemia.

doi:10.1300/5683_11

Only a few studies have been carried out to evaluate the effect of the drugs on complications of diabetes mellitus, such as nephropathy, neuropathy, and retinopathy, which need to be addressed especially since synthetic oral hypoglycemic agents and insulin, which form the mainstay of treatment of diabetes by controlling hyperglycemia, nonetheless have serious side effects and fail to alter the course of diabetic complications. *Eugenia jambolana and Momordica charantia* have been shown to yield good results in the amelioration of diabetic complications such as diabetic nephropathy,[5] fructose-induced insulin resistance,[6] and cataract[7] in experimental animals. The two plants also partially prevented diabetic neuropathy[8] in small animals. There are conflicting reports on the hypoglycemic activity of some plants that may be attributed to a number of factors such as botanical identity of the drugs, time and place of collection, method of preparation, mode of administration, and type of experimental animal used.[2]

Clinical data is generally of preliminary nature. There are roughly seven single plants, which have been studied in some detail, and these are covered here. Work on other potentially useful single drugs for which exploratory clinical work is available is presented in brief. Also discussed are a few plants used clinically to treat diabetic complications.

NOTES

1. Govind Reddy R, Diabetes management: Ayurvedic line and dietetics. *Express Pharma Pulse* (August 23): 21 (2001).

2. Nagarajan S, Jain HC, Aulakh GS. Indigenous plants used in the control of diabetes. In Atal CK, Kapur BM (eds.), *Cultivation and utilization of medicinal plants* (pp. 584-604). Jammu: Regional Research Laboratory, 1982.

3. Handa SS, Chawla AS, Maninder. Hypoglycemic plants—A review. *Fitoterapia* 60:195-224 (1989).

4. Grover JK, Yadav S, Vats V. Medicinal plants of India with anti-diabetic potential. *J Ethnopharmacol* 81:81-100 (2002).

5. Grover JK, Vats V, Rathi SS, Dawar R. Traditional Indian anti-diabetic plants attenuate progression of renal damage in streptozotocin induced diabetic mice. *J Ethnopharmacol* 76:233-238 (2001).

6. Vats V, Grover JK, Tandon N, Rathi SS, Gupta N. Treatment with extracts of *Momordica charantia* and *Eugenia jambolana* prevents hyperglycemia and hyperinsulinemia in fructose fed rats. *J Ethnopharmacol* 76:139-143 (2001).

7. Rathi SS, Grover JK, Vats V, Biswas NR. Prevention of experimental diabetic cataract by Indian Ayurvedic plant extracts. *Phytother Res* 16:774-777 (2002).

8. Grover JK, Rathi SS, Vats V. Amelioration of experimental diabetic neuropathy and gastropathy in rats following oral administration of plant *(Eugenia jambolana, Mucuna pruriens* and *Tinospora cordifolia)* extracts. *Indian J Exp Biol* 40:273-276 (2002).

MAIN PLANTS

Azadirachta indica *A Juss. (Family: Meliaceae)*

Latin: *Melia azadirachta* Linn.	Hindi: Neem, Nimb
Sanskrit: Nimba	Tamil: Veppan, Vembu
English: Margosa	

Azadirachta indica or the *neem* is a large evergreen tree found growing throughout India. It is also cultivated widely. The *neem* tree has been used since antiquity in India for a variety of ailments. Since the tree is found growing everywhere, it often serves to provide twigs that are used as chewing sticks for cleaning the teeth and gums; leaves that are used for skin problems and during infections such as measles, chicken pox, etc. to help soothe itch. In addition, young leaves are plucked and chewed as a medicine to control blood sugar and to improve immunity. Flowers of the *neem* tree serve to control blood pressure and the seed kernel serves as an antifeedant for controlling insect attack. Leaves, seed oil, and bark of the tree have been used to treat diabetes. Traditionally, *neem* has been used for the treatment of skin diseases, fevers including malaria and rheumatism and other inflammations.[1] Every part of the *neem* tree is thus used for numerous indications.

A very large number of substances have been isolated from different parts of the *neem* tree. These have been terpenoids—diterpenoids, tetranortriterpenoids (liminoids), and triterpenoids—steroids, coumarins, fatty acids, flavonoids, fatty acid derivatives, hydrocarbons, and sulfur compounds.[1,2]

The aqueous leaf extract has been shown to produce hypoglycemia in small animals when administered orally at 200 mg·kg^{-1} (10 percent w·v^{-1} aqueous leaf extract)[3] and at 0.15 ml·kg^{-1} (50 percent w·v^{-1} aqueous leaf extract) when administered intravenously[4] to dogs. However, in another study, oral aqueous leaf extract, prepared by decocting the leaf, seed oil, and the compound nimbidin, was tested at dose levels of 1, 5, and 10 ml·kg^{-1} body weight and it failed to reduce blood glucose levels, whereas seed oil at 2.5 ml·kg^{-1} and nimbidin at 200 mg·kg^{-1} body weight were active and exhibited significant hypoglycemic effect in both normoglycemic-fasted rabbits and glucose-fed animals in glucose tolerance test.[5]

Aqueous fraction of alcoholic[6,7] and methanolic extracts[8] of *neem* leaves exhibited hypoglycemic and antihyperglycemic effect in adrenaline-induced, glucose-fed,[6] and streptozotocin diabetic rats. [7, 8] Fractions exhibiting hypoglycemic activity were found to be rich in flavonoid glycosides.[7] An evaluation of the leaves of four Ayurvedic medicinal plants—*Azadirachta indica, Gymnema sylvestre, Catharanthus roseus,* and *Ocimum sanctum*— in normal and streptozotocin-diabetic rats for blood sugar lowering activity showed that *A. indica* leaf had the most potent blood sugar–lowering activity and the best safety margin.[9]

In addition, *neem* leaf extract or seed oil exert their hypoglycemic effect in rabbits both when given as pretreatment before alloxan or after induction of diabetes suggesting that *neem* could be useful for control of blood sugar in diabetes, and also for helping to retard or to prevent onset of the disease.[10] *Neem* oil has been shown to reduce blood glucose levels in several experimental models in rabbits,[11] and in both normal and alloxan-diabetic rats.[12]

A series of studies have been carried out to elucidate the mechanism of action. It has been suggested that *neem* extract is an effective hypoglycemic agent only in animals having residual and healthy beta cells and it can act only in the presence of a stimulus, such as an external glucose load. *Neem* increases peripheral glucose utilization by blocking the effect of epinephrine on glucose metabolism.[13] However, in an in vitro experiment *neem* extract did not enhance glucose uptake or glycogen synthesis in isolated rat hemidiaphragm.[14] *Neem* leaf extract also blocks in a significant fashion the serotonin inhibition of insulin secretion mediated by glucose.[15]

In an exploratory clinical trial, 5 g of fresh tender *A. indica* leaf paste or an equivalent amount of dried leaf powder filled in capsules given to type I diabetics enabled five out of seven patients to reduce their insulin dosage by 30-50 percent, while maintaining their blood glucose values.[16]

In an open uncontrolled study on 85 patients of type II diabetes, who were on conventional allopathic drugs, 5-10 drops per day of *neem* seed oil in soft gelatin capsules was given in two divided doses along with the prescribed treatment. *Neem* oil was found to act in a synergesic manner to conventional drugs, and it was possible to reduce the dosage of other oral antidiabetic drugs and insulin, based on the response of the blood glucose levels of patients to treatment.[17]

In an open preliminary study, patients with secondary diabetes were given varying doses of *neem* oil depending upon severity of diabetes: those with mild diabetes received 5 drops, those with moderate diabetes received 10 drops, and those with severe diabetics receiving 15 drops of *neem* oil twice a day. Patients experienced relief in symptoms such as itching, dyspepsia, fatigue, and muscular pain. In addition, patients had improved wound healing. The oil was evaluated as useful in mild and moderate diabetes, and was found to have 50 percent effect on patients with severe diabetes.[18]

Considering the preliminary but promising nature of results, further work is required in studying the material being used in the clinical trials and in using larger patient numbers for evaluation. Also to be evaluated is the safety of the preparations.

The use of tender *neem* leaves for health and in diabetes is recommended in traditional medicine, not only in the geriatric population, but also in the pediatric age group of infants. After a review of literature, including various toxicity studies, the leaf, bark extract, and isolated liminoids were considered to have a wide margin of safety.[1] In another review of literature, the leaf extract had experimental LD_{50} values ranging from 10 to 13 $g \cdot kg^{-1}$ bodyweight.[19] *Neem* seed oil has shown toxicity, which, as suggested, may be due to contamination with seeds of Persian lilac or *Melia azedarach*,[1] or due to aflatoxins. However, purified *neem* oil obtained by debittering, deodorizing, and decolorizing is nontoxic,[20] suggesting the importance of developing chemical profiles of raw materials and isolated compounds, which could help in evaluating the possible toxic effect of a preparation by identifying its toxic compounds.

Coccinia grandis *Linn. (Family: Cucurbitaceae)*

Latin: *Coccinia indica* Wight & Arn, *Cephalandra indica* (Naud)	Hindi: Kanduri, Kundru
Sanskrit: Bimbi, Bimba	English: Ivy Gourd
Tamil: Kovakai	

Coccinia indica is a climbing or prostrate perennial herb found growing throughout India and the Indian subcontinent. All parts of the plant are used, including leaves, stem, fruits, and roots. The drug has traditionally been used for the treatment of skin problems, respiratory disorders, and for diabetes. *Coccinia indica* is well known in Bengal for the treatment of diabetes, where it is reputed to be an Indian substitute for insulin. It is considered to be very effective in reducing urine sugar levels.[21] There are two varieties recorded—the wild variety with greenish bitter nonedible fruits and the cultivated edible variety *C. indica* var. *palmata* that is sold in the market as a vegetable. Fruits of *C. indica* var. *palmata* have been shown to have more potent hypoglycemic activity and are preferred over the wild variety for treatment of diabetes,[22] although usually the wild bitter variety is preferred for use in medicine.[23]

From the aerial parts of *C. indica* var. *palmata,* heptacosane, triacontane, cephalandrol, β-sitosterol, and the alkaloids—cephalandrines A and B—have been isolated. From the fruits, lupeol, β-amyrin, and its acetate—cucurbitacin B and pectin—have been isolated.[24] The fruit pectin has been shown to produce significant reduction in blood glucose levels.[25]

The different parts of the plant have shown a varied response when tested for hypoglycemic activity. Root extracts, either aqueous or alcoholic, have shown significant hypoglycemic effect in alloxan-diabetic rabbits[26,27] and rats,[28] and in glucose loaded[29,30] and fasted rats.[30]

Alcoholic extract of the fruits inhibited in rats, though not significantly, the hyperglycemic effect caused by anterior pituitary extract[31]—corticotropin and somatropin.[32] Decoction of fruits of *C. indica* W & A at 20 ml·kg^{-1} showed significant hypoglycemic activity in glucose-fed fasted rabbits. The edible fruits of *C. indica* var. *palmata* was found to be more potent than that of *C. indica* W & A. Thus the fruit juice of the wild variety did not show any activity whereas the fruit juice of *C. indica* var *palmata* at 20 ml·kg^{-1} showed very significant activity (*p < 0.001*) at the end of the fifth hour.[22] The pectin isolated from the fruits at 200 mg per 100 g body weight has been shown to reduce blood glucose levels in normal rats by enhanced glycolysis, glycogenesis, and decreased glycogenolysis.[25]

Alcoholic extract of leaves of *bimbi* reduced blood sugar levels in guinea pigs[33] and streptozotocin-induced diabetic rats.[34,35] Depressed synthesis of blood glucose was due to depression of the enzymes glucose-6-phosphatase,[34,35] fructose-1,6-bisphosphatase, and enhanced glucose oxidation.[34]

In a double-blind clinical trial, tablets made from freeze-dried leaves of *C. indica* were tried on 16 patients with uncontrolled maturity-onset diabetes in the treatment group, and 16 patients in the placebo group received placebo tablets made from chlorophyll. Patients received 3 tablets, weight of tablet not mentioned,[37] twice daily for 6 weeks. Ten patients on the drug showed significant improvement in glucose tolerance (*p < 0.001*), whereas none of the placebo group showed such marked improvement.[36,37] Maximum effect was seen after 3 weeks, and no adverse effects were observed.

In an open trial, 41 patients with diabetes mellitus were treated with either *C. indica* powder or juice. Of these 24 were given 3 g of the powder twice daily with water before food for 5 weeks and 17 were given 30 ml drug juice, prepared from a fresh plant, twice daily before food. Response was seen within 7 days, evaluated based on reduction of blood sugar levels and relief of classical symptoms such as excessive urine, thirst, hunger, fatigue, numbness, and blurred vision. Excellent response was seen in 80 percent of the patients on powder and 47 percent on juice. No side effects were seen.[38]

Along with the normal diet 50-100 g of *C. indica* powder per day was given to 100 hyperglycemic patients, in the age group of 25-70 years, and 60 healthy volunteers. Significant results were seen from the first week. Lowering of blood cholesterol, low-density lipoproteins, and serum triglycerides were seen with an increase in high-density lipoproteins.[39]

Coccinia indica showed glycemic control in noninsulin-dependent diabetic patients, who did not respond to diet therapy alone. The drug showed moderate blood sugar lowering property that increased with use in subsequent months.[40]

Dried aqueous extract of fresh leaves of *C. indica* was made into 3 g pellets, which were again oven dried and 1 pellet was given twice a day before food to 25 NIDDM patients. Group 1 was a control group of 15 healthy controls, Group 2 consisted of 30 untreated patients, and Group 3 consisted of 25 patients treated with *C. indica* and 15 with the oral drug "Diabenese" (chlorpropamide) for comparison. Diet was restricted and follow-up was done at 6-week intervals for two consecutive periods. The herbal drug was found to be effective in controlling both hyperglycemia and hyperlipidemia at the end of 6 weeks. Reduction of blood sugar in the *C. indica* group was comparable to Diabetese.[41]

To study the influence of *C. indica* on certain enzyme levels, dried extract of 50 mg·kg⁻¹ body weight·day⁻¹ of *C. indica* was given twice a day before food to 30 diabetic patients both IDDM and NIDDM for 6 weeks. Treatment significantly restored the reduced activity of lipoprotein lipase (LPL), and lowered the levels of glucose-6-phosphatase and lactate dehydrogenase (LDH), which are raised in severe diabetics. The authors postulate that the ingredients of *C. indica* extract act like insulin to correct the elevated levels of glucose-6-phosphatase and LDH in the glycolytic pathway, and restore the LPL in the lipolytic pathway with the control of hyperglycemia in diabetes.[42]

Considering the positive results obtained, further trials are needed with a larger number of patients. In addition, the composition should be standardized in order to obtain consistent results. *C. indica* belongs to the Cucurbitaceae family. The fruits of the cultivated variety of *C. indica* are commonly eaten as a vegetable and therefore considered safe to use. In the clinical trials no side effects and toxicity were observed.[37,38]

Gymnema sylvestre *R. Br. (Family: Asclepediaceae)*

Sanskrit: Meshashringi	Tamil: Sirukurinja
Hindi: Gurmar	English: Periploca of the woods

Gymnema sylvestre (see Plate 11 in color gallery) is a woody climber found growing extensively in the southern and central parts of India. The leaves of the plant when chewed have the peculiarity of numbing the tongue so that one is not able to recognize sweet or bitter tastes. Hence the Hindi name *gurmar* that means destroyer of sweet (*gur:* sweet; *mar:* destroyer). This has been shown in humans to be owing to the presence of triterpene acids known as gymnemic acids and in rats due to a 35-amino acid peptide called gurmarin.[43] The leaves have been used for the treatment of diabetes for a long time. The plant is considered a stomachic, a stimulant, a diuretic, and a laxative. It is said to be useful in cough, biliousness, and sore eyes.[44]

From the leaves of *Gymnema* several oleanane and dammarane triterpene saponins have been isolated and characterized. The best known of the oleanane triterpenoid saponins are the gymnemic acids that have been isolated from the aqueous extracts. Fractions containing gymnemic acids have shown hypoglycemic activity. Gymnemic acid IV has been shown to increase the plasma insulin levels in streptozotocin-diabetic mice.[45] Apart from these compounds flavones, anthraquinones, hentriacontane, pentatriacontane, resins, inositol, d-quercitol, lupeol, β-amyrin, stigmasterol, and some acids, for example, tartaric acid, formic acid, and butyric acid have been isolated and their structure determined.[46]

There are a number of animal studies regarding the beneficial effect of *Gymnema* on diabetes. Administration of *gurmar* leaf powder to alloxan-diabetic animals regulates blood sugar levels[47,48] inducing protracted longevity.[48] In addition to blood glucose homeostatis, enzyme activity controlling glucose utilization by insulin-dependent pathways was also increased.[47]

In glucose-fed streptozotocin-diabetic rats glucose homeostatis was observed[49-51] by feeding leaf extracts possibly because of increased serum insulin levels[50] caused by regeneration of the islets of

Langerhans[51] and/or by increasing cell permeability.[52] It has been suggested that extracts containing gymnemic acids suppress elevation of blood glucose levels by inhibiting glucose uptake in the intestine.[49,53] Gymnemic acid IV, but not gymnemic acid I-III or gymnemasaponin V, at dose levels of 3.4-13.4 mg·kg^{-1} reduced blood glucose levels by 13.5-60 percent 6 hours after administration in a manner similar to glibenclamide. Also at 13.4 mg·kg^{-1}, plasma insulin levels were increased in streptozotocin-diabetic rats suggesting that this may contribute to the antihyperglycemic activity of the leaves.[45]

Lipid abnormalities found in alloxan-diabetic animals was restored to near normalcy by feeding with the hypoglycemic leaf extract of *Gymnema sylvestre.*[54] This activity of the leaf extract given at 100 mg·kg^{-1} in hypolipidemic rats for 2 and 10 weeks[55,56] was found to reduce triglyceride and total cholesterol levels[55,56] similar to clofibrate.[55] Gymnemic acid fractions containing 363.3 mg·g^{-1} of gymnemagenin[57] and leaf extract[58] have been shown to increase excretion of fecal cholesterol and cholic acid-derived bile acids. In addition, gymnemic acids potently inhibit absorption of oleic acid in the intestine.[59] Increased glycoprotein levels, which are considered the major cause of nephropathy, neuropathy, and retinopathy and found elevated in streptozotocin-diabetic rats, were brought under control by administration of leaf extract GS$_4$.[60]

Clinical studies have been conducted using the leaf powder and concentrates from the leaves containing gymnemic acids. In an early exploratory trial, ten healthy normal persons and six diabetics with mild-to-moderate hyperglycemia were given an aqueous decoction of powdered leaf of *gurmar* at a concentration of 10 g per 100 ml. The dose was 2 g thrice daily for 10 days. After 10 days, there was a definite fall in blood glucose levels after glucose tolerance test, which was significant only in diabetics. Fasting blood glucose levels had fallen significantly both in normal and diabetic patients.[61]

The two studies used the concentrate named GS$_4$ obtained by extraction of the leaves with 50 percent aqueous ethanol[51,60] precipitation with hydrochloric acid followed by recrystallization of the crystals with aqueous ethanol. In 22 NIDDM patients on conventional therapy, oral hypoglycemic drugs were supplemented for 18-20 months with 400 mg·kg^{-1} of GS$_4$. During supplementation with GS$_4$, patients showed a significant reduction in blood glucose, glycosylated hemo-globin, and glycosylated plasma proteins because of which the dosage of conventional drugs glibenclamide or tolbutamide could be de-creased or stopped. Thus 5 of the 22 patients could stop conventional therapy and manage with GS_4 alone. During supplementation most of the patients reported a sense of well-being, better alertness, and less ex-haustion when doing work.[62]

GS_4 was administered orally to 27 IDDM patients along with their daily insulin injection for varying periods ranging from 2 to 30 months. None of the patients had symptoms of renal damage, retinopathy, or car-diovascular damage. These patients were compared with a control group of 37 patients on insulin therapy alone. Patients on GS_4 were able to reduce their insulin dose with reduction of blood glucose lev-els, glycosylated hemoglobin, and glycosylated plasma protein lev-els. Plasma lipid levels came back to near normal levels. In addition, there was a sense of well-being, an improved ability to do work to-gether, and increased mental alertness. In the control group on insulin therapy alone, there was no significant decrease in blood lipid levels, fasting blood glucose, glycosylated hemoglobin, and glycosylated plasma proteins or serum amylase levels. Therapy with the *Gymnema sylvestre* extract GS_4 appears to enhance endogenous insulin, accord-ing to the authors, by regeneration or revitalization of the residual beta cells.[63]

In another open trial, the hypoglycemic activity of *Gymnema sylvestre* leaf powder, at a dose of 10 g per day when administered for 7 days to 16 normal persons and 43 mild diabetics, was studied. After 7 days, 36 diabetics received tolbutamide, whereas the remaining seven diabetics received *Gymnema sylvestre* powder alone for 2 more weeks. Fasting blood sugar levels of the seven diabetics on *gurmar* powder for 3 weeks showed improved glucose tolerance. Lipid levels in normal per-sons remained unchanged, whereas in diabetics there was a significant decrease in total cholesterol, serum triacylglycerol, and free fatty acids. *Gymnema sylvestre* also showed a definite hypoglycemic effect in both normal subjects and in diabetic patients, and the effect in diabetics was evaluated as comparable to that of tolbutamide.[64]

The water-soluble portion GS of the alcoholic extract of *Gymnema sylvestre* leaves, containing gymnemic acids (A-D) along with potassium and magnesium ions obtained by fractionation of the extract using bioassay, was given orally at dose levels of 120-360 mg daily to 61 diabetic patients in the age group of 23-60 years. In 70 percent of the cases glucose homeostatis could be achieved using GS with results being seen in 2-4 weeks. The authors concluded that GS is useful in NIDDM patients who are poorly controlled by standard therapy. There was no abnormality in the biochemical investigations, such as blood count, hemoglobin, liver function tests, and nonprotein nitrogen, when carried out after 1 year of therapy.[65]

Gymnema sylvestre leaves and stem are extensively used in Gujarat, India, for the treatment of diabetes.[66] Preparations of the leaves and extracts are widely available in Japan as health foods in the form of tea bags, tablets, beverages, and confectionary.[57] The leaves and stems have been considered nontoxic to human beings.[66] In a trial with *Gymnema sylvestre* extract known as GS$_4$ there were no undesirable side effects, such as nausea, vomiting, lassitude, or other gastrointestinal disturbances. Patients reported an increased sense of well-being and a few female patients experienced relief of pain in the limbs.[63] In a 1-year clinical trial, consumption of GS fraction from *Gymnema sylvestre* by type II diabetic patients showed no abnormality in blood count, hemoglobin, liver function test, and nonprotein nitrogen.[65] Rats that were fed extract powder of *Gymnema sylvestre* for 1 year in graded amounts ranging from 0.01 to 1 percent of diet were examined weekly up to 12 weeks, then at 26, and finally at 52 weeks showed no toxic effects at 1-percent level in the diet as seen from hematological, biochemical, and histological examination. In addition, there was no change in food consumption and in body weight.[67]

Momordica charantia *Linn. (Family: Cucurbitaceae)*

Sanskrit: Karabella	Tamil: Pavakka
Hindi: *Karela*	English: Bitter Gourd, Bitter Melon

Momordica charantia is a slender climber with yellow flowers found growing throughout India. It is also cultivated countrywide for its fruits, as it is a commonly eaten vegetable despite its bitter taste. The plant bears gherkin-shaped fruits with protuberances that are sold in the market when green, and there are several types available in different sizes big and small and shades of green.[68] The green fruits are sliced and dried in the sun to preserve them, in order to be consumed during the off season. The fruits are also popularly used for the treatment of diabetes, for which the cultivated variety of big fruits is used; the small fruits variety is generally preferred in medicine.[69] However, a study with two varieties of *karela* showed that the bigger fruits were more effective than the small, oval, dark-green fruits in alloxan-diabetic rabbits with mild ketosis.[70] The fruits, leaves, and roots have been commonly used as a folk remedy for diabetes. The fruits are considered a cooling bitter tonic, useful as a stomachic and carminative. They are also used for the liver and spleen and for gout and rheumatism.[68]

A large number of compounds have been isolated from the fruits of *Momordica charantia*.[71] The saponins and proteins are found to be important for the hypoglycemic activity. Of these the polypeptide known as p-insulin,[72] (which has 17-amino acids and 166 residues, and has the same amino acid composition except for an extra methionine residue when compared to bovine insulin) and charantin,[73] (which is a steroidal glycoside mixture of sitosterol and 5, 25- stigmastadien-3-β-ol glucosides), and the triterpene glycosides—oleanolic acid 3-O-glucuronide and momordicin Ic[74] are considered responsible for the hypoglycemic activity although p-insulin itself does not act orally. Also contributing to the hypoglycemic activity is the pyrimidine nucleoside vicine,[75] which is found in the seeds. Other steroidal glycosides found in the fruit are momordicines and the cucurbitin glycosides—momordicosides.[71]

The hypoglycemic activity of the fruit and seeds has been studied extensively in different animal models[76-85] and the work was reviewed in 1996.[71] Fruit juice causes glucose tolerance in alloxan-diabetic rabbits but not in normal animals. P-insulin has been shown to be a very effective hypoglycemic agent when administered subcutaneously to gerbils, langurs, and humans.[72] Charantin was found to produce a lowering of blood glucose concentration when administered either orally or intravenously.[73,86] Oleanolic acid 3-O-glucuronide and momordicin 1 c exhibit hypoglycemic activity by suppressing the transfer of glucose from the stomach to the small intestine, and by inhibiting glucose transport.[74] Intraperitoneal administration of vicine caused a hypoglycemic response in fasting albino rats.[75]

Fruit juice causes significant ($p < 0.004$) increase in the number of beta cells in streptozotocin-induced diabetic mice,[87] although an earlier study reported lack of any significant effect on the ability to tolerate external glucose load in diabetic mice by administration of 10 ml·kg^{-1} fruit juice for 30 days, which was attributed to the lack of viable beta cells capable of secreting insulin upon stimulation in order to exert its oral hypoglycemic effect.[88]

Fruit juice of *Momordica charantia* has also been shown to be a potent scavenger of superoxide and hydroxyl radicals.[89] Four different preparations of *karela*—fruits, juice, seed extract, freeze-dried juice, and commercially available capsules showed that in healthy rats the hypoglycemic activity of fruit juice, freeze-dried fruit juice, and seed extract were comparable and they showed significant improvement in the ability to tolerate an oral glucose load, whereas commercial capsules did not significantly improve glucose tolerance.[90]

Studies of rats with diets supplemented with 0.5-3.5 percent of freeze-dried powder of fruit for 14 days both in the presence and absence of dietary cholesterol showed that there was a marked reduction of hepatic total cholesterol, triglyceride levels, and an increase in HDL-cholesterol.[91] In streptozotocin-diabetic rats, long-term feeding for 10 weeks of fruit extract brought elevated lipid levels back to near-normal values.[92]

Fruit extracts of *Momordica charantia* when fed at 4 g·kg·day^{-1} per rat to murine alloxan-diabetic rats retarded the formation of cataract. The *karela*-treated diabetic mice developed cataract in 140-180 days, whereas controls receiving 0.9 percent sodium chloride solution developed cataract in 90-100 days.[93] *Karela* extracts (200 mg·kg^{-1}) fed daily prevented, to a significant extent ($p < 0.05$), renal hypertrophy in diabetic rats.[94] Aqueous extracts of *karela* at 400 mg·day^{-1} prevented, substantially, hyperglycemia and hyperinsulinemia induced by a high fructose diet.[95]

Experimental evidence obtained so far suggests that *karela* exhibits its hypoglycemic activity through inhibition of glucose absorption[96] and also tends to be extrapancreatic, independent of glucose absorption in the intestine.[80] Thus also seen in the experimental studies are increased utilization of glucose by the liver,[83,97] inhibition of glucose synthesis while increasing glucose oxidation,[98] and decreased insulin resistance by increasing the amounts[84] of the transporter protein GLUT.[84] The depressed carbohydrate enzyme levels in the liver of diabetic mice were partially restored to normal,[99] whereas oxidative stress was reduced by normalizing disturbed glutathione S-transferase distribution.[100] Momordicin Ic and oleonolic acid-3-O-glucuronolide inhibit transfer of glucose from the stomach to the intestine, and inhibit glucose transport to the brush border of the small intestine.[74] In addition, *karela* is shown to cause regeneration of beta cells in streptozotocin-diabetic rats[86] and exhibit an insulinomimetic or insulinogogue effect.[101-103]

An experimental study in different animal models, using different doses, was carried out to find out the scope of use of *karela* in diabetes of varying intensity. The study showed that *karela* is best used for controlling hyperglycemia in mild-to-moderate noninsulin-dependent diabetics only. The extracts had no adverse effect on various hematological parameters. *Karela* extracts were found to differ from insulin in four ways—oral administration; a delayed onset with a sustained duration of action; increase in the peripheral utilization of action even in tissues that are insulin dependent, for example decrease of glycogen even in the kidney; and a longer duration of action.[99]

Momordica charantia has been studied in small groups of patients by Vaclad, who noticed that blood sugar was significantly lowered in patients administered fresh fruit juice or tablets prepared from fruit powder.[104-106]

Inspired by reports of use of *karela* in diabetes[107,108] and of its possible effect on the other drugs being consumed by diabetics, a study was carried out on nine NIDDM patients of Asian origin. Coadministration of a water-soluble extract of the fruits during a 50 g glucose tolerance test significantly reduced blood glucose concentrations without any influence on the insulin levels. Since *karela* is often eaten in the form of curry as part of the diet, the addition of fried *karela* fruits to the daily diet for 8 to 11 weeks was also investigated. This produced a small but significant improvement in the glucose tolerance with no increase in insulin levels. In addition, there was a significant reduction in glycosylated hemoglobin levels.[109]

Similarly a beneficial effect was seen in eight NIDDM patients given daily powdered *karela* fruit for 7 weeks. Improvement in glucose tolerance and fasting blood glucose levels was observed.[110] There was a significant glucose tolerance in 73 percent of maturity-onset diabetic patients, who were administered fruit juice of *karela,* whereas the remaining 27 percent failed to respond.[111]

Aqueous extract of fruit given for 3-7 weeks resulted in a significant fall in postprandial blood sugar levels. There was a marked fall in both the blood sugar and the urine sugar levels; the hypoglycemic effect takes place in a cumulative and gradual manner unlike that when using insulin. The aqueous extract, with a fall in blood sugar of 54 percent, was found to be more effective than the dried-fruit powder, with a fall in blood sugar of 25 percent, after 3 weeks of therapy. There was also significant reduction of glysoylated hemoglobin at the end of the trial.[112]

The effect of aqueous homogenized suspension of the green fruit pulp of *M.charantia,* given to 100 moderate NIDDM patients 2 hours after the intake of 75 g of glucose, was studied. There was a significant reduction ($p < 0.001$) in postprandial serum glucose levels in 86 percent of the patients and fasting glucose levels in 5 percent of the cases.[113]

In an open study in Germany, 41 NIDDM patients took a 500 mg capsule of *Momordica charantia* extract, containing at least 10 percent charantin, twice a day prior to the two main meals, for 24 weeks. In the group of patients considered to have moderate diabetes, with fasting glucose $\leqslant 200$ mg·dl^{-1} and HbA$_{lc}$ $\leqslant 8.0$ percent, the blood glucose levels fell by 25 percent and the HbA$_{lc}$ by 0.5 percent bringing them into the classification of patients with glucose intolerance, and therefore less prone to late complications of diabetes. No adverse effects were noted during the course of the trial.[114]

P-insulin administered subcutaneously led to a significant hypoglycemic fall in six IDDM, one NIDDM, and two asymptomatic diabetics.[115] In another study, subcutaneous p-insulin led to a significant fall in blood glucose levels in 11 IDDM patients; however, no significant effect was seen in eight NIDDM patients. A single IDDM patient could be maintained on p-insulin for 5 months.[72]

Momordica charantia fruits are commonly eaten as a vegetable in India with no untoward effects. However, it can cause loose motions and stomachache[114] when consumed in large quantities, probably because of its bitter taste and its known laxative and emetic action.[116] In a clinical trial to evaluate the safety and efficacy of an extract of *Momordica charantia,* no adverse effects were observed, leading the authors to conclude that the extract at the dose employed was a safe nutraceutical without any toxic side effects.[114] Some adverse effects in animals have been reported, for example, changes in testicular function in dogs[114] and uterine hemorrhage in pregnant rats,[117] emphasizing the need for caution in use in pregnancy and supervision by a physician when coadministered with other drugs for diabetes in the context of the known synergesic effect with other antidiabetic drugs.[108,114,118]

Pterocarpus marsupium *Roxb. (Family: Fabaceae)*

Sanskrit: Asana, Beejaka	Tamil: Vengai
Hindi: Vijayasar, Bijasal, Bija	English: Indian Malabar Kino

Pterocarpus marsupium is a moderate-to-large-sized deciduous tree found commonly in the hills in south and central India. The tree yields one of the most important timbers of India. *Pterocarpus marsupium* is well-known for its use in skin diseases and in diabetes. The sapwood is pale-yellowish white to white and the heartwood is golden-yellowish brown in color, which stains yellow when it is moist;[119] the yellow color is probably indicative of the flavonoids present in the wood. The heartwood of *Pterocarpus marsupium* is considered to be useful for diabetes and has been the subject of a multicentric clinical study undertaken by the Indian Council of Medical Research (ICMR) to establish its efficacy. (See later in this chapter.) In many parts of India, tumblers made of the heartwood of *Pterocarpus marsupium* are sold in the market, and diabetics drink water stored overnight in these tumblers to control blood sugar levels. This folkloric use has been corroborated by a small clinical trial.[120]

The heartwood is a rich source of flavonoids and other phenolic compounds.[121] From the alkali-soluble portion of the heartwood were isolated isoliquiritigenin, liquiritigenin, and pterostilbene, and from the sapwood, pterostilbene.[122] Other compounds from the heartwood are marsupin, pterosupin,[121] marsupol, carsupin, propterol, and propterol B.[122] The bark contains epicatechin and pterostilbene.[122] Among the compounds considered to have hypoglycemic activity are epicatechin, marsupin, and pterostilbene. Pterosupin and liquiritigenin have been shown to be effective in reducing total cholesterol and lipid, and lipoprotein levels.[121]

The oral hypoglycemic activity of *Pterocarpus marsupium* has been studied in a number of experimental models, using aqueous infusion of *vijaysar* in acute hyperglycemic response caused by anterior pituitary extract in glucose-fed albino rats,[123] in alloxan-induced diabetic rats,[124] in normal,[125-127] and alloxan-diabetic rabbits.[125] The aqueous extract was found to be more active than the alcoholic extract, and also found to be active in both acute and chronic experiments in normal rabbits. In addition, the aqueous extract showed a more potent hypoglycemic effect than *Gymnema sylvestre* and *C. indica.*[125] Administration of aqueous extract of *vijaysar* for 15 days resulted in reduced glucose absorption from the gastrointestinal tract, which was attributed to the action of tannates.[128] Other workers also reported similar findings of blood sugar lowering.[129,130]

Pterostilbene from *vijaysar,* when administered intravenously to dogs, led to a fall in blood sugar at 10 mg·kg^{-1}, whereas higher doses led to an initial hyperglycemia followed by hypoglycemia. It also caused a fall in the blood pressure of anesthetized dogs and was found to be toxic at 30 mg·kg^{-1}.[131] The flavonoid fraction and the pure component (-)-epicatechin of *Pterocarpus marsupium* was shown to cause regeneration of the beta cells of the pancreas, which was considered to explain its hypoglycemic action.[132-134] Some other authors were unable to repeat these studies[135-138]; however, later studies have shown that (-)-epicatechin has insulogenic as well as insulin-like properties.[139,140] In addition, epicatechin has been shown in vitro to enhance insulin release by conversion of proinsulin to insulin, which was more pronounced in immature rat islets.[141] Marsupin and ptero-stilbene on i.p. administration to streptozotocin-hyperglycemic rats significantly lowered blood glucose levels, the effect being comparable to metformin (1,1-dimethylbiguanide).[142]

In order to work out a dose-response relationship, aqueous extract of *vijaysar* bark was administered to normal rats, glucose-fed hyperglycemic rats, and alloxan-induced diabetic rats. At 1 g·kg^{-1} given orally there was significant ($p > 0.001$) reduction in blood sugar 2 hours after the administration of aqueous extract. In alloxan-diabetic rats, the aqueous extract of *vijaysar* on daily administration for 3 weeks produced a significant ($p < 0.001$) lowering of blood glucose levels, which is slow in onset, starting from the first week and progressing till the third week.[143] In addition, the aqueous extract has also been shown to exert an anticataract effect in alloxan diabetic rats. [144]

The decoction of *vijaysar* bark extract showed hypocholesterolemic effect in rabbits.[145] The ethyl acetate extract of *vijaysar* administered for 14 days to rats with hyperlipidemia produced a significant reduction of serum triglyceride, total cholesterol, and LDL- and VLDL-cholesterol levels. Among the active constituents of the *vijaysar* bark extract are liquiritigenin and pterosupin.[121]

There have been a number of exploratory studies with small groups of patients. Only one open, multicentric trial has been reported by the Indian Council for Medical Research (ICMR) in 1998, which concluded that *vijaysar* was useful in the treatment of newly diagnosed or mild, untreated NIDDM patients.

In a preliminary open clinical trial, 1 dram of heartwood extract of *vijaysar* was given thrice a day, after the main meals, to 14 diabetic patients on insulin. After a washout period of 5 days, only one patient showed significant hypoglycemic activity. No side effects were observed. However, as part of the same study, the activity of *vijaysar* was compared with that of powdered seeds of *Eugenia jambolana* and it was found that 42 percent of patients responded at a dose level of 1 dram three times a day of *Eugenia jambolana* as compared to 7 percent patients responding to *vijaysar.*[146] It appears that *vijaysar* is not useful in IDDM patients.

The decoction of the bark extract of *vijaysar* was administered to 22 diabetic patients at different dose levels. Glucose tolerance improved in 12 patients after 7 days of treatment.[147] In another open study, 250 mg capsules of dried aqueous extract, prepared by decocting the heartwood, was given to 35 diabetic patients. A favorable response was found only with respect to urine sugar, with little effect on blood sugar levels.[148] In another trial, 20 NIDDM patients were divided into two groups of ten patients each. After a washout period of 10 days, ten patients who were earlier on standard drugs such as chlorpropamide, tolbutamide, or phenformin had the drugs withdrawn and the patients were given 5 g *vijaysar* granules made from dried aqueous extract of *vijaysar* heartwood powder thrice a day for 3 weeks, whereas the other group of ten patients, who were freshly diagnosed with diabetes, were started straightaway on *vijaysar.* Both groups showed significant lowering of blood sugar. No major side effects were observed but two patients taking *vijaysar* had loose motions and gastric upset, controlled by reduction in the dosage.[149]

Water stored overnight in a tumbler made of *vijaysar* heartwood is commonly used as a remedy for diabetes, as mentioned earlier. A small clinical trial was carried out with ten patients, who were given 200 ml of the water, which was stored in the tumbler overnight, twice a day for 1 month, taken after lunch, whereas water stored for the whole day was drunk after dinner. There was encouraging reduction of blood sugar from the second week of treatment and this hypoglycemic activity continued as long as the heartwood water was given.[120]

In an open trial with two groups, patients were administered either 500 mg of *Saussurea lappa* extract twice a day or 100 ml of *Pterocarpus marsupium* decoction twice a day after meals for 30 days. Both drugs were found effective in the management of diabetes and no side effects were observed. There was a decrease in the mean postprandial blood sugar from the initial 283 mg percent to 241 mg percent after the treatment period, in patients treated with *Pterocarpus marsupium.* There was only a slight decrease in cholesterol levels.[150]

An open, multicentric trial involving four centers and three dosage levels was carried out for 12 weeks to evaluate the efficacy of *vijaysar* in 97 newly diagnosed or untreated NIDDM patients. The aqueous extract, prepared by decocting the bark extract and evaporating it to dryness, was administered to patients. Patients were assessed based on blood glucose and glycosylated hemoglobin levels. It was found that by 12 weeks, control of both fasting and postprandial blood glucose levels was attained in 67 of 97 (69 percent) patients studied. Blood sugar was controlled with an extract dose of 2 g in about 73 percent of patients, with 3 g in 16 percent of patients, and with 4 g in 10 percent of the patients. Four of the patients had to be withdrawn from the trial owing to excessively high postprandial blood glucose levels. The fall in both fasting and postprandial levels by 32 and 45 mg·dl^{-1}, respectively, after 12 weeks of treatment was significant ($p < 0.001$) starting from initial values of 151 and 216 mg·dl^{-1}. There was also a significant decrease ($p < 0.001$) in the glycosylated hemoglobin levels from 9.8 to 9.4 percent. There was no significant change in mean lipid levels. No side effects were seen and all other laboratory parameters remained stable during the treatment period. As a result of the trial it was concluded that *vijaysar* is useful in newly diagnosed cases of diabetes mellitus.[151]

Thus the drug seems to be effective with an adequate dosage and careful selection of patients—either newly diagnosed or untreated NIDDM patients. The drug requires further investigation. In clinical trials with *Pterocarpus marsupium* no side effects have been noticed,[149-151] except for loose motions and gastric upset.[149] In small animals, extracts of *Pterocarpus marsupium* showed no untoward effect in doses used to elicit hypoglycemic effect.[126,132]

Salacia *spp. (Family: Celastraceae)*

Latin: *Salacia reticulata* Wight	Malayalam: Ekanayakam, Ponkoranti, Koranti
Sanskrit: Vairi, Pitika	
Latin: *Salacia oblonga* Wall ex Wight & Arn	Malayalam: Ponkoranti
Latin: *Salacia prinoides* DC, *S.chinensis* Linn., *S.latifolia* Wall. ex M. Laws.	Malayalam: Cherukuranti. Trade name: Saptrangi
Latin: *Salacia macrosperma* Wight.	Malayalam: Anakoranti
Latin: *Salacia fruticosa*	

The genus Salacia is a group of climbing or creeping shrubs or small trees of which 18 species are found in India.[152] Over five species are used in Ayurveda and Siddha for the treatment of diabetes—*Salacia prinoides, S. macrosperma, S. oblonga, S. fruticosa,* and *S. reticulata,* that have varied locational distribution.[152-154] Of these, the three most commonly used are *S. prinoides* (=*chinensis; latifolia*), *S. oblonga,* and *S. reticulata. S. reticulata* is also one of the most widely used plants for diabetes in Sri Lanka.[155] Preparations of *S. reticulata* are sold in Japan as a food supplement for obesity and diabetes.[156] It is not certain from a study of literature whether carefully identified species have been used and, therefore, whether there are problems in the interpretation of results. Roots and root bark of *Salacia* species have been used in Ayurvedic medicine for the treatment of diabetes. Apart from this, the root has been used for treating itch, rheumatism, and venereal diseases, such as gonorrhea. [152]

The xanthone mangiferin has been isolated from the roots of several Salacia species—*S. reticulata,*[157,158] *S. oblonga, S. chinensis,* and *S. prinoides.*[158] However, *S. chinensis* is considered a synonym for *S. prinoides.*[152] Also isolated from *S. reticulata* are catechin and catechin dimers. Potent alpha-glucosidase inhibitors, salacinol and kotalanol, have been isolated from both *S. reticulata*[159,160] and *S. oblonga.*[161] Several compounds—xathone,[158] triterpenoids,[161] diterpenoids,[161] and flavonoids—with inhibitory effect on rat lens aldose reductase have been isolated from stems of *S. reticulata, S. oblonga,* and *S. chinensis.*[158,161,162]

S. prinoides

The hypoglycemic activity of infusion and decoction of root bark of *S. prinoides* was studied in detail at different dose levels: $1 g \cdot kg^{-1}$ bodyweight of infusion showed hypoglycemic activity comparable to tolbutamide.[163] Of the three Salacia species—*S. prinoides, S. macrosperma,* and *S. fruticosa,* the infusion of *S. prinoides* was found to exhibit maximum hypoglycemic activity at a dose of $1 g \cdot kg^{-1}$ bodyweight. *S. fruticosa* did not have potent hypoglycemic activity, although *S. macrosperma* exhibited some degree of hypoglycemic activity.[164]

S. oblonga

Two fractions derived from the petroleum ether extract of the root bark of *S. oblonga* showed 60 and 76 percent hypoglycemic activity of an equal dose of tolbutamide (250 mg·kg^{-1}) in albino rats.[165] *S. oblonga* root bark has significant blood sugar lowering activity and antioxidant property. Petroleum ether extract of root bark has also been shown to prevent streptozotocin-induced hyperglycemia and hyperinsulinemia, and produce a significant decrease in peroxidation products in streptozotocin-diabetic rats.[166] Aqueous methanolic extracts of *S. oblonga* inhibited the increase of serum glucose level in sucrose- and maltose-loaded rats. The aqueous portion of this extract containing potent alpha-glucosidase inhibitors salacinol and kotalanol, along with nine other sugars, inhibited alpha-glucosidase, whereas the ethyl acetate extract containing known di- and triterpenes and a new triterpene kotalagenin-16-acetate exhibited potent aldose reductase activity.[161]

S. reticulata

Salacia reticulata aqueous extract decoction of root bark fed at 1 ml per rat per day to fasting rats caused a 30-percent reduction of blood glucose levels, 3 hours after administration of the extract.[155] Aqueous extract of *S. reticulata* (0.5-5 g·kg^{-1}) reduced plasma glucose concentration in streptozotocin-induced diabetic rats; the effect being maximum at 1-5 hours after administration of extract.[167]

Among the active constituents isolated is the xanthone mangiferin that has been shown to lower blood glucose levels in KK-Ay mice, an animal model for type 2 diabetes. Mangiferin has also been shown to improve hyperinsulinemia, possibly by decreasing insulin resistance,[168] and to exhibit alpha-glucosidase and aldose reductase–inhibitory activities.[158] Other active ingredients include salacinol and kotalanol, which are potent alpha-glucosidase inhibitors.[159-161]

In India, *Salacia reticulata* is usually one ingredient of multiplant preparations in most products. Preparations of *S. reticulata* are available as herbal supplements for the treatment of obesity and diabetes in Japan. The extract, obtained by extraction of the roots with hot water have been shown to prevent postprandial increase in blood sugar in humans.[169] In addition, it decreased fasting blood sugar, glycosylated hemoglobin, and body mass index in mild NIDDM patients.[170]

As a single ingredient *Salacia prinoides* has undergone preliminary exploratory clinical evaluation and has been found to possess both hypolipidemic and hypoglycemic activity. Tablets of root bark of *S. prinoides (Ekanayakam)* 500 mg were given to 18 NIDDM patients (fasting serum glucose levels of 120-160 mg·dl^{-1}) at a dose level of 2.5, 3.5, and 5 g per day (six patients at each dose level), while six patients were kept as control with restricted diet just as the drug group. There was efficient lowering of blood glucose, mean serum cholesterol, and triglyceride levels, and increase in HDL-cholesterol levels without any side effects with *Salacia* treatment.[171]

In another open trial, 42 NIDDM patients were given either 500 mg tablets of *Salacia prinoides* alone or a 500 mg tablet of 1:1 mixture of *Salacia prinoides* and *Strychnos potatorum* for 2 months. A control group was managed with diet restrictions. Hypoglycemic and hypocholesterolemic activities were observed. There was a significant reduction in blood glucose levels; however, reduction in blood glucose levels was greater in patients who were on *Salacia prinoides* alone.[172]

In another study, 25 patients were treated with 500 mg of *S. prinoides* (= *chinensis*) powder along with *triphala* tablets 2.5 g thrice a day for 6 months, which brought down blood sugar and urine sugar levels.[173] *Triphala* is a well-known Ayurvedic preparation containing, in equal proportions, dried fruits of *Terminalia chebula*, *T. belerica*, and *Phyllanthus emblica* and used as a bowel tonic.

There is an urgent need to conduct well-planned clinical trials to evaluate these potentially promising Ayurvedic drugs, and also to evaluate the relative efficacy of the different species.

Preparations with *Salacia reticulata* are available in the Japanese market, and as a combination drug with other plants in India. The safety profile of the hot-water extract of *Salacia reticulata* in terms of acute and subacute toxicity, mutagenicity, antigenicity, and phototoxicity have been carried out.[174-176] In pregnant rats root extract of *S. reticulata* at a dose level of 10 g·kg^{-1} significantly increased postimplantation losses, leading the authors to recommend that it should not be used in pregnancy.[177] However, the dose levels used seem to be high. The safety evaluation of hot-water extract of *Salacia oblonga* at ten times the normal intake for 2 weeks did not change the clinical chemistry or produce histological changes in rats.[178]

Syzygium cuminii *(L.) Skeels. (Family: Myrtaceae)*

Latin: *Eugenia jambolana* Lam. *E. cuminii* Druce	Hindi: Jaman, Jam, Jamun
Sanskrit: Jambu	Tamil: Naval
English: Black Plum, Black Berry	

Syzygium cuminii is a large evergreen tree found throughout India in the plains up to an elevation of 1,800 m,[179] that bears a large crop of subacidic, astringent fruits, which consist of an inner seed covered by a pink-to-purple pulp that can be eaten, that are sold in the market. Seeds of *jambu* have been used in India for a very long time for the treatment of diabetes although the fruit pulp and leaves are also used in other parts of the world. It is also a very common household remedy for diabetes, especially in the villages in South India either by itself or in combination with *Gymnema sylvestre.*

The bark extract decoction is used in gargling for sore throat, spongy gums and stomatitis, and for dysentry and diarrhea. Leaves are used for diarrhea, especially in children. The vinegar made from the fruits is used as a stomachic, a carminative, and a diuretic drug. The seeds of the fruit are used in diabetes, where it is considered to reduce the quantity of sugar in the urine and to allay thirst.[179-181]

The seeds contain several phenolic compounds including gallic acid, ellagic acid, corilagin, substituted galloyl glucoses, caffeic acid, ferulic acid, quercetin, and the glycoside jamboline.[182-184]

There have been a number of studies on the hypoglycemic effect caused by seeds and seed extracts of *jambu.* Oral administration of seeds of *jambu* reduced blood sugar levels in different animal models[185,186] comparable to chlorpropamide at doses ranging from 170 to 510 mg per rat,[185] and comparable to phenformin at a dose of 1 g·kg^{-1} in casein diet in streptozotocin-induced diabetes in rabbits.[186] In addition, there was significant decrease in postmeal values of cholesterol, free fatty acids, and triglycerides comparable to phenformin.[186] Also observed was an increase of cathepsin B activity both by plant extract and chlorpropamide reflecting possible proteolytic conversion of proinsulin to insulin.[185] An aqueous suspension of seeds of *jambu* was tested for hypoglycemic activity at different dose levels ranging from 1 g to 6 g·kg^{-1} body weight in rabbits. The maximum hypoglycemic effect of 42.64 percent, which was shown at 4 g·kg^{-1} dose level 3 hours after intake.[187] Aqueous, alcoholic, and acetone extracts of *jambu* seeds fed to albino rats at different doses for periods from 15 to 45 days produced significant hypoglycemic effect. The acetone extracts also reduced cholesterol and serum urea levels. In addition, blood sugar levels once lowered continued to be stable even for a fortnight after the treatment was stopped.[188] Oral administration of aqueous extracts of seeds of *jamun (jambu)* to alloxan-diabetic rats at a dose of 2.5 g and 5 g·kg^{-1} body weight but not at the 7.5 g level for 6 weeks resulted in significant reduction of blood glucose levels, which was greater than glibenclamide. The extract also showed antioxidant activity but not at the 7.5 g level.[189] At 2.5 g·kg^{-1} there was an increase in hepatic hexokinase activity and a decrease of glucose-6-phosphatase in alloxan-diabetic animals.[190]

Free radical scavenging activity of the methanolic extract of *jambu* seeds and of the major constituent of the extract, gallic acid, showed free radical scavenging activity greater than ascorbic acid while that of the methanolic extract was comparable to ascorbic acid. The authors suggest that this free radical scavenging activity could be useful in prevention of cataract.[191] This has been confirmed by another study that feeding lyophilized aqueous extract of the seeds at 200 mg·kg·day^{-1} for 4 months prevented murine alloxan-diabetic cataract in rats.[192]

Daily administration for 21 to 120 days of lyophilized aqueous extract of *jambu* seeds at 200 mg·day^{-1} showed significant antihyperglycemic activity in mild-to-moderate degree of hyperglycemia, partially restoring altered skeletal and hepatic glycogen content and enzyme levels. Some degree of activity was also exhibited in severely diabetic mice (>400 mg·dl^{-1}).[193] At 400 mg·day^{-1} for 15 days *jambu* extract prevented hyperglycemia and hyperinsulinemia induced by a diet high in fructose.[194] Renal hypertrophy was also prevented when fed at 200 mg·kg^{-1} for 40 days when compared to diabetic controls.[195]

Despite the popular usage of *jambu* seeds there are only a few open clinical trials. In an early trial on 28 patients 4-24 g of *jambu* seed powder was given thrice a day. Twenty patients showed significant fall in fasting and postprandial blood sugar, seven showed decreases in postprandial blood sugar and an increase in fasting blood sugar, whereas one patient showed increases in both parameters. In addition, patients showed improvement in signs and symptoms of the disease. While there was no observable toxicity in the liver, kidney, and blood, side effects seen were nausea, diarrhea, and epigastric pain.[196]

In an open clinical trial, 30 NIDDM patients were treated with 12 g of *jambu* powder given in three divided daily doses for 3 months. There was good control of blood sugar along with relief in symptoms that increased with duration of treatment. A control group of six patients were kept on chlorpropamide. Results with *Eugenia jambolana* were assessed as comparable to chlorpropamide. No side effects were observed.[197]

A compound herbal preparation, consisting of 2 g each of powdered *Gymnema sylvestre* leaves and *Syzygium cuminii* seeds, was taken by 20 patients thrice daily for 6 weeks. Ten patients on restricted diets served as control. Seventy percent of the patients were found to have responded well, based on biochemical parameters and relief of symptoms such as frequency and quantity of urine, feeling of well-being, numbness and tingling of hand and feet, and itching. In addition, the response was considered good in 13.33 percent of patients, whereas the response was considered poor in 16.67 percent of patients. No side effects or toxicity was observed in rats.[198]

The fruits of *Syzygium cuminii* are commonly and widely consumed in India; however, large quantities are not consumed because of the astringent nature of the fruits. In one clinical trial with *Syzygium cuminii* seeds, there were two cases of nausea, two of diarrhea, and one of epigastric pain.[196] Another trial, however, did not show any side effects and the drug was well tolerated.[197] Thus, clinical trials with standardized material and larger patient numbers are needed to obtain a clear picture of the safety and efficacy of the herb.

Trigonella foenum-graecum *Linn. (Family: Fabaceae)*

Sanskrit: Methika	Tamil: Vendium
Hindi: Methi	English: Fenugreek

Trigonella foenum-graecum is an annual herb found growing wild in Punjab, Kashmir, and the upper Gangetic plains. It is also cultivated extensively throughout India. Two types are known—a dwarf type used for culinary purposes and a tall type used for fodder. The seeds are common ingredients of curry, and the leaves are cooked and eaten as a vegetable. Dried leaves are sold in the market to add flavor and nutrition to food. The seeds are a common spice and also used medicinally. The seeds are aromatic, bitter, carminative, tonic, and a galactagogue. Internally it is used for inflammation of the gastrointestinal tract, for diarrhea, and dysentry probably because of the mucilage present in the seeds.[199]

The seeds are a rich source of dietary fiber with 45-60 percent total carbohydrates, mostly as soluble fiber present as mucilage, 20-30 percent protein, and 10 percent of fixed oil. There are also several steroidal saponins in the seeds. The bitter taste of the seeds is because of the presence of furostanol saponins. Also present are sterols, flavonoids, alkaloids such as trigonelline, 0.015 percent of an essential oil,[200] and amino acids including the novel insulin secreting amino acid 4-hydroxyisoleucine.[201]

A number of studies have been carried out in small animals to find out the scope of hypoglycemic activity. An antidiabetic effect has been shown in rats, dogs, and mice.[202-204] In alloxan-diabetic rats fenugreek extract[205,206] and its major alkaloid trigonelline[206] produced a significant hypoglycemic effect. Pretreatment with fenugreek prior to production of diabetes by streptozotocin improved both blood glucose and lipid levels.[207] The antidiabetic and hypocholesterolemic activity of fenugreek has been reviewed in 1998.[208]

Fenugreek seeds brought back altered creatinine kinase activity in the heart, skeletal muscle, and liver of diabetic rats back to normal values.[209] Changes in hepatic and renal glucose[210,211] and lipid metabolizing enzymes[211] were also normalized. Fenugreek seeds have been shown to have an antioxidant effect.[212] The hypocholesterolemic activity has been reported by several authors.[213-217] Fenugreek is considered to exert its antidiabetic effect in different ways—through its fiber content in a manner similar to guar gum both being rich in galactomannans,[208,220] through inhibition of intestinal glucosidase[218] and through insulin release by 4-hydroxyisoleucine.[201] Trigonelline was subsequently shown not to be active by administration in amounts present in fenugreek.[219]

A number of small clinical trials have been conducted to evaluate the hypoglycemic activity of fenugreek. The hypoglycemic activity of fenugreek seeds and leaves was tested in normal subjects and diabetic patients. In an acute study on healthy volunteers, a single dose of various forms of fenugreek were tried out—25 g seeds, 5 g gum isolate, or 150 g leaves being given, the seeds being administered in four different forms—as whole seeds, defatted seeds, degummed seeds, and cooked seeds. Although the gum isolate and leaves showed no hypoglycemic effect, maximal reduction of blood glucose was shown by whole seeds. Therefore, in NIDDM patients 25 g of fenugreek seed powder in two divided doses was mixed with their usual diet for 21 days. There was significant reduction in blood glucose levels and insulin response. In addition, there was significant reduction ($p < 0.05$) in 24-hour urinary glucose output and in cholesterol levels.[220]

In type I diabetics, 100 g of defatted fenugreek, given in divided doses at lunch and dinner for 10 days, significantly reduced fasting blood sugar, improved glucose tolerance, reduced 24-hour urinary glucose excretion by 54 percent, and also showed a significant hypolipidemic effect.[221] A similar study in 15 NIDDM patients, who were fed randomly meals in cross-over design and incorporated with or without 100 g of defatted fenugreek seed powder, produced similar results.[222] Also in type II diabetics, fed with 15 g of fenugreek seed powder soaked in water per day, there was postprandial lowering of blood sugar level.[223]

In a cross-over study to determine whether the improved glucose tolerance was owing to the effect of fenugreek on the absorption or metabolism of glucose, the diet was either randomly incorporated with 25 g of fenugreek seed or left out in ten NIDDM patients as pretreatment for 15 days prior to intravenous glucose load. Results showed that the addition of fenugreek to the diet significantly reduced the area under the plasma glucose curve and increased glucose clearance, suggesting that improved peripheral glucose utilization contributes to improved glucose tolerance. Fenugreek also significantly increased molar insulin binding sites of erythrocytes.[224]

Studies have also been conducted to observe the hypolipidemic effect of fenugreek seeds in diabetic patients, who are known to be at risk of developing cardiovascular disease. An open long-term study was carried on 60 NIDDM patients to study the effect of fenugreek on lipid levels. There was an initial control period of 7 days followed by an experimental period of 24 weeks when patients consumed 25 g of fenugreek seed powder in two divided doses as soup in water before lunch and dinner. The was a significant fall in total cholesterol, LDL, and VLDL cholesterol, and also in triglyceride levels.[225]

A double-blind placebo-controlled study was conducted in order to evaluate the effects of fenugreek on glycemic control and insulin resistance in newly diagnosed mild-to-moderate NIDDM patients. In the treatment group, 12 patients received 1 g·day^{-1} of aqueous alcoholic extract of fenugreek seeds, whereas the control group of 13 patients received placebo capsules for 2 months along with diet and exercise. Patients were randomly assigned either to treatment group or to placebo group. Both groups were checked to make sure they had similar baseline values. At the end of 2 months both the fasting and after meal blood sugar levels were comparable in the two groups. However, area under curve of blood glucose and insulin was significantly ($p < 0.001$) lower in the treatment group. There was also a decrease in insulin resistance and a significant decrease in triglyceride and increase in HDL cholesterol.[226]

Fenugreek seeds are a commonly used spice in Indian cooking and the leaves are used as a vegetable. In clinical trials, generally, no side effects have been reported at lower dosage levels of 15-25 g seed;[223,224] however, with 100 g of fenugreek four patients complained of diarrhea and flatulence.[221] In subsequent trials, a few patients had GI disturbances even at 25 g.[225,226] In a long-term study lasting 24 weeks, on diabetic patients who were administered 25 g of fenugreek seeds per day, there was no toxicity in the liver and kidney and no abnormality in blood parameters.[227]

No toxicity was observed in a short-term study of 90 days when rats were fed with equivalent of two and four times the human dosage of 25 g of fenugreek seeds, which is generally used in NIDDM patients to improve glucose tolerance and lipid levels. Liver function tests were normal as were liver histology and blood picture.[228]

NOTES

1. van der Nat JM, van der Sluis WG, de Silva KTD, Labadie RP. Ethno-pharmacognostical survey of *Azadirachta indica* A. Juss (Meliaceae). *J Ethnopharmacol* 35:1-24 (1991).

2. Chawla AS, Kumar M, Bansal I. Chemical constituents and biological activity of *"neem"*—A review. *Indian Drugs* 32:57-64 (1995).

3. Luscombe DK, Taha SA. Pharmacological studies on the leaves of *Azadirachta indica. J Pharmacy Pharmacology* 26 (suppl.):111 (1974).

4. Murty KS, Rao DN, Rao DK, Murty LBG. A preliminary study of the hypoglycaemic and antihyperglycaemic effects of *Azadirachta indica. Indian J Pharmacol* 10:247-250 (1978).

5. Pillai NR, Santhakumari G. Hypoglycaemic activity of *Melia azadirachta* Linn. *(neem). Indian J Med Res* 74:931-933 (1981).

6. Chattopadhyay R, Chattopadhyay RN, Nandy AK, Poddar G, Maitra SK. Preliminary report on antihyperglycemic effect of a fraction of fresh leaves of *Azadirachta indica* (Beng *neem*). *Bull Calcutta School Trop Med* 35(1-4):29-33 (1987).

7. Chakrabortty T, Verotta L, Poddar G. Evaluation of *Azadirachta indica* leaf extract for hypoglycaemic activity in rats. *Phytother Res* 3:30-32 (1989).

8. Mandal SC, Pal (Dutta) S, Kumar CKA, Lakshmi SM. A study on the hypoglycaemic activity of the methanolic extract of *Azadirachta indica (neem)* leaves. *Indian J Nat Prod* 16(1):8-11 (2000).

9. Chattopadhyay RR. A comparative evaluation of some blood sugar lowering agents of plant origin. *J Ethnopharmacol* 67:367-372 (1999).

10. Khosla P, Bhanwara S, Singh J, Seth S, Srivastava RK. A study of hypoglycemic effects of *Azadirachta indica (neem)* in normal and alloxan diabetic rabbits. *Indian J Physiol Pharmacol* 44:69-74 (2000).

11. Sharma MK, Khare AK, Feroz H. Effect of *neem* oil on blood levels of normal, hyperglycemic and diabetic animals. *Nagarjun* 26:247-250 (1983).

12. Dixit VP, Sinha R, Tank R. Effect of *neem* seed oil in the blood glucose concentration of normal and alloxan diabetic rats. *J Ethnopharmacol* 17:95-98 (1986).

13. Chattopadhyay RR. Possible mechanism of antihyperglycemic effect of *Azadirachta indica* leaf extract. Part IV. *General Pharmacol* 27:431-434 (1996).

14. Chattopadhyay R, Chattopadhyay RN, Nandy AK, Poddar G, Maitra SK. The effect of a fraction of fresh leaves of *Azadirachta indica* (Beng: *neem*) on glucose uptake and glycogen content in the isolated rat hemidiaphragm. *Bull Calcutta School Trop Med* 35(1-4):8-11 (1987).

15. Chattopadhyay RR. Possible mechanism of antihyperglycemic effect of *Azadirachta indica* leaf extract Part V. *J Ethnopharmacol* 67:373-376 (1999).

16. Shukla R, Singh S, Bhandari CR. Preliminary clinical trials on antidiabetic actions of *Azadirachta indica. Med Surg* 13:11-12 (1973).

17. Bhargava AK. A note on the use of *neem* oil *(Azadirachta indica)* as antihyperglycaemic agent in human volunteers of secondary diabetes. *J Vet Physio Allied Sci* 5:45-48 (1986).

18. Jha SN. Effect of *neem* oil *(Azadirachta indica)* as antihyperglycaemic agent. *Indian Med J* 84:331 (1990).

19. Ross IA. *Medicinal plants of the world* (vol. 2, pp. 81-118). Totowa, NJ: Humana Press, 2001.

20. Chinnasamy N, Harishankar N, Kumar PV, Rukmani C. Toxicological studies on debitterized *neem* oil *(Azadirachta indica)*. *Food Chem Toxicol* 31:297-301 (1993).

21. Nadkarni AK. *Dr KM Nadkarnis's Indian materia medica* (vol. I, pp. 300-302). Bombay: Popular Prakashan, 1976.

22. Pillai NR, Ghosh D, Uma R, Anandakumar A. Hypoglycaemic activity of *Coccinia indica* W & A. *Bull Medico Ethno Res* 1:234-242 (1980).

23. Pandey G. *Dravyaguna vijnana* (materia medica—vegetable drugs) (1st edn., vol. 1, pp. 424-429). Varanasi: Krishnadas Academy, 1998.

24. Malhotra SC. (ed.), *Phytochemical investigation of certain medicinal plants used in Ayurveda* (pp. 191-192). New Delhi: Central Council for Research in Ayurveda and Siddha, 1990.

25. Pressanna Kumar G, Sudheesh S, Vijayalakshmi NR. Hypoglycaemic effect of *Coccina indica:* Mechanism of action. *Planta Med* 59:330-332 (1992).

26. Brahmachari HD, Augusti KT. Orally effective hypoglycaemic principles of *Coccinia indica* Wight and Arn. *J Pharm Pharmacol* 15:411-412 (1963).

27. De UN, Mukherjee B. Effect of *Coccinia indica* Wight & Arn on alloxan diabetes in rabbits—A preliminary note. *Indian J Med Sci* 7:665-672 (1953).

28. Mukherjee SK, De UN, Mukherjee B. Contribution in the field of diabetes research in the last decade. *Ind Med Gazz* 3:97-104 (1963).

29. Mukherjee B, Chandrasekar B, Mukherjee SK. Blood sugar lowering effect of *Coccinia indica* root and whole plant in different experimental rat models. *Fitoterapia* 59:207-210 (1988).

30. Chandrasekar B, Mukherjee B, Mukherjee SK. Blood sugar lowering potentiality of selected Cucurbitaceae plants of Indian origin. *Indian J Med Res.* 90:300-305 (1989).

31. Gupta SS. Experimental studies of pituitary diabetes Part III. Effect of indigenous antidiabetic drugs against acute hyperglycaemic response of anterior pituitary extract in glucose fed albino rats. *Indian J Med Res* 51:716-724 (1963).

32. Gupta SS, Variyar MC. Experimental studies of pituitary diabetes. Part IV. Effect of *Gymnema sylvestre* and *Coccinia indica* against the hyperglycaemic response of somatropin and corticotropin hormones. *Indian J Med Res* 52:200-207 (1964).

33. Mukherjee K, Ghosh NC, Datta T. *Coccinia indica* Linn. as potential hypoglycaemic agent. *Indian J Exp Biol* 10:347-349 (1972).

34. Shibib BA, Khan LA, Rahman R. Hypoglycaemic activity of *Coccinia indica* and *Momordica charantia* in diabetic rats: Depression of the hepatic gluconeogenic enzymes glucose 6-phosphatase and fructose-1,6-bisphosphatase and elevation of both liver and red-cell shunt enzyme glucose-6-phosphate dehydrogenase. *Biochem J* 292:267-270 (1993).

35. Hossain MZ, Shibib MA, Rahman R. Hypoglycemic effects of *Coccinia indica:* Inhibition of key gluconeogenic enzyme, glucose-6-phosphatase. *Indian J Exp Biol* 30:418-420 (1992).

36. Khan AKA, Akhtar S, Mahtab H. *Coccinia indica* in the treatment of patients with diabetes mellitus. *Bangladesh Med Res Counc Bull* 5(2):60-66 (1979).

37. Khan AKA, Akhtar S, Mahtab H. Treatment of diabetes mellitus with *Coccinia indica. Br Med J* 280 (6220):1044 (1980).

38. Shaw BP, Gupta S. A clinical study of *bimbi (Coccinia indica)* in the treatment of *madhumeha* (Diabetes mellitus). *Nagarjun* 25(2):24-26 (1981).

39. Ghosal J, Ray A, Ray R. Influence of *Cephalandra indica* Naud *(Telakucha)* on serum lipids and lipoproteins in the humans of different age groups (pp. 110-111). Calcutta: International Seminar—Traditional Medicine, 1992.

40. Banerjee A, Ray P, Ray A, Ray R. Clinical evaluation of *Cephalandra indica* Naud *(Telakucha)* in diabetes mellitus. (p. 135). Calcutta: International Conference on Current Progress in Medicinal and Aromatic Plants Research, 1995.

41. Kamble SM, Jyotishi GS, Kamalakar PL, Vaidya SM. Efficacy of *Coccina indica* W & A in diabetes mellitus *J Res Ayur Siddha* XVII(1-2):77-84 (1996).

42. Kamble SM, Kamalakar PL, Vaidya S, Bambole VD. Influence of *Coccinia indica* on certain enzymes in glycolytic and lipolytic pathway in human diabetes. *Indian J Med Sci* 52:143-146 (1998).

43. Kurihara Y. Characteristics of antisweet substances, sweeet proteins, and sweetness inducing proteins. *Crit Rev Food Sci Nutr* 32:231-252 (1992).

44. *The wealth of India, raw materials* (vol. IV, pp. 276-277). New Delhi: Publications and Information Directorate, CSIR, 1956.

45. Sugihara Y, Nojima H, Matsuda H, Murakami T, Yoshikawa M, Kimura I. Antihyperglycemic effects of gymnemic acid IV, a compound derived from *Gymnema sylvestre* leaves in streptozotocin-diabetic mice. *J Asian Nat Prod Res* 2:321-327 (2000).

46. Agarwal SK, Singh SS, Verma S, Lakshmi V, Sharma A, Sushil Kumar. Chemistry and medicinal uses of *Gymnema sylvestre (gur-mar)* leaves—A review. *Indian Drugs* 37:354-360 (2000).

47. Shanmugasundaram KR, Paneerselvam C, Samudram P, Shanmugasundaram ERB. Enzyme changes and glucose uitization in diabetic rabbits: The effect of *Gymnema sylvestre* R. Br. *J Ethnopharmacol* 7:205-234 (1983).

48. Srivastava Y, Bhatt HV, Jhala CI, Nigam SK, Kumar A, Verma Y. Oral *Gymnema sylvestre* R. Br. leaf extracts inducing protracted longevity and hypoglycaemia in alloxan diabetic rats: Review and experimental study. *Int J Crude Drug Res* 24:171-176 (1986).

49. Okabayashi Y, Tani S, Fujisawa T, Koide M, Hasegawa H, Nakamura T, Fujii M, Otsuki M. Effect of *Gymnema sylvestre* R. Br. on glucose homeostatis in rats *Diabetes Res Clin Pract* 9:143-148 (1990).

50. Chattopadhyay RR, Medda C, Das S, Basu TK, Poddar G. Hypoglycemic and antihyperglycemic effect of *Gymnema sylvestre* leaf extract in rats. *Fitoterapia* LXIV:450-454 (1993).

51. Shanmugasundaram ERB, Gopinath KL, Shanmugasundaram KR, Rajendran VM. Possible regeneration of the islets of Langerhans in streptozotocin-diabetic rats given *Gymnema sylvestre* leaf extracts. *J Ethnopharmacol* 30:265-279 (1990).

52. Persaud SJ, Al-Majed H, Raman A, Jones PM. *Gymnema sylvestre* stimulates insulin release *in vitro* by increased membrane permeability. *J Endocrinol* 163:207-212 (1999).

53. Shimizu K, Iino A, Nakajima J, Tanaka K, Nakajyo S, Urakawa N, Atsuchi M, Wada T, Yamashita C. Suppression of glucose absorption by some fractions extracted from *Gymnema sylvestre* leaves. *J Vet Med Sci* 59:245-251 (1997).

54. Rathi NA, Shanmugasundaram KR. Glycemic control in the development of vascular disease in diabetes mellitus. Effect of *Gymnema sylvestre* R. Br. *Biomedicine* 7(2):39-44 (1987).

55. Bishayee A, Chatterjee M. Hypolipidemic and antiatherosclerotic effects of oral *Gymnema sylvestre* R. Br. leaf extract in albino rats fed on high fat diet. *Phytother Res* 8:118-120 (1994).

56. Shigematsu N, Asano R, Shimosaka M, Okazaki M. Effect of long term administration with *Gymnema sylvestre* R. Br. on plasma and liver lipid in rats. *Biol Pharm Bull* 24:643-649 (2001).

57. Nakamura Y, Tsumura Y, Tonogai Y, Shibata T. Fecal steroid excretion is increased in rats by oral administration of gymnemic acids contained in *Gymnema sylvestre* leaves. *J Nutr* 129:1214-1222 (1999).

58. Shigematsu N, Asano R, Shimosaka M, Okazaki M. Effect of administration with the extract of *Gymnema sylvestre* R. Br. leaves on lipid metabolism in rats. *Biol Pharm Bull* 24:713-717 (2001).

59. Wang LF, Luo H, Miyoshi M, Imoto T, Hiji Y, Sasaki T. Inhibitory effect of gymnemic acid on intestinal absorption of oleic acid in rats. *Can J Physiol Pharmacol* 76:1017-1023 (1998).

60. Shanmugasundaram ERB, Venkatasubrahmanyam M, Vijendran N, Shanmugasundaram KR. Effect of an isolate from *Gymnema sylvestre* R. Br. in the control of diabetes mellitus and the associated pathological changes. *Ancient Sci of Life* VII:183-194 (1988).

61. Khare AK, Tondon RN, Tewari JP. Hypoglycaemic activity of an indigenous drug *(Gymnema sylvestre, "Gurmar")* in normal and diabetic persons. *Indian J Physiol Pharm* 27:257-258 (1983).

62. Baskaran K, Ahamath BK, Shanmugasundaram KR, Shanmugasundaram ERB. Antidiabetic effect of a leaf extract from *Gymnema sylvestre* in non-insulin-dependent diabetes mellitus patients. *J Ethnopharmacol* 30:295-305 (1990).

63. Shanmugasundaram ERB, Rajeswari G, Baskaran K, Rajesh Kumar BR, Shanmugasundaram KR, Ahmath BK. Use of *Gymnema sylvestre* leaf extract in the control of blood glucose in insulin-dependent diabetes mellitus. *J Ethnopharmacol* 30:281-294 (1990).

64. Balasubramaniam K, Arasaratnam V, Nageswaran A, Anushiyanthan S, Mugunthan N. Studies on the effect of *Gymnema sylvestre* on diabetics. *J Nat Sci Council of Sri Lanka* 20(1):81-89 (1992).

65. Chakrabortty T. Studies on the development of new medicines from indigenous plants (pp. 5-14). Darjeeling, India: Procs Fifth Internatl Soc Horticultural Science Symposium on Medicinal, Aromatic and Spice Plants, February 23-26,1985.

66. Mukherjee SK, Saxena AM, Shukla G. *Progress of diabetes research in India during the 20th century* (pp. 13-16). New Delhi: National Institute of Science Communication, CSIR, 2002.

67. Ogawa Y, Sekita K, Umemurra T, Saito M, Ono A, Kawaskai Y, Uchida O, Matsushima Y, Inoue T, Kanno J. [*Gymnema sylvestre* leaf extract: A 52-week dietary toxicity study in Wistar rats]. *Shokuhin Eiseigaku Zasshi* 45:8-18 (2004).

68. *The wealth of India, raw materials* (vol. VI, pp. 408-411). New Delhi: Publications and Information Directorate (CSIR), 1962.

69. Sivarajan VV and Balachandran I. *Ayurvedic drugs and their plant sources* (pp. 220-222). New Delhi: Oxford and IBH Publishing Co Pvt Ltd., 1994.

70. Chatterjee KP. On the presence of an antidiabetic principle in *Momordica charantia. Indian J Physio Pharmacol* 7:240 (1963).

71. Raman A and Lau C. Anti-diabetic properties and phytochemistry of *Momordica charantia* L. (Cucurbitaceae). *Phytomedicine* 2:349-362 (1996).

72. Khanna P, Jain SC, Panagariya A, Dixit VP. Hypoglycemic activity of polypeptide p from a plant source. *J Nat Prod* 44:648-655 (1981).

73. Lotlikar MM, Rajarama Rao MR. Note on a hypoglycemic principle isolated from the fruits of *Momordica charantia. J University Bombay* 29:223-224 (1962).

74. Matsuda H, Li Y, Murakami T, Matsumura N, Yamahara J, Yoshikawa M. Antidiabetic principles of natural medicines III. Structure-related inhibitory activity and action of oleanolic acid glycosides on hypoglycemic activity. *Chem Pharm Bull* (Tokyo) 46:1399-1403 (1998).

75. Handa G, Singh J, Sharma ML, Kaul A, Neerja, Zafar R. Hypoglycemic principle of *Momordica charantia* seeds. *Indian J Nat Prod* 6(1):16-19 (1990).

76. Sharma VN, Sogani RK, Arora RB. Some observations on hypoglycemic activity of *Momordica charantia. Indian J Med Res* 48:471-477 (1960).

77. Gupta SS, Seth CB. Effect of *Momordica charantia* Linn *(karela)* on glucose tolerance in albino rats. *J Indian Med Assn* 39:581-584 (1962).

78. Jose MP, Cheeran JV, Nair KPD. Effect of selected indigenous drugs on the blood sugar level in dogs. *Indian J Pharm* 8:86 (1976).

79. Karunanayake EH, Welihinda J, Sirimanne SR, Sinnadorai G. Oral hypoglcemic activity of some medicinal plants of Sri Lanka. *J Ethnopharmacol* 11:223-231 (1984).

80. Day C, Cartwright T, Provost J, Bailey CJ. Hypoglycemic effect of *Momordica charantia* extracts. *Planta Med* 56:426-429 (1990).

81. Ali L, Khan AKA, Mamun MIR, Moshihuzzaman M, Nahar N, Nur-e-Alam M, Rokeya B. Studies on hypoglycemic effects of fruit pulp, seed, and whole plant of *Momordica charantia* on normal and diabetic model rats. *Planta Med* 59:408-412 (1993).

82. Cakici I, Hurmoglu C, Tunctan B, Abacioglu N, Kanzik I, Sener B. Hypoglycemic effect of *Momordica charantia* extracts in normoglycemic or cyproheptadine-induced hyperglycemic mice. *J Ethnopharmacol* 44:117-121 (1994).

83. Sarkar S, Pranava M, Marita R. Demonstration of the hypoglycemic action of *Momordica charantia* in a validated animal model of diabetes. *Pharmacol Res* 33:1-4 (1996).

84. Muira T, Itoh C, Iwamoto N, Kato M, Kawai M, Park SR, Suzuki I. Hypoglycemic activity of the fruit of the *Momordica charantia* in type 2 diabetic mice. *J Nutr Sci Vitaminol* (Tokyo) 47:340-344 (2001).

85. Matsuda H, Murakami T, Shimada H, Matsumura N, Yoshikawa M, Yamahara J. Inhibitory mechanisms of oleanolic acid 3-O-monodesmosides on glucose absorption in rats. *Biol Pharm Bull* 20:717-719 (1997).

86. Lotlikar MM, Rao MRR. Pharmacology of a hypoglycaemic principle isolated from the fruits of *Momordica charantia* Linn. *Indian J Pharm* 28(5):129-133 (1966).

87. Ahmed I, Adeghate E, Sharma AK, Pallot DJ, Singh J. Effects of *Momordica charantia* fruit juice on islet morphology in the pancreas of the streptozotocin-diabetic-rat. *Diab Res Clin Pract* 4(3):145-151 (1998).

88. Karunanayake EH, Jeevathayaparan S, Tennekoon KH. Effect of *Momordica charantia* fruit juice on streptozotocin-induced diabetes in rats. *J Ethnopharmacol* 30:199-204 (1990).

89. Sreejayan, Rao MNA. Oxygen free radical scavenging activity of the juice of *Momordica charantia* fruits. *Fitoterapia* 62:344-346 (1991).

90. Jeevathayaparan S, Tennekoon KH, Karunanayake EH, Jayasinghe SA. Oral hypoglycemic activity of different preparations of *Momordica charantia*. *J Nat Sci Counc Sri Lanka* 19(1):19-24 (1991).

91. Jayasooriya AP, Sakano M, Yukizaki C, Kawano M, Yamamoto K, Fukuda N. Effects of *Momordica charantia* powder on serum glucose levels and various lipid parameters in rats fed with cholesterol-free and cholesterol-enriched diets. *J Ethnopharmacol* 72:331-336 (2000).

92. Ahmed I, Lakhani MS, Gillett M, John A, Raza H. Hypotriglyceridemic and hypocholesterolemic effects of anti-diabetic *Momordica charantia (karela)* fruit extract in streptozotocin-induced diabetic rats. *Diabetes Res Clin Pract* 51:155-161 (2001).

93. Srivastava Y, Bhatt HV, Verma Y. Effect of *Momordica charantia* Linn. pomous aqueous extract on cataractogenesis in murine alloxan diabetics. *Pharmacol Res Commun* 20:201-209 (1988).

94. Grover JK, Vats V, Rathi SS, Dawar R. Traditional Indian anti-diabetic plants attenuate progression of renal damage in streptozotocin induced diabetic mice. *J Ethnopharmacol* 76:233-238 (2001).

95. Vikrant V, Grover JK, Tandon N, Rathi SS, Gupta N. Treatment with extracts of *Momordica charantia* and *Eugenia jambolana* prevents hyperglycemia and hyperinsulinemia in fructose fed rats. *J Ethnopharmacol* 76:139-143 (2001).

96. Meir P, Yaniv Z. An *in vitro* study on the effects of *Momordica charantia* on glucose uptake and glucose metabolism in rats. *Planta Med* 50:12-16 (1985).

97. Welihinda J, Karunanayake EH. Extra pancreatic effects of *Momordica charantia* in rats. *J Ethnopharmacol* 17:247-255 (1986).

98. Shibib BA, Khan LA, Rahman R. Hypoglycaemic activity of *Coccinia indica* and *Momordica charantia* in diabetic rats: Depression of the hepatic gluceogenic enzymes glucose 6-phosphatase and fructose 1,6-bisphosphatase and elevation of both liver and red-cell shunt enzyme glucose-6-phosphate dehydrogenase. *Biochem J* 292:267-270 (1993).

99. Rathi SS, Grover JK, Vats V. The effect of *Momordica charantia* and *Mucuna pruriens* in experimental diabetes and their effect on key metabolic enzymes involved in carbohydrate metabolism. *Phytother Res* 16:236-243 (2002).

100. Raza H, Ahmed I, John A. Tissue specific expression and immuno-histochemical localization of glutathione S-transferase in streptozotocin induced

diabetic rats: Modulation by *Momordica charantia (karela)* extract. *Life Sci* 74:1503-1511 (2004).

101. Welihinda J, Arvidson G, Gylfe E, Hellman B, Karlsson E. The insulin-releasing activity of the tropical plant *Momordica charantia. Acta Biol Med Ger* 41:1229-1240 (1982).

102. Higashino H, Suzuki A, Tanaka Y, Pootakham K. [Hypoglycemic effects of Siamese *Momordica charantia* and *Phyllanthus urinaria* extracts in streptozotocin-induced diabetic rats]. *Nippon Yakurigaku Zasshi, Folia Pharmacological Japon* 100:415-421 (1992).

103. Ali L, Khan AKA, Hassan Z, Mamun MIR, Mosihuzzaman M, Nahar N, Nur-e-Alam M, Rokeya B . Insulin releasing properties of fractions from *Momordica charantia* fruit on isolated rat islets. *Diabetologia* 36(1):181 (1993).

104. Vad BG. Oral treatment of diabetes mellitus with special reference to *karela* fruit. *Maharashtra Med J* 5:569-591 (1959).

105. Vad BG. Place of *Momordica charantia* in the treatment of diabetes mellitus. *Maharashtra Med J* 6:733-745 (1960).

106. Vad BG. *Momordica charantia* in the treatment of diabetes mellitus. *Indian J Pharm* 23(5):115 (1961).

107. Pons JA, Stevenson DS. The effect of *Momordica charantia* in diabetes mellitus. *Puerto Rico J Public Health Trop Med* 19:196-215 (1943).

108. Aslam M, Stockley IH. Interaction between curry ingredient *(karela)* and drug (chlorpropamide). *Lancet* I:607 (1979).

109. Leatherdale BA, Panesar RK, Singh G, Atkins TW, Bailey CJ, Bignell AHC. Improvement in glucose tolerance due to *Momordica charantia (karela). Brit Med J* 282:1823-1824 (1981).

110. Akhtar MS. Trial of *Momordica charantia* Linn. *(karela)* powder in patients with maturity-onset diabetes. *J Pak Med Assoc* 32:106-107 (1982).

111. Welihinda J, Karunanayake EH, Sheriff MHR, Jayasinghe KSA. Effect of *Momordica charantia* on the glucose tolerance in maturity onset diabetes. *J Ethnopharmacol* 17:277-282 (1986).

112. Srivastava Y, Bhatt HV, Verma Y, Venkaih K, Raval BH. Antidiabetic and adaptogenic properties of *Momordica charantia* extract: An experimental and clinical evaluation. *Phytother Res* 7:285-289 (1993).

113. Ahmad N, Hassan MR, Halder H, Bennoor KS. Effect of *Momordica charantia (Karolla)* extracts on fasting and postprandial serum glucose levels in NIDDM patients. *Bangladesh Med Res Counc Bull* 25:11-13 (1999).

114. Zänker KS, Gottschalk G, Hans S. Sicherheits-und Wirsamkeitsstudie mit einem Extrakt aus *Momordica charantia* bei Patienten mit Typ-2-Diabetes. *Z Phytother* 24:163-169 (2003).

115. Baldwa VS, Bhandari CM, Pangaria A, Goyal RK. Clinical trial in patients with diabetes mellitus of an insulin-like compound obtained from plant source. *Ups J Med Sci* 82:39-41 (1977).

116. Nadkarni AK. *Dr KM Nadkarni's Indian materia medica* (vol. 1, pp. 805-807). Bombay: Popular Prakashan, 1976.

117. Mukherjee SK, Saxena AM, Shukla G. *Progress of diabetes research in India during the 20th century* (pp. 17-21). New Delhi: National Institute of Science Communication, 2002.

118. Basch E, Gabardi S, Ulbricht C. Bitter melon *(Momordica charantia)*: A review of efficacy and safety. *Am J Health Syst Pharm* 60:356-359 (2003).

119. *The wealth of India, raw materials* (vol. VIII, pp. 302-305). New Delhi: Publications and Information Directorate, CSIR, 1969.

120. Kedar P, Chakrabarti CH. Blood sugar, blood urea, and serum lipids as influenced by *Gurmar* preparation, *Pterocarpus marsupium* and *Tamarindus indica* in diabetes mellitus. *Maharashtra Med J* 28:165-169 (1981).

121. Jahromi MAF, Ray AB, Chansouria JPN. Antihyperlipidemic effect of flavonoids from *Pterocarpus marsupium*. *J Nat Prod* 56:989-994 (1993).

122. Satyavati GV, Gupta AK, Tandon N (eds.). *Medicinal plants of India* (vol. 2, pp. 530-539). New Delhi: Indian Council of Medical Research, 1987 and references cited therein.

123. Gupta SS. Experimental studies on pituitary diabetes. Part III. Effect of indigenous antidiabetic drug against the acute hyperglycemic response of anterior pituitary extract in glucose fed albino rats. *Indian J Med Res* 51:716-724 (1963).

124. Pandey HC, Sharma PV. Hypoglycemic effect of bark of *Pterocarpus marsupium* Roxb. *(Bijaka)* on alloxan induced diabetes. *Med Surg* 16(7):9 (1976).

125. Trivedi CP. Observations on the effect of some indigenous drugs on blood sugar level of normal and diabetic rabbits. *Indian J Physiol Pharmacol* 7:811-812 (1963).

126. Shah DS. A preliminary study of the hypoglycemic action of heartwood of *Pterocarpus marsupium* Roxb. *Indian J Med Res* 55:166-168 (1967).

127. Saifi AQ, Shinde S, Kavishwar WK, Gupta SR. Some aspects of phytochemistry and hypoglycemic actions of *Pterocarpus marsupium* (Papilionaceae). *J Res Ind Med* 6:205-207 (1971).

128. Joglekar GV, Chaudhary NY, Aiman R. Effect of indigenous plant-extracts on glucose absorption in mice. *Indian J Physiol Pharmacol* 3:76 (1959).

129. Gupta SS. Effect of *Gymnema sylvestre* and *Pterocarpus marsupium* on glucose tolerance in albino rats. *Indian J Medical Sci* 17:501-505 (1963).

130. Khandare SS, Rajwade GG, Jangle SN. A study of the effect of *bija* and *jamun* seed extract on hyperglycemia induced by glucose load. *Maharashtra Med J* 30:117-118 (1983).

131. Haranath PSRK, Rao KR, Anjaneyulu CR, Ramanathan JD. Studies on the hypoglycemic and pharmacological actions of some stilbenes. *Indian J Med Sci* 12:85-89 (1958).

132. Chakravarthy BK, Gupta S, Gambhir SS, Gode KD. Pancreatic beta cell regeneration. A novel antidiabetic mechanism of *Pterocarpus marsupium* Roxb. *Indian J Pharmacol* 12:123-127 (1980).

133. Chakravarthy BK, Gupta S, Gode KD. Functional beta-cell regeneration in the islets of pancreas in alloxan induced diabetic rats by (-) epicatechin. *Life Sci* 31:2693-2697 (1982).

134. Chakravarthy BK, Gupta S, Gode KD. Antidiabetic effect of (-) epicatechin. *Lancet* 2:272-273 (1982).

135. Kolb H, Kiesel U, Greulich B, van der Bosch J. Lack of antidiabetic effect of (-) epicatechin. *Lancet* I (8284):1303 (1982).

136. Sheehan EW, Zemaitis MA, Slatkin DJ, Schiff PL. A constituent of *Pterocarpus marsupium*, (-) epicatechin, as a potential antidiabetic agent. *J Nat Prod* 46:232-234 (1983).

137. Sheehan EW, Stiff DD, Duah F, Slatkin DJ, Schiff PL Jr, Zemaitis MA. The lack of effectiveness of (-) epicatechin against alloxan induced diabetes in Wistar rats. *Life Sci* 33:593 (1983).

138. Ryle PR, Barker J, Gaines PA, Thomson AD, Chakraborty J. Alloxan-induced diabetes in the rat-protective action of (-) epicatechin? *Life Sci* 34:591-595 (1984).

139. Ahmad F, Khalid P, Khan MM, Rastogi AK, Kidwai JR. Insulin like activity in (-) epicatechin. *Acta Diabetol Lat* 26:291-300 (1989).

140. Rizvi SI, Zaid MA, Suhail M. Insulin-mimetic effect of (-) epicatechin on osmotic fragility of human erythrocytes. *Indian J Exp Biol* 33:791-792 (1995).

141. Ahmad F, Khan MM, Rastogi AK, Chaubey M, Kidwai JR. Effect of (-) epicatechin on cAMP content, insulin release and conversion of proinsulin to insulin in immature and mature rat islets *in vitro*. *Indian J Exp Biol* 29:516-520 (1991).

142. Manickam M, Ramanathan M, Jahromi MA, Chansouria JP, Ray AB. Antihyperglycemic activity of phenolics from *Pterocarpus marsupium*. *J Nat Prod* 60:609-610 (1997).

143. Vats V, Grover JK, Rathi SS. Evaluation of anti-hyperglycemia and hypoglycemic effect of *Trigonella foenum-graecum* Linn, *Ocimum sanctum* Linn and *Pterocarpus marsupium* Linn in normal and alloxanized diabetic rats. *J Ethnopharmacol* 79:95-100 (2002).

144. Vats V, Yadav SP, Biswas NR, Grover JK. Anti-cataract activity of *Pterocarpus marsupium* bark and *Trigonella foenum-graecum* seeds extract in alloxan diabetic rats. *J Ethnopharmacol* 93:289-294 (2004).

145. Pandey MC, Sharma PV. Hypocholesterolemic effect of bark of *Pterocarpus marsupium* Roxb. *(Bijaka)*—An experimental study. *J Res Indian Med Yoga Homeopath* 13(1):137 (1978).

146. Sepaha GC and Bose SN. Clinical observations on the antidiabetic properties of *Pterocarpus marsupium* and *Eugenia jambolana*. *J Indian Med Assoc* 27:388-391 (1956).

147. Pandey MC, Sharma PV. Hypoglycemic effect of bark of *Pterocarpus marsupium* Roxb. (Bijaka). A clinical study. *Med Surg* 25(11):21 (1975).

148. Rajasekharan S, Tuli SN. *Vijaysar, Pterocarpus marsupium* in the treatment of *madhumeha* (diabetes mellitus)—A clinical trial. *J Res Indian Med Yoga Homeo* 11(2):9-15 (1976).

149. Ojha JK, Bajpai HS, Sharma PV. Hypoglycemic effect of *Pterocarpus marsupium* Roxb. *(vijaysar)*. *J Res Indian Med Yoga Homeo* 13(4):12-16 (1978).

150. Singh DC, Sharma BP. Management of *madhumeha* (diabetes mellitus) by indigenous drugs—*Bijaysar* and *Kustha*. *Aryavaidyan* 4(1):21-23 (1990).

151. Indian Council of Medical Research (ICMR) Collaborating Centres, New Delhi. Flexible dose open trial of *vijaysar* in cases of newly diagnosed non-insulin-dependent diabetes mellitus. *Indian J Med Res* 108:24-29 (1998).

152. *The wealth of India, raw materials* (vol. IX, pp.168-169). New Delhi: Publications and Information Directorate, CSIR, 1972.

153. Rastogi RP, Mehrotra BN. *Compendium of Indian medicinal plant* (vol. 1, pp. 356-357). Lucknow: Central Drug Research Institute and New Delhi: Publications and Information Directorate, 1993.

154. Rastogi RP, Mehrotra BN. *Compendium of Indian medicinal plants* (vol. 2, pp. 600-602). Lucknow: Central Drug Research Institute and New Delhi: Publications and Information Directorate, 1993.

155. Karunanayake EH, Welihinda J, Sirimanne SR, Sinnadorai G. Oral hypoglycaemic activity of some medicinal plants of Sri Lanka. *J Ethnopharmacol* 11:223-231 (1984).

156. Yoshikawa M, Shimoda H, Nishida N, Takada M, Matsuda H. *Salacia reticulata* and its polyphenolic constituents with lipase inhibitory and lipolytic activities have mild antiobestiy effects in rats. *J Nutr* 132:1819-1824 (2002).

157. Karunanayake EH, Sirimanne SR. Mangiferin from root bark of *Salacia reticulata*. *J Ethnopharmacol* 13:227-228 (1985).

158. Yoshikawa M, Nishida N, Shimoda H, Takada M, Kawahara Y, Matsuda H. [Polyphenol constituents from *Salacia* species: Quantitative analysis of mangiferin with alpha-glucosidase and aldose reductase inhibitory activities]. *Yakugaku Zasshi* 121:371-378 (2001).

159. Yoshikawa M, Morikawa T, Matsuda H, Tanabe G, Muraoka O. Absolute streostructure of potent alpha-glucosidase inhibitor, salacinol, with unique thiosugar sulfonium sulfate inner salt structure from *Salacia reticulata*. *Bioorg Med Chem* 10:1547-1554 (2002).

160. Yoshikawa M, Murakami T, Yashiro K, Matsuda H. Kotalanol, a potent alpha-glucosidse inhibitor with thiosugar sulfonium sulfate structure, from antidiabetic ayurvedic medicine *Salacia reticulata*. *Chem Pharm Bull* (Tokyo) 46: 1339-1340 (1998).

161. Matsuda H, Murakami T, Yashiro K, Yamahara J, Yoshikawa M. Antidiabetic principles of natural medicines IV. Aldose reductase and alpha-glucosidase inhibitors from the roots of *Salacia oblonga* Wall. (Celastraceae): Structure of a new friedelane-type triterpene, kotalagenin 16-acetate. *Chem Pharm Bull* (Tokyo) 47:1725-1729 (1999).

162. Matsuda H, Morikawa T, Toguchida T, Yoshikawa M. Structural requirements of flavonoids and related compounds for aldose reductase inhibitory activity. *Chem Pharm Bull* 50:788-795 (2002).

163. Pillai NR, Seshadri C, Santhakumari G. Hypoglycaemic activity of root bark of *Salacia prenoides*. *Indian J Exp Biol* 17:1279-1280 (1979).

164. Nair RB, Bhatt AV, Santhakumari G. Comparative study of the hypoglycaemic activity of the *Salacia* species. *J Res Ayur Siddha* III(1&2):53-68 (1980).

165. Augusti KT, Joseph P, Babu TD. Biologically active principles isolated from *Salacia oblonga* Wall. *Indian J Physiol Pharmacol* 39:415-417 (1995).

166. Krishnakumar K, Augusti KT, Vijayammal PL. Hypoglycaemic and antioxidant activity of *Salacia oblonga* Wall. extract in streptozotocin-induced diabetic rats. *Indian J Physiol Pharmacol* 43:510-514 (1999).

167. Serasinghe S, Sersinghe P, Yamazaki H, Nishiguchi K, Hombhanje F, Nakanishi S, Sawa K, Hattori M, Namba T. Oral hypoglycemic effect of *Salacia*

reticulata in the streptozotocin-induced diabetic rat. *Phytother Res* 4:205-206 (1990).

168. Muira T, Ichiki H, Hasimoto I, Iwamoto N, Kato M, Kubo M, Ishihara E, Komatsu Y, Okada M, Ishida T, Tanigawa K. Antidiabetic activity of a xanthone compound, mangiferin. *Phytomedicine* 8:85-87 (2001).

169. Shimoda H, Kawamori S, Kawahara Y. Effects of an aqueous extract of *Salacia reticulata,* a useful plant in Sri Lanka, on postprandial hyperglycemia in rats and human. *J JPn Soc Nutr Food Sci* 51:279-287 (1998).

170. Kajimoto O, Kawamori S, Shimoda H, Kawahara Y, Hirata H, Takahashi T. Effects of a diet containing *Salacia reticulata* on mild type 2 diabetes in humans. *J JPn Soc Nutr Food Sci* 53:199-205 (2000).

171. Kowsalya S, Chandrasekhar U, Geetha N. Development and evaluation of a hypoglycaemic tablet with the herb *Salacia prinoides (Ekanayakam)*. *Indian J Nutr Diet* 32(2):33-39 (1995).

172. Kowsalya S, Chandrasekhar U, Sharmila JB. Development and evaluation of hypoglycaemic tablets from selected herbs. *Indian J Nutr Diet* 33 (9):208-215 (1996).

173. Sivaprakasam K, Rao KK, Yasodha R, Veluchamy G. Siddha remedy for diabetes mellitus. *J Res Ayur Siddha* V (1-4):25-32 (1984).

174. Shimoda H, Fujimura T, Makino K, Yoshijima K, Naitoh K, Ihota H, Miwa Y. Safety profile of extractive from trunk of *Salacia reticulata* (Celastraceae). *J Food Hyg Soc Jpn* 40:198-205 (1999).

175. Shimoda H, Asano I, Yamada Y. [Antigenicity and phototoxicity of water soluble extract from *Salacia reticulata* (Celastraceae)]. *J Food Hyg Soc Jpn* 42:144-147 (2001).

176. Shimoda H, Furahashi T, Naitoh K, Nagase T, Okada M. Thirteen week repeat dose oral toxicity study of *Salacia reticulata* extract in rats. *Jpn J Med Pharm Sci* 46:527-540 (2001).

177. Ratnasooriya WD, Jayakody JR, Premakumara GA. Adverse pregnancy outcome in rats following exposure to a *Salacia reticulata* (Celastraceae) root extract. *Braz J Med Biol Res* 36:931-935 (2003).

178. Wolf BW, Weisbrode SE. Safety evaluation of an extract from *Salacia oblonga*. *Food Chem Toxicol* 41:867-874 (2003).

179. *The wealth of India, raw materials* (vol. X, pp. 100-104). New Delhi: Publications and Information Directorate, CSIR, 1976.

180. Chopra RN, Nayar SL, Chopra IC. *Glossary of Indian medicinal plants* (p. 238). New Delhi: Publications and Information Directorate, CSIR, 1956.

181. Nadkarni AK. *Dr KM Nadkarni's Indian materia medica* (3rd edn., vol. 1, pp. 516-518). Bombay: Popular Prakashan, 1976.

182. Bhatia IS, Bajaj KL. Chemical constituents of the seeds and bark of *Syzygium cumini*. *Planta Med* 28:346-352 (1975).

183. Bhatia IS, Bajaj KL. Tannins in black plum *Syzygium cuminii* L. seeds. *Biochem J* 128:56 (1972).

184. Central Council for Research in Ayurveda and Siddha. *Phytochemical investigations of certain medicinal plants used in Ayurveda* (pp.100-102). New Delhi: Central Council for Research in Ayurveda and Siddha, 1990 and references cited therein.

185. Bansal R, Ahmad N, Kidwai JR. Effects of oral administration of *Eugenia jambolana* seeds and chloropropamide on blood glucose level and pancreatic cathepsin B in rat. *Indian J Biochem Biophys* 18:377 (1981).

186. Kedar P, Chakrabarti CH. Effects of jambolan seed treatment on blood sugar, lipids and urea in streptozotocin induced diabetes in rabbits. *Ind J Physio Pharmacol* 27:135-140 (1983).

187. Nair RB, Santakumari G. Antidiabetic activity of the seed kernel of *Syzygium cumini* Linn. *Ancient Sci Life* VI:80-84 (1986).

188. Singh N, Tyagi SD, Garg V, Joneja S, Agarwal SC, Asthana A. Extract of long term feeding of different extracts of *Syzygium cumini* seeds on alloxan induced diabetes in albino rats. *Agr Biol Res* 6(2):80-88 (1990).

189. Prince PSM, Menon VP, Pari L. Hypoglycaemic activity of *Syzygium cumini* seeds: Effect on lipid peroxidation in alloxan diabetic rats. *J Ethnopharmacol* 61:1-7 (1998).

190. Prince PSM, Menon VP, Pari L. Effect of *Syzygium cumini* extracts on hepatic hexokinase and glucose-6-phosphatase in experimental diabetes. *Phytother Res* 11:529-531 (1997).

191. D'mello PM, Jadhav MA, Jolly CI. Free radical scavenging activity of *Syzygium cumini* and *Ficus bengalensis*—Plants used in Ayurveda for diabetes mellitus. *Indian Drugs* 37:518-520 (2000).

192. Rathi SS. Grover JK, Vats V, Biswas NR. Prevention of experimental diabetic cataract by Indian Ayurvedic plant extracts. *Phytother Res* 16:774-777 (2002).

193. Grover JK, Vats V, Rathi SS. Anti-hyperglycemic effect of *Eugenia jambolana* and *Tinospora cordifolia* in experimental diabetes and their effects on key metabolic enzymes involved in carbohydrate metabolism. *J Ethnopharmacol* 73:461-470 (2000).

194. Vikrant V, Grover JK, Tandon N, Rathi SS, Gupta N. Treatment with extracts of *Momordica charantia* and *Eugenia jambolana* prevents hyperglycemia and hyperinsulinemia in fructose fed rats. *J Ethnopharmacol* 76:139-143 (2001).

195. Grover JK, Vats V, Rathi SS, Dawar R. Traditional Indian anti-diabetic plants attenuate progression of renal damage in streptozotcin induced diabetic mice. *J Ethnopharmacol* 76:233-238 (2001).

196. Srivastava Y, Bhatt HV, Gupta OP, Gupta PS. Hypoglycaemia induced by *Syzygium cuminii* Linn seeds in diabetes mellitus. *Asian Med J* 26:489-491 (1983).

197. Kohli KR, Singh RH. A clinical trial of *Jambu (Eugenia jambolana)* in non-insulin dependent diabetes mellitus. *J Res Ayur Siddha* 14(3-4):89-97 (1993).

198. Jain AK, Shaw BP. Effect of herbal compound on maturity onset diabetes. *Ancient Sci Life* VII(1):12-16 (1987).

199. *The wealth of India, raw materials* (vol. X, pp. 299-306). New Delhi: Publications and Information Directorate, CSIR, 1976.

200. Bisset NG, Wichtl M (eds.). *Herbal drugs and phytopharmaceuticals* (2nd edn, pp. 203-205). Stuttgart: Medpharm Scientific Publishers and Boca Raton: CRC Press, 2001.

201. Sauvaire Y, Petit P, Broca C, Manteghetti M, Baissac Y, Fernandez-Alvarez J, Gross R, Royce M, Leconte A, Gomis R, Ribes G. 4-Hydroxylisoleucine: A novel amino acid potentiator of insulin secretion. *Diabetes* 47: 206-210 (1998).

202. Madar Z. Fenugreek *(Trigonella foenum–graecum)* as a means of reducing postprandial glucose level in diabetic rats. *Nutr Rep Int* 29:1267-1273 (1984).

203. Ribes G, Sauvaire Y, Baccou JC, Valette G, Chenon D, Trimble ER, Loubatières-Mariani MM. Effects of fenugreek seeds on endocrine pancreatic secretions in dogs. *Ann Nutr Metab* 28(1):37-43 (1984).

204. Ajabnoor MA, Tilmisany AK. Effect of *Trigonella foenum graecum* on blood glucose in normal and alloxan-diabetic mice. *J Ethnopharmacol* 22:45-49 (1988).

205. Khosla P, Gupta DD, Nagpal RK. Effect of *Trigonella foenum-graecum* (fenugreek) on blood glucose in normal and diabetic rats. *Indian J Physiol Pharmacol* 39:173-174 (1995).

206. Shani J, Goldschmied A, Ahronson Z, Sulman FG. Hypoglycemic effect of *Trigonella foenum-graecum* and *Lupinus termis* (Leguminosae) seeds and their major alkaloids in alloxan diabetic and normal rats. *Arch Int Pharmacodyn Ther* 210:27-36 (1974).

207. Amin R, Abdul-Ghani AS, Suleiman MS. Effect of fenugreek and lupin seeds on the development of experimental diabetes in rats. *Planta Med* 54:286-290 (1988).

208. Al-Habori M, Raman A. Antidiabetic and hypocholesterolaemic effects of fenugreek. *Phytother Res* 12:233-242 (1998).

209. Genet S, Kale RK, Baquer NZ. Effects of vanadate, insulin and fenugreek *(Trigonella foenum-graecum)* on creatinine kinase levels in tissues of diabetic rat. *Indian J Exp Biol* 37:200-202 (1999).

210. Gupta D, Raju J, Baquer NZ. Modulation of some gluconeogenic enzyme activities in diabetic rat liver and kidney: Effect of antidiabetic compounds. *Indian J Exp Biol* 37:196-199 (1999).

211. Raju J, Gupta D, Rao AR, Yadava PK, Baquer NZ. *Trigonella foenum-graecum* (fenugreek) seed powder improves glucose homeostatis in alloxan diabetic rat tissues by reversing the altered glycolytic, gluconeogenic and lipogenic enzymes. *Mol Cell Biochem* 224(1-2):45-51 (2001).

212. Ravikumar P, Anuradha CV. Effect of fenugreek seeds on blood lipid peroxidation and antioxidants in diabetic rats. *Phytother Res* 13:197-201 (1999).

213. Singhal PC, Gupta RK, Joshi LD. Hypocholesterolaemic effect of *Trigonella foenum-graecum* (methi). *Curr Sci* 51:136-137 (1982).

214. Sharma RD. Hypocholesterolaemic activity of fenugreek (T. *foenum-graecum*): An experimental study in rats. *Nutr Rep Int* 30:221-231 (1984).

215. Valette G, Sauvaire Y, Baccou JC, Ribes G. Hypocholesterolaemic effect of fenugreek seeds in dogs. *Atherosclerosis* 50:105-111 (1984).

216. Stark A, Madar Z. The effect of an ethanol extract derived from fenugreek *(Trigonella foenum-graecum* L.) on bile acid absorption and cholesterol levels in rats. *Br J Nutr* 69:277-287 (1993).

217. Khosla P, Gupta DD, Nagpal RK. Effect of *Trigonella foenum-graecum* (fenugreek) on serum lipids in normal and diabetic rats. *Indian J Pharmacol* 27:89-93 (1995).

218. Riyad MA, Abdul-Salam SA, Mohammad SS. Effect of fenugreek and lupine seeds on the development of experimental diabetes in rats. *Planta Med* 54:286-290 (1988).

219. National Institute of Nutrition. *Annual report* (p. 11). Hyderabad, India: Indian Council of Medical Research, 1987.

220. Sharma RD. Effect of fenugreek seeds and leaves on blood glucose and serum insulin responses in human subjects. *Nutr Res* 6:1353-1364 (1986).

221. Sharma RD, Raghuram TC, Rao NS. Effect of fenugreek seeds on blood glucose and serum lipids in type I diabetes. *Eur J Clin Nutr* 44:301-306 (1990).

222. Sharma RD, Raghuram TC. Hypoglycaemic effect of fenugreek seeds in non-insulin dependent diabetic patients. *Nutr Res* 10:731-739 (1990).

223. Madar Z, Abel R, Samish S, Arad J. Glucose lowering effect of fenugreek seed in non-insulin dependent diabetics. *Eur J Clin Nutr* 42:51-54 (1988).

224. Raghuram TC, Sharma RD, Sivakumar B, Sahay BK. Effect of fenugreek seeds on intravenous glucose disposition in non-insulin dependent diabetic patients. *Phytother Res* 8:83-86 (1994).

225. Sharma RD, Sarkar A, Hazra DK, Misra B, Singh JB, Maheshwari BB, Sharma SK. Hypolipidaemic effect of fenugreek seeds: A chronic study in non-insulin dependent diabetic patients. *Phytother Res* 10:332-334 (1996).

226. Gupta A, Gupta R, Lal B. Effect of *Trigonella foenum-graecum* (fenugreek) seeds on glycaemic control and insulin resistance in type 2 diabetes mellitus: a double blind placebo controlled study. *J Assoc Physicians India* 49: 1057-1061 (2001).

227. Sharma RD, Sarkar A, Hazar DK, Misra B, Singh JB, Maheshwari BB. Toxicological evaluation of fenugreek seeds: A long term feeding experiment in diabetic patients. *Phytother Res* 10:519-520 (1996).

228. Rao US, Sasikaran B, Rao SP. Short term nutritional and safety evaluation of fenugreek. *Nutr Res* 16:1495-1505 (1996).

OTHER PLANTS

Cinnamomum tamala *Nees & Eberm.*
(Family: Lauraceae)

Sanskrit: Tamalapatra, Tejpatra	Tamil: Talishapattiri
Hindi: Tejpat	English: Indian Cassia Lignea

Cinnamomum tamala leaves known as *tejpatra* are used in Indian kitchens to add flavor to rice dishes, such as pulav. In a study on 32 NIDDM patients with mild to moderate diabetes, two heaped teaspoons of *C. tamala* leaf powder was given orally four times a day 0.5 hour before breakfast, lunch, tea, and dinner to find the effect on fasting blood sugar, glucose tolerance, and immediate response to intake of the drug. Eight patients were kept as control with no treatment except for a restricted diet of 1,800 calories. After 1 month, the control group showed a minor significant rise ($p < 0.01$) in blood sugar levels, whereas there was a significant fall in fasting blood sugar ($p < 0.001$), in the treated group. It was also possible to show that the drug lowers blood sugar level after glucose load.

In a third experiment on seven patients to see the immediate effect of 20 g of *C. tamala* on fasting blood sugar, the drug was given after collection of fasting blood samples. It was seen that the fall in blood sugar started half an hour after the intake of *Cinnamomum tamala,* and the decrease continued upto 2 hours. The fall was significant at all points ($p < 0.01$).[1] A radioimmunoassay study on five patients, to determine insulin levels in addition to fasting blood sugar levels, showed that fasting blood sugar dropped from 186±42.34 mg percent before intake to 129.9±25.39 mg percent at the end of 2 hours, whereas insulin levels changed from 16.83 before intake to 31 $\mu u \cdot g^{-1}$ at the end of 2 hours. When two heaped teaspoons of the drug were taken for 15 days there was a significant fall in blood sugar levels (168.4±25.25 to 111.8±17.6 mg percent) after treatment. There was also a rise in insulin levels, which was not significant.[2]

Experimentally a 50-percent ethanolic extract of the leaves of *C. tamala* significantly reduced the plasma glucose levels both in normal and streptozotocin-diabetic rats. In addition, the extract was able to prevent rise in cholesterol and triglycerides in diabetic rats.[3]

Clerodendron phlomidis *Linn. (Family: Verbenaceae)*

Latin: *Clerodendrum multiflorum* (Burm. f) O. Kuntze Clerodendrum phlomidis Linn. f	Tamil: Thaludalai, Takkari
Sanskrit: Tarkaari, Vaijayanti	Hindi: Arni

In a study, 23 patients were divided into four groups. In the first group a 1:4 decoction prepared from 15-30 g of *Clerodendron phlomidis* was administered to 13 diabetic patients in daily divided doses for 5 weeks. In the second group of three patients, 500 mg of tolbutamide was given every day. The third group was given 30 units of insulin daily, whereas the fourth group was kept as control with no medication and controlled diet. *C.phlomidis* treatment led to a response in 46 percent of the patients. There was a reduction of blood sugar, urine sugar, and improvement in symptoms and in glucose tolerance. The mean percentage fall of blood sugar with *C.phlomidis* as compared to tolbutamide was 7.1 versus 11 percent, whereas the fall in urine sugar was 18.2 versus 22.2 percent. No side effects were observed.[4]

Phyllanthus amarus *Schum & Thonn.*
(Family: Euphorbiaceae)

Sanskrit: Bhumiyamalaki, tamalaki	Tamil: Keelanelli
Hindi: Bhuiavala	

In a clinical study on 25 patients with moderate to severe diabetes (250-400 mg per 100 ml) 1 g of *Phyllanthus amarus* led to statistically significant lowering of blood sugar levels when given thrice a day for 3 months.[5] In another study, a preparation of whole plant of *Phyllanthus amarus* was given for 10 days to nine mild hypertensives, four of whom were diabetic. There was a significant reduction in systolic blood pressure in nondiabetic hypertensives and in women. Also blood glucose levels was significantly reduced in the treated group.[6]

NOTES

1. Chandola HM, Tripathi SN, Udupa KN. Hypoglycaemic response of *C. tamala* in patients of maturity onset (Insulin independent) diabetes. *J Res Ayur Siddha* I:275-290 (1980).

2. Chandola HM, Tripathi SN, Udupa KN. Effect of *C.tamala* on plasma insulin vis-a-vis blood sugar in patients of diabetes mellitus. *J Res Ayur Siddha* I:345-357 (1980).

3. Sharma SR, Dwivedi SK, Swarup D. Hypoglycaemic and hypolipidemic effects of *Cinnmomum tamala* Nees leaves. *Indian J Exp Biol* 34:372-374 (1996).

4. Chaturvedi GN, Subramaniyam PR, Tiwari SK, Singh KP. Experimental and clinical studies on diabetes mellitus evaluating the efficacy of an indigenous oral hypoglycaemic drug—*arani (Clerodendron phlomidis)*. *Ancient Sci Life* III:216-224 (1984).

5. Sivaprakasam K, Yasodha R, Sivanandam G, Veluchamy G. Clinical evaluation of *Phyllanthus amarus* Schumm. & Thonn. in diabetes mellitus (p. 17). New Delhi: Sem Res Ayurveda and Siddha, CCRAS, March 20-22, 1995.

6. Srividya N, Periwal S. Diuretic, hypotensive and hypoglycaemic effect of *Phyllanthus amarus. Indian J Exp Biol* 33:861-864 (1995).

DIABETIC COMPLICATIONS

Diabetic foot

One of the late complications of diabetes is the "diabetes foot," which arises due to diabetic neuropathy, and not as thought earlier due to arterial complications, and results in a nonhealing, painless foot ulcer, which wrongly treated can lead to amputation.

Rubia cordifolia *Linn. sensu Hook.* f *(Family: Rubiaceae)*

Sanskrit: Manjistha	Tamil: Manjitti
Hindi: Manji, Majit	English: The Indian Madder

Rubia cordifiolia or *manjistha* has traditionally been used both internally and externally for the treatment of burns, wounds, fractures, bruises, insect bites, etc. *Rubia cordifolia* has potent antioxidant and anti-inflammatory activity. This has been made use of in the treatment of nonhealing diabetic foot ulcers (DFU).

In an open comparative clinical study, 100 patients, with nonhealing DFU of 20-30 months duration, were divided into two groups of 50 each. Group I was given oral antibiotics for systemic use along with antiseptics for topical use together with pentoxyfilline 400 mg thrice a day. Group II was treated by dipping the ulcer in *Rubia cordifiolia* extract and also by applying it topically as ointment. In addition, 500 mg of *Rubia cordifiolia* and *Bauhinia variegeta (kanchanara)* was given orally thrice a day for 3-4 months. General health, arterial circulation, ulcer margin measurements, radiological, biochemical, and microbiological assessments were done every month.

Recovery in group I on antibiotics was moderate and 60 percent underwent amputation, whereas group II showed very good recovery with only 10 percent partial amputation.[1]

Diabetic neuropathy

In patients of confirmed diabetic neuropathy, *Sida cordifolia* was given and found to help in the management of diabetic nerve problems. Further details are not available.[2]

Diabetic retinopathy

Asparagus racemosus *Willd. (Family: Liliaceae)*

Another complication of diabetes is the effect on the vision or diabetic retinopathy. *Asparagus racemosus* or *shatavari*, which was described earlier in Chapter 3 for use in peptic ulcer, is also considered in Ayurveda to improve the vision *(chakshushya)*. In an exploratory open trial, 30 diabetic patients were daily given 3 g of *Asparagus racemosus* root powder with water for 3 months, in addition to the antidiabetic treatment they were taking. It was found that there was absorption of vitriol and retinal hamorrhages, as well as soft and hard exudates. There was also improvement in parameters, such as venous dilation, microaneurysm, and neovascularization. According to the authors the drug had helped reduce changes of diabetic retinopathy and also helped in preventing further development of lesions as a result of diabetic retinopathy.[3]

NOTES

1. Ohja JK, Dwivedi KN. Effect of plant extract on non-healing diabetic foot ulcers. *Sachitra Ayurved* 48:870-874 (1996).

2. Hazra J, Ojha JK, Srikanth N, Chopra KK. Effect of *Bala (Sida cordifolia)* on diabetic neuropathy (p. 79). Chennai: Proc Internatl Congress Ayurveda "Ayurveda 2000," January 28-30, 2000.

3. Sharma S, Shrikant, Sahu M. Effect of *shatavari* on diabetic retinopathy (pp. 85-86). Chennai: Proc Internatl Congress Ayurveda "Ayurveda 2000," January 28-30, 2000.

Chapter 12

Central Nervous System Agents

The importance of the psyche in the cause of disease and in the maintenance of health has been recognized in Ayurveda, and plants have often been used to treat the Central Nervous System (CNS) disorders and retain mental ability even at a ripe old age. There is a sophisticated system of classification in Ayurveda based on pharmacological properties, and there are several categories described, including some with no equivalents in modern pharmacology.[1] Among the several kinds of CNS drugs described in Ayurveda, the most important and closely related to the Ayurvedic categories are—neuroleptics, hypnotics, analgesics, antipyretics, anxiolytics, memory enhancers, etc.[2] About 85 drugs have been listed under different groups and some in more than one.[3]

NOTES

1. Vaidya ADB. The status and scope of Indian medicinal plants acting on central nervous system. *Indian J Pharmacol* 29:S340-S343 (1997).

2. Dhawan BN. Development of new centrally acting drugs from Ayurveda. In Ravindranath V, Brady L, Vaidya ADB, Coelho GV, Nityanand, Koslow SH (eds.). *Allopathic and Ayurvedic medicine and mental health* (pp. 16-24). Proceedings of Indo-US workshop on Traditional Medicine and Mental Health, October 13-17, 1996. Mumbai: Bharatiya Vidya Bhawan, 2003.

3. Satyavati GV. Leads from Ayurveda on medicinal plants acting on the nervous system. In Koslow SH, Murthy RS, Coelho GV (eds.). *Decade of the brain, India/USA research in mental health and neurosciences* (pp. 185-189). Rockville, MD: National Institutes of Health, 1995.

doi:10.1300/5683_12

MEMORY AND LEARNING ENHANCERS

Unique to Ayurveda are the so-called *medhya rasayana,* which were used to enhance memory and intellect, and to reduce anxiety due to stress. The Sanskrit *medhya* is derived from *medha* meaning intellect and therefore promoting mental function. *Rasayanas* are considered to be rejuvenators used to maintain health and modify the ill effects of aging. Several such plants that promote memory and learning have been described in Ayurveda. A few of them have been investigated to some extent and are described in the following section.

Bacopa monnieri *(Linn.) Pendell (Family: Scophulariaceae)*

Latin: *Bacopa monniera* (Linn.) Wettst, *Herpestis monnieria* (Linn.) HBK	Hindi: Brahmi
Sanskrit: Brahmi	English: Thyme-Leaved
Tamil: Nirparami	Gratiola, Water Hyssop

Bacopa monnieri is a small herb with pale lilac flowers found growing throughout India in moist areas. The name *brahmi* probably refers to Brahma's wife Brahmi—the Goddess of Learning—Saraswati—and therefore to its traditional use in improving retention and enhancing memory, and thereby intellect. Two plants often go under the name *brahmi*—*Bacopa monnieri* and *Centella asiatica,* and the two plants are the most commonly used *medhya rasayana* or mental rejuvenators; however, *Bacopa monnieri* is considered more powerful since it is used in the treatment of epilepsy and insanity, whereas *Centella asiatica,* known as *mandukaparni* in Sanskrit, is considered a general mental tonic because it is also used in small amounts as a vegetable[1,2] in food items such as salads, chutneys, and tea. *Bacopa monnieri* whole plant has the official status in the *Indian Herbal Pharmacopoeia,* 2002, as a brain tonic.[3]

Chemical investigation of *Bacopa monnieri* has led to the isolation of several triterpenoid saponins of which Bacoside A, which is a mixture of several saponins and Bacoside B, are considered to be the active constituents responsible for the memory-enhancing properties of the herb.[3,4] Bacoside A is a mixture of Bacoside A_1—a minor component—Bacoside A_2, and Bacoside A_3—which has been shown to be a potent inhibitor of superoxide.[5,6] Other components include hersaponin, betulic acid, alkaloids, flavonoids, and phytosterols[3]—a number of other constituents have been isolated from the plant as well.

Initial experimental studies focused on the antianxiety effects of the herb, which acting as tranquilizer led to improved mental functioning and better retention.[7,8] Subsequent studies conducted with the alcoholic extract of the plant or with a standardized extract have demonstrated improved learning performance of rats in various stressful conditions.[4,9] In addition, *Bacopa monnieri* mitigates the amnesic effect of stressors, for example scopolamine, stress, electroconvulsive shock,[10] phenytoin,[11] and morphine.[12] In aged rats *Bacopa monnieri* slows down memory loss at 1 mg per 100 g body weight taken once a day,[13] and in animal models of Alzheimer's disease, it has a memory-promoting effect.[14] Several groups of authors and researchers have demonstrated the antioxidant properties of *Bacopa monnieri*.[15-17] In addition, the free radical scavenging and protective effect of *Bacopa monnieri* is suggested to be mediated through the reduction of high concentrations of nitric oxide produced by astrocytes in Alzheimer's disease, ischemia, and epilepsy.[18] Among the active constituents, Bacoside A_3 has been shown to be a potent inhibitor of superoxide with Bacopasaponin C showing less potent activity, whereas the two other remaining mixtures after isolation were not active.[6] A standardized extract of *Bacopa monnieri* has been shown to exhibit antistress activity[19] by modulation of expression of cells involved in the brain.[20] Also *Bacopa monnieri* extract exhibits an antidepressant effect in experimental models of depression in rats.[21]

It is only in recent years that the interest in *Bacopa monnieri* has increased with more information becoming available. Initial clinical trials were carried out in the 1980s on the antianxiety effect on patients with anxiety neurosis.

In an open trial, 35 patients with anxiety neurosis were daily given 30 ml of *Bacopa monnieri* made into syrup in two divided doses (equivalent to 12 g crude drug) for 1 month. Patients were assessed weekly based on clinical relief, psychological, physiological, and biochemical changes. Treatment resulted in the reduction in anxiety levels apart from significant reduction in symptoms, resulting in improved mental function, assessed as mental fatigue and immediate memory span. There was also reduction in the levels of urinary vanillyl mandelic acid (VMA) and corticosteroids being excreted.[22]

In another open trial, 36 subjects were divided into two groups: 18 normal subjects and 18 patients with anxiety neurosis. All subjects received one 500 mg capsule containing *Bacopa monnieri* extract equivalent to 2.5 g of dried drug thrice a day for 4 weeks. Treatment with the drug led to significant improvement in anxiety levels and depression, mental fatigue, and memory span, apart from effects on systolic blood pressure and rate of expiration. Patients also reported significant improvement in nervousness, palpitation, headache, and insomnia. Response to the drug was more pronounced in patients than in healthy volunteers.[23]

In a safety and tolerability study conducted in a double-blind placebo-controlled noncross-over manner in 31 healthy human volunteers, single doses of 20-30 mg of Bacosides A and B, as well as multiple doses of 100-200 mg, were well tolerated. No untoward reactions or side effects were seen.[24]

In another study carried out in double-blind placebo-controlled independent group design in order to examine the acute effects of *Bacopa monniera* extract on cognitive function in 38 healthy humans, the subjects were assigned to one of the two kinds of treatment: either 300 mg *Bacopa monniera* extract ($n = 18$) or placebo ($n = 20$). Testing, carried out before the intake of drug and 2 hours after, showed that there was no acute effect at the dose given.[25]

In a similar double-blind placebo-controlled independent group design, the chronic effects of administration of 300 mg of *Bacopa monniera* extract or placebo for 5 weeks and 12 weeks was studied. Neuropsychological testing done at baseline, after 5 weeks and after 12 weeks showed significant improvement in the speed of visual information processing, enhanced learning rate, and memory consolidation, and improved anxiety state in the *Bacopa monniera* extract group as compared with the placebo group. Improvement was maximal at 12 weeks suggesting that *Bacopa monniera* exerts a favorable influence on learning and memory.[26]

In a double-blind randomized placebo-controlled trial, the chronic effects of administration of *Bacopa monnieri* extract was studied in 76 adults enrolled in the trial. Testing of various memory functions and the level of anxiety was done at baseline, at the end of 3 months of the trial, and 6 weeks after the end of trial. The results showed that the rate of learning was unaffected, but there was a decrease in the rate of forgetting newly learned matter.[27]

In a single-blind trial, 40 children aged between 6 and 8 years were divided into two groups. One group of 20 children were given 1.05 g *Bacopa monnieri* drug made into syrup (1 teaspoon containing equivalent of 350 mg *Bacopa monnieri*) thrice a day for 3 months, whereas the other group received placebo syrup. At the end of the treatment period, there was improvement in immediate memory and perception, and in the children's general performance.[28]

In a study to test the safety and tolerability of Bacosides A and B, no side effects were seen, and the drug was well tolerated.[24] Further the effect of acute[25] and chronic[26] administration (12 weeks) of 300 mg of *Bacopa monnieri* extract on cognitive function in healthy volunteers was studied in a double-blind placebo-controlled manner. Adverse effects in the chronic study were not very different from placebo, only a greater percentage in the *Bacopa monniera* group reported dry mouth, nausea, and fatigue.[26]

Centella asiatica *Urban (Linn.)* (Family: Apiaceae)

The use of *Centella asiatica* (see Plate 8 in color gallery) in chronic venous insufficiency is covered in Chapter 6, "Cardiovascular drugs" and for wound healing in Chapter 9, "Dermatological agents." However, the herb is best known in India as a *medhya rasayana* or mental rejuvenator, which improves memory and retention. *Medhya rasayana* reduce the negative impact of stress by their mild tranquilizing action and by improving memory span and "intelligence."[29] The plant is also considered a rejuvenator or *rasayana* helping to maintain youthful vigor and vitality. It is used in the treatment of epilepsy, senility, and premature aging.[30] The leaves and the plant have been used for this purpose for a very long time, often taken in food in the form of spiced paste of the leaves known as chutneys, in salads, or as tea to improve vigor, and as a brain tonic. Interestingly, it is given to children learning the *Vedas* in *Veda Patashalas,*[31] or the traditional schools, where the *Vedas* are taught in the traditional manner of memorizing the vast number of *Vedic* verses solely by loud repetition and memorization. It is also a favorite, nowadays, with school children as examinations approach, to help in building memory and retaining the studied material. It is an official drug in the *Indian Herbal Pharmacopoeia,* 2002, as a brain tonic and sedative.[32]

As with other *medhya* drugs, the first experimental studies investigated the sedative and antianxiety effects of the herb; since a calm mind helped in learning. Thus, the saponin fraction containing brahmoside and brahminoside was shown in rats to act as a mild tranquilizer.[33] Several extracts, including the alcoholic[34-36] and aqueous extracts, showed potentiation of barbiturate or phenobarbitone hypnosis.[34] An experimental study in rats on the effect of 100 mg per 100 g body weight of an alcoholic extract of *Centella asiatica* on various neurotransmitters showed decreased levels of acetylcholine and increased levels of histamine and catecholamines, relative to a control group, suggesting that this may contribute to the antianxiety effect seen clinically.[36] In addition, the alcoholic extract showed a dose-dependent increase in gamma amino butyric acid (GABA) levels in rats that was blocked by the specific $GABA_A$ blocker—bicuculline methiodide.[37] In vitro *Centella asiatica* has shown affinity for $GABA_B$ receptor, which may contribute to memory enhancement.[38] The aqueous extract of *Centella asiatica* (25 mg·kg^{-1} i.p.) showed, in small animals, an antianxiety effect comparable to diazepam[39] and the alcoholic extract injected intraperitoneally showed a mild sedative effect.[40]

An experimental study on the effect of an aqueous extract of fresh *Centella asiatica* leaf was studied in small animals (albino rats) using a two-compartment passive avoidance task. In drug-treated animals, there was a significant improvement in 24-hour retention when compared to controls treated with saline. A study of the levels of central neurotransmitters norepinephrine, dopamine, and 5-hydroxytryptamine and their metabolites showed a significant decrease in the drug-treated group suggesting that these neurotransmitters help in the learning process mainly through inhibition. In addition, there is a decrease in the urinary level of the metabolites homovanillic acid and 5-hydroxyl indole acetic acid.[41] *Centella asiatica* aqueous extract has cognition-enhancing effect[42] by virtue of its antioxidant activity.[42,43] The aqueous extract has also been shown to reduce the amnesic effects of pentylenetetrazole.[44] In an animal model for Alzheimer's disease, the aqueous extract of *Centella asiatica* was able to prevent cognitive deficits and oxidative stress.[45]

In a double-blind placebo-controlled study, 30 mentally retarded children were administered 0.5 g per day of the plant powder for 12 weeks. There was significant improvement in the general ability of the children and also in their behavioral pattern.[46] In a 6-month, double-blind trial in 30 mentally retarded children aged between 7 and 18 years given one 500 mg tablet of *Centella asiatica* (part not mentioned, probably whole plant powder as used by the same group in other trials) daily for 6 months, there was a significant increase in the general mental ability, overall adjustment, and mental concentration seen at the end of 6 months. This improvement in general behavior was maintained up to 1 year after withdrawal of the drug.[47] In a double-blind study, 57 normal children with an IQ between 90 and 110 were given 0.5 g of the plant powder for 1 year. There were 14 dropouts and data from 43 children was evaluated. It was found that there was no significant improvement in the intelligence quotient.[48]

In another open trial with 12 educable, mentally retarded children, in the age group of 8-12 years, were given 100 mg·kg^{-1} body weight of powder of *Centella asiatica* in two divided doses for 6 months and followed up for 1 year. Posttreatment values on Malin's Intelligence scale for Indian Children (MISIC), Bender's Gestalt Test, and Raven Matrices showed modifications at various mental levels. There was a very significant improvement in the academic performance of eight children.[49]

In a double-blind placebo-controlled trial to test the anxiolytic activity, subjects were randomly assigned to receive either a single dose of 12 g of *Centella asiatica* ($n = 20$) or placebo ($n = 20$), and the acoustic startle response (ASR) was tested 30 and 60 minutes after the treatment when *Centella asiatica* was found to attenuate the ASR, suggesting that it has an anxiolytic effect.[50]

Further clinical studies are needed to fully delineate the usefulness of this very promising plant and also to establish its effect on other body systems and side-effect profile. The plant is generally considered safe and is commonly used in food. However, it is traditionally consumed only in moderate amounts; larger amounts are considered to cause headache and dizziness.[51] There are also reports of photosensitivity when consumed. In animal experiments on mice no mortality was observed up to 5 g·kg^{-1}. The alcoholic extract was found nontoxic up to 350 mg·kg^{-1}intraperitoneally.[52]

Celastrus paniculatus *Willd. (Family Celastraceae)*

Sanskrit: Jyotishmati	Tamil: Valuluvai
Hindi: Malkanguni	English: Black Oil Plant, Climbing Staff Tree, Intellect Tree

Celastrus paniculatus is a large, woody climber bearing yellow fruits found growing almost all over India up to 1,800 m. The fruits are capsules containing 3-6 seeds with an unpleasant odor and taste, enclosed in a red aril. The seed oil, known as *Celastrus* oil or *malkanguni* oil varies in color depending upon the method of processing: pale yellow—on cold expression, dark brown—when obtained by extraction with hexane, or black—if heat is used in the extraction process.[53,54] In Ayurveda, the seeds and seed oil of *Celastrus paniculatus* are most commonly used in mental disorders and are considered to enhance memory and comprehension.[54] The fruits, including the seeds, have an official status in the *Indian Herbal Pharmacopoeia,* 2002, as a tranquilizer.[55]

The seed contains 42-45 percent of fatty oil consisting of palmitic, oleic, linoleic, and linolenic acids and their glycerol esters. Also present in minor amounts are sesquiterpene polyesters—of which malkangunin is the major component—sesquiterpene alkaloids, and triterpenoids.[55] Experimental studies have shown sedative and tranquilizing action[56,57]of the seed oil. The effects of the seed extract on the brain of albino rats have been studied[58] and found to significantly increase the number of lipids and phospholipids in the brain. Rats fed with 1 ml of 5 percent seed oil emulsion for 3-7 days showed improved learning and memory.[59,60] In another experimental model involving a two-compartment avoidance task, albino rats that were fed seed oil showed improved cognitive ability compared to saline controls and decreased levels of norepinephrine, dopamine, and serotonin, and their metabolites in the brain and in urine suggesting that these aminergic systems are involved in the memory and learning process.[61] Seed oil 50-400 mg·kg^{-1} for 14 days was able to prevent amnesic effect of scopolamine in navigational memory performance in rats.[62] Both the methanol extract of the herb[63] and the aqueous extract of the seed[64,65] showed significant protective effect against free radical damage suggesting that the antioxidant activity may be responsible for its cognitive-enhancing properties and also could offer protection against a host of neurodegenerative diseases. In an animal model of Alzheimer's disease, aqueous extract of *Celastrus paniculatus* was effective in protecting against ICV streptozotocin-caused cognitive impairment.[66]

The seed oil is widely used in psychiatric practice with promising results.[67] A recent study reported the use of *Celastrus paniculatus* in depressive illness. In a controlled clinical study 55 patients with depression were divided into three groups—group A (24 patients) received two 500 mg tablets of *Jyotishmati* (made from leaves and small stems) thrice daily for 6 weeks, group B (18 patients) received the same dose of *Jyotishmati* in addition to modern treatment (not specified), while group C (13 patients) received placebo. There was statistically significant reduction of symptoms such as sadness, lack of interest, insomnia and psychomotor retardation, and a significant reduction in the degree of depression based on HDRS (Hamilton Depression Rating Scale) in both the treatment groups with respect to placebo, with an additive effect in group B. Similar dropout rates were seen (group A—6, B—4, and C—4).[68] However, an early double-blind study in mentally deficient patients showed that the seeds had no effect on learning.[69] In mentally retarded children chronic treatment with *Celastrus paniculatus* oil produced improvement in IQ scores and decreased the content of catecholamine metabolites.[70]

Products from *Celastrus paniculatus* are reported to have low toxicity. However larger doses can cause burning of the skin.[71] In an acute toxicity study the seed oil was given in doses from 0.5 to 5 g·kg^{-1} body weight to rats. No toxic manifestation, behavioral changes, and mortality were seen even at the highest dose. In a rotorod test, rats given the seed oil could stay on the rotorod for more than 3 minutes showing no loss of motor coordination. Thus *Celastrus* oil does not have any acute neurotoxic effects.[61]

Convolvulus pluricaulis *Chois. (Family: Convolvulaceae)*

Latin: *Convolvulus microphyllus* Sieb. Ex Spreng, *Convolvulus prostratus* Forsk	Hindi: Sankahul
Sanskrit: Shankapushpi	

Covolvulus pluricaulis is a small, diffuse herb covered with white hairs and bearing white or pale pink flowers from mid-winter to mid-spring found throughout India in the hotter regions.[72] Like other plants dealt with in this chapter, this plant is also a *medhya rasayana* drug or mental rejuvenator. It was considered by Caraka to be one of the best in this category of mental rejuvenators;[73] however, it has not been scientifically investigated to any great degree.

Several alkaloids—convolvine, convolamine, phyllabine, convolidine, confoline, subhirsine, convosine, scopoline, and convolvidine have been isolated from the plant, in addition to the ubiquitous sterol—β-sitosterol.[74] The whole plant is used as the drug.

In small animals, *Convolvulus pluricaulis* has been shown to have tranquilizing activity.[75,76] The alcoholic extract of the plant and various fractions derived from it have also been shown to have potentiate barbiturate hypnosis[77,78] using diazepam as a standard; maximum activity being seen in the water-soluble portion of the chloroform extract[78] and exhibited by the leaves and flowers,[79] especially in the spring when the flowering is at its peak.[80] The activity in the barbiturate hypnosis was better than *Centella asiatica.*[81] The effect of the drug was also tested on the levels of acetylcholine, catecholamine, serotonin, and histamine in normal and stressed rats, and found to act as a tranquilizer, also enhancing cognitive function.[82] In addition, feeding of *Convolvulus pluricaulis* increased protein synthesis in the hippocampus[83] and also influenced GABA levels in the brain tissue and blood.[84] Furthermore, the ethanolic extract showed some degree of antioxidant activity, which was not significant.[85]

In an open trial on 30 patients with anxiety neurosis, the drug was given daily in the form of a syrup in 30 ml of divided doses, each dose corresponding to 10 g of crude drug, for a period of 1 month. Patients showed significant symptomatic relief—reduction in anxiety levels, increased work output, decreased stress hormone levels, and lowered blood pressure and pulse rate—apart from a significant reduction in mental fatigue rate after 1 month of therapy.[86]

More scientific work on the chemical, pharmacological, and clinical aspects is required to understand the high esteem in which it was held by Caraka. At this point it may be pertinent to mention that this plant is one of the controversial drugs in Ayurveda and there are discussions as to the identity of this plant, although it has been generally agreed upon by scholars that *Convolvulus pluricaulis* is the accepted source of the drug.

Withania somnifera *Dunal. (Family: Solanaceae)*

Other aspects of the use of *Withania somnifera* have been covered in Chapter 8, "Antirheumatic agents." There are several chemotypes of the plant available with varying amounts of the various sitoindosides. The roots have been considered an important mental rejuvenator *(medhya rasayana)* in Ayurveda for 3,000 years, and as being useful in the treatment of various nervous disorders, in improving memory, and being helpful in conditions such as epilepsy and insanity. The drug also helps in the rejuvenation of the nervous system and protects it against environmental influences, improves cognitive deficits due to age, stress, or drugs, and builds nonspecific host defense.[87]

The alcoholic extract of *Withania somnifera* root showed sedative effects in rats, potentiating barbiturate hypnosis, improving learning behavior, and reducing acetylcholine and catecholamine levels, while increasing 5-hydroxytryptamine and histamine levels in the whole brain tissue.[88] The methanolic extract of *Withania somnifera* showed a GABA mimetic activity.[89] Defined extracts of *Withania somnifera* consisting of mixtures of Sitoindosides VII-X and Withaferin A prepared by combination of equimolar amounts of the compounds taken from *Withania somnifera* induced an increase in the cortical muscarinic acetylcholine capacity, which may partly explain the cognition-enhancing effects seen both in animals and humans.[90] The bioactive withanolides, as a defined mixture described above, administered orally once daily to rats in a dose of 20 and 50 mg·kg⁻¹ for 5 days showed an anxiolytic effect comparable to 0.5 mg·kg⁻¹ lorazepam given intraperitoneally and an antidepressant effect comparable to imipramine (10 mg·kg⁻¹, ip).[87] This same mixture of sitoindosides and withaferin A when given orally to rats at 20-50 mg·kg⁻¹ in an experimental model of Alzheimer's disease was found at 50 mg·kg⁻¹ to significantly reverse amnesic effect of ibotenic acid and reduce cholinergic markers after 2 weeks of treatment,[91] in addition to demonstrating free-radical scavenging activity and antioxidant activity in chronic footshock-induced stress.[92] *Withania somnifera* extract at 50, 100, and 200 mg·kg⁻¹ has also been shown to improve retention in a passive avoidance task in a stepdown test, and also shown to significantly reverse amnesic effects of scopolamine (0.3 mg·kg⁻¹). In another experiment, the amnesic effect of electric shock treatment was significantly reversed by daily administration of *Withania somnifera* extract for 6 days.[93] Sitoindosides IX and X have been shown in a stepdown test to improve both short- and long-term memory in mice after oral intake.[94] In addition, the methanol extract of *Withania somnifera* has been shown to promote formation of dendrites in human neuroblastoma cells;[95] more specifically the axons were extended by withanolide A and dendrites by withanosides IV and VI.[96] These compound plus a few other similar ones have also displayed significant neurite outgrowth at 1 μM concentration in human neuroblastoma cell line.[97] In addition, a different extract significantly reduced degenerating cells in the hippocampal region of stressed rats.[98] Thus, although there is considerable experimental evidence for the possible cognitive-enhancing effects of *Withania somnifera,* there is very little clinical evidence in the form of formal trials, only a single trial in patients of anxiety neurosis is available. However, the drug is extensively used in Ayurveda both as a single drug, and in combination, for various nervous conditions, and needs to be clinically studied.

In an open trial, 30 patients of anxiety neurosis were administered 40 ml of an alcoholic extract of *ashwagandha* in the form known in Ayurveda as *arista,* which is obtained by extraction of the roots of *Withania somnifera* by self-generated alcohol to yield an extract containing 15 percent alcohol; 40 ml of preparation corresponds to 12 g of dried roots. This preparation was given in divided doses for 1 month and patients were evaluated every week for clinical symptoms such as nervousness, palpitation, tremors, headache, anorexia, insomnia, lack of concentration, dyspepsia, fatigue, and irritability. In addition, various psychological tests were conducted to determine anxiety levels, adjustment level, mental fatigue, and immediate memory span and biochemical determination of stress hormones. After 1 month of treatment there was significant decrease in intensity of symptoms, maximum improvement being seen in nervousness scores. Mental fatigue rate was significantly reduced, assessed in terms of fewer mistakes committed and greater work output after 1 month of treatment. The immediate memory span also increased significantly. Other changes included increased body weight and breath-holding time. In addition, there was reduced urinary excretion of cortisol and catecholamines. There was no change in blood pressure and respiration rate.[99]

In a double-blind placebo-controlled study, the effect of *Withania somnifera* on psychomotor performance of healthy men and women was compared with *Panax ginseng*. Volunteers were divided into three groups. Group 1 received standardized ginseng extract, group 2 volunteers were given 250 mg *Withania somnifera* root powder twice a day for 40 days, and group 3 was given lactose in capsules as placebo. At the end of the treatment period, volunteers on *Withania somnifera* were tested and found to perform better in tasks involving logical thinking, problem solving, and reaction time than the group receiving *Panax ginseng*.[100]

Information on the safety of *Withania somnifera* has been covered in Chapter 8, "Antirheumatic drugs."

NOTES

1. Sivarajan VV, Balachandran I. *Ayurvedic drugs and their plant sources* (pp. 97-99). New Delhi: Oxford and IBH Publishing Co Pvt Ltd., 1994.

2. Singh RH, Sinha BN. *Brahmi* versus *mandukaparni:* A study on the identification of two *medhya rasayana* drugs. *J Res Ind Med Yoga Homeo* 13(4):65-68 (1978).

3. *Indian herbal pharmacopoeia* (rev. new edn., pp. 70-78). Mumbai: Indian Drug Manufacturers' Association, 2002.

4. Singh HK, Dhawan BN. Neuropsychopharmacological effects of the Ayurvedic nootropic *Bacopa monniera* Linn. *(brahmi)*. *Indian J Pharmacol* 29:S359-S365 (1997).

5. Dhawan BN. Development of new centrally acting drugs from Ayurveda. In Ravindranath V, Brady L, Vaidya ADB, Coelho GV, Nityanand, Koslow SH (eds.). *Allopathic and Ayurvedic medicine and mental health* (pp. 16-24). Procs of Indo-US workshop on Traditional Medicine and Mental Health, October 13-17, 1996. Mumbai: Bharatiya Vidya Bhawan, 2003.

6. Pawar R, Gopalakrishnan C, Bhutani KK. Dammarane triterpene saponin from *Bacopa monniera* as the superoxide inhibitor in polymorphonuclear cells. *Planta Med* 67:752-754 (2001).

7. Singh RH, Singh L, Sen SP. Studies on the anti-anxiety effect of the *medhya rasayana* drug, *brahmi* (*Bacopa monnieri* Linn.). Part II. Experimental *Studies. J Res Ind Med Yoga Homeo* 14(3):1-6 (1979).

8. Singh RH, Sinha BN, Sarkar FH, Udupa KN. Comparative biochemical studies on the effect of four *medhya rasayana* drugs described by Charaka on some central neurotransmitters in normal and stressed rats. *J Res Ind Med Yoga Homeo* 14 (3):7-14 (1979).

9. Singh HK, Dhawan BN. Effect of *Bacopa monniera* Linn. *(brahmi)* extract on avoidance responses in rat. *J Ethnopharmacol* 5:205-214 (1982).

10. Dhawan BN, Singh HK, *World pschyiatric association-section meeting. International convention on biological psychiatry; theme: Future mental health care and biological psychology, pharmacology of the Ayurvedic nootropic* Bacopa monniera (abstract NR 59). Mumbai: Internl Convention Biol Psychiatr, 1996.

11. Vohora D, Pal SN, Pillai KK. Protection from phenytoin-induced cognitive deficit by *Bacopa monnieri*, a reputed Indian nootropic plant. *J Ethnopharmacol* 71:383-390 (2000).

12. Sumathy T, Govindasamy S, Balakrishna K, Veluchamy G. Protective role of *Bacopa monniera* on morphine-induced mitochondrial enzyme activity in rats. *Fitoterapia* 73:381-385 (2002).

13. Gupta BS, Gupta U, Dixit SP, Dubey GP. *Brahmi (Bacopa monnieri) slows down memory loss in aged rats* (abstract A-21). Varanasi: Institute of Medical Sciences, Banaras Hindu University, Internl Sem Free Radical Mediated Diseases & Ayurveda, September 2-4, 1996.

14. Bhattacharya SK, Kumar A, Ghosal S. Effect of *Bacopa monniera* on animal models of Alzheimer's disease and perturbed central cholinergic markers of cognition in rats. In Mori A, Satoh T (eds.). *Emerging drugs, Vol. 1: Molecular aspects of Asian medicines* (pp. 21-32). Westbury, NY: PJD Publications, 2001.

15. Tripathi E, Tripathi YB. *Effect of* Bacopa monniera and Nardostachys jatamansi *in rat brain homogenate: A comparative study* (abstract A-36). Varanasi: Faculty of Ayurveda, Institute of Medical Sciences, Banaras Hindu University, Internl Sem Free Radical Mediated Diseases & Ayurveda, September 2-4, 1996.

16. Bhattacharya SK, Bhattacharya A, Kumar A, Ghosal S. Antioxidant activity of *Bacopa monnieri* in rat frontal cortex, striatum and hippocampus. *Phytother Res* 14:174-179 (2000).

17. Russo A, Izzo AA, Borelli F, Renis M, Vanella A. Free radical scavenging capacity and protective effect of *Bacopa monniera* L. on DNA damage. *Phytother Res* 17:870-875 (2003).

18. Russo A, Borrelli F, Campisi A, Acquaviva R, Raciti G, Vanella A. Nitric oxide-related toxicity in cultured astrocytes: Effect of *Bacopa monniera. Life Sci* 73:1517-1526 (2003).

19. Rai D, Bhatia G, Palit G, Pal R, Singh S, Singh HK. Adaptogenic effect of *Bacopa monniera (brahmi). Pharmacol Biochem Behav* 75:823-830 (2003).

20. Chaudhri DK, Parmar D, Kakkar P, Shukla R, Seth PK, Srimal RC. Antistress effects of bacosides of *Bacopa monnieri:* Modulation of Hsp 70 expression, superoxide dismutase and cytochrome P 450 activity in rat brain. *Phytother Res* 16:639-645 (2002).

21. Sairam K, Dorababu M, Goel RK, Bhatacharya SK. Antidepressant activity of standardized extract of *Bacopa monniera* in experimental models of depression in rats. *Phytomedicine* 9:207-211 (2002).

22. Singh RH, Singh L. Studies on the anti-anxiety effect of the *medhya rasayana* drug, *brahmi* (*Bacopa monniera* Wettst.)—Part I. *J Res Ayur Siddha* 1(1):133-148 (1980).

23. Yadava RK, Singh RH. A clinical and experimental study on *medhya* effect of *Aindri* (*Bacopa monnieri* Linn.) *J Res Ayur Siddha* 17(1-2):1-15 (1996).

24. Asthana OP, Srivastava JS, Ghatak A, Gaur SPS, Dhawan BN. Safety and tolerability of Bacosides A and B in healthy human volunteers. *Indian J Pharmacol* 28:37 (1996).

25. Nathan PJ, Clarke J, Lloyd J, Hutchinson CW, Downey L, Stough C. The acute effects of an extract of *Bacopa monniera (brahmi)* on cognitive function in healthy normal subjects. *Human Psychopharmacol* 16:345-351 (2001).

26. Stough C, Lloyd J, Clarke J, Downey LA, Hutchinson CW, Rodgers T, Nathan PJ. The chronic effects of an extract of *Bacopa monnieri (brahmi)* on cognitive function in healthy human subjects. *Psychopharmacol* 156:481-484 (2001).

27. Roodenrys S, Booth D, Bulzomi S, Phipps A, Micallef C, Smoker J. Chronic effects of *brahmi (Bacopa monnieri)* on human memory. *Neuropsychopharmacol* 27:279-281 (2002).

28. Sharma R, Chaturvedi C, Tewari PV. Efficacy of *Bacopa monnieri* in revitalizing intellectual functions in children. *J Res Edu Indian Med* 6(1-2):1-10 (1987).

29. Handa SS, Rasayana Drugs, Part II, *Pharmatimes* (March):17-25 (1994).

30. Lad V, Frawley D. *The yoga of herbs* (pp.170-172). New York: Lotus Press, 1986.

31. Late Dr. Krishnan PK, retired medical officer and unit head, personal communication. Chennai, India: Arignar Anna Government Hospital, 1987.

32. *Indian herbal pharmacopoeia* (rev. new edn., pp. 123-133). Mumbai: Indian Drug Manufacturers' Association, 2002.

33. Ramaswamy AS, Periyasamy SM, Basu N. Pharmacological studies on *Centella asiatica* Linn. *(Brahma manduki). J Res Indian Med* 4:160-173 (1970).

34. Shukla SP. A study on barbiturate hypnosis potentiation effect of different fraction of indigenous plant drug *mandukaparni* (*Hydrocotyle asiatica* Linn.). *Bull Med Ethnobot Res* 10 (3-4):119-123 (1980).

35. Agrawal SS. Some CNS effects of *Hydrocotyle asiatica* Linn. *J Res Ayur Siddha* 2(3):144-149 (1981).

36. Singh RH, Shukla SP, Mishra BK. The psychotropic effect of the *medhya rasayana* drug, *mandukaparni (Hydrocotyle asiatica)*: An experimental study. Part II. *J Res Ayur Siddha* 2(1):1-10 (1981).

37. Chatterjee TK, Chakraborty A, Pathak M, Sengupta GC. Effects of the plant extract *Centella asiatica* (Linn.) on cold restraint stress ulcer in rats. *Indian J Exp Biol* 30:889-891 (1992).

38. Dev S. Ancient modern concordance in Ayurvedic plants: Some examples. *Environ Health Perspectives* 107:783-789 (1999).

39. Diwan PV, Karwande I, Singh AK. Anti-anxiety profile of *manduk parni (Centella asiatica)* in animals. *Fitoterapia* LXII:253-257 (1991).

40. Adesina SK. Some plants used as anticonvulsants in American, Indian and African traditional medicine. *Fitoterapia* 53:147-162 (1982).

41. Nalini K, Aroor AR, Karanth KS, Rao A. Effect of *Centella asiatica* fresh leaf aqueous extract on learning and memory and biogenic amine turnover in albino rats. *Fitoterapia* LXIII:232-237 (1992).

42. Veerendra Kumar MH, Gupta YK. Effect of different extracts of *Centella asiatica* on cognition and markers of oxidative stress in rats. *J Ethnopharmacol* 79:253-260 (2002).

43. Jadhav HR, Bhutani KK. Antioxidant properties of Indian medicinal plants. *Phytother Res* 16:771-773 (2002).

44. Gupta YK, Veerendra Kumar MH, Srivastava AK. Effect of *Centella asiatica* on pentylenetetrazole-induced kindling, cognition and oxidative stress in rats. *Pharmacol Biochem Behav* 74:579-585 (2003).

45. Veerendra Kumar MH, Gupta YK. Effect of *Centella asiatica* on cognition and oxidative stress in an intracerebroventricular streptozotocin model of Alzheimer's disease in rats. *Clin Exp Pharmacol Physiol* 30:336-342 (2003).

46. Appa Rao MVR, Srinivasan K, Koteswara Rao T. The effect of *mandukaparni (Centella asiatica)* on the general mental ability *(medhya)* of mentally retarded children. *J Res Indian Med* 8(4):9-15 (1973).

47. Appa Rao MVR, Srinivasan K, Koteswara Rao T. The effect of *Centella asiatica* on the general mental ability of mentally retarded children. *Indian J Psychiatry* 19:54-59 (1977).

48. Kupparajan K, Srinivasan K, Janaki K. A double blind study of effect of *mandookaparni* on general mental ability of normal children. *J Res Indian Med Yoga Homeo* 13(1):37-41 (1978).

49. Sharma R, Jaiswal AN, Kumar S, Chaturvedi C, Tewari PV. Role of *bhrahmi (Centella asiatica)* in educable mentally retarded children. *J Res Edu Ind Med* 4(1-2): 55-57 (1985).

50. Bradwejn J, Zhou Y, Koszycki D, Shlik J. A double blind, placebo-controlled study on the effects of *gotu kola (Centella asiatica)* on acoustic startle response in healthy subjects. *J Clin Psychopharmacol* 20:680-684 (2000).

51. Nadkarni AK. *Dr KM Nadkarni's Indian materia medica* (vol. 1, pp. 662-666). Bombay: Popular Prakashan, 1976.

52. *Selected medicinal plants of India. A monograph on identity, safety and clinical usage* (pp. 83-86). Bombay: Chemexcil. Basic Chemicals, Pharmaceuticals and Cosmetics Export Promotion Council, 1992.

53. *The wealth of India, raw materials* (vol. 3, pp. 412-413). New Delhi: Publications and Information Directorate, CSIR, 1992.

54. Gogte VM. *Ayurvedic pharmacology & therapeutic uses of medicinal plants* (pp. 378-379). Trans. SPARC, Mumbai: Bharatiya Vidya Bhawan, 2000.

55. *Indian herbal pharmacopoeia* (rev. new edn., pp. 114-122). Mumbai: Indian Drug Manufacturers' Association, 2002.

56. Gaitonde BB, Raiker KP, Shroff FN, Patel JR. Pharmacological studies with *malakanguni*—An indigenous tranquillizing drug (preliminary report). *Current Med Pract* 1:619-621(1957).

57. Sheth UK, Vaz A, Deliwala CV, Bellare RA. Behavioural and pharmacological studies of a tranquillising fraction from the oil of *Celastrus paniculatus* (*malkanguni* oil). *Arch Int Pharmacodyn Ther* 144:34-50 (1963).

58. Bidwai PP, Wangoo D, Bhullar NK. Effect of *Celastrus paniculatus* seed extract on the brain of albino rats. *J Ethnopharmacol* 21:307-314 (1987).

59. Karanth KS, Haridas KK, Gunasundari S, Guruswami MN. Effect of *Celastrus paniculatus* on learning process. *Arogya J Health Sci* 6:137-139 (1980).

60. Karanth KS, Padma TK, Gunasundari MN. Influence of *Celastrus* oil on learning and memory. *Arogya J Health Sci* 7:83-86 (1981).

61. Nalini K, Karanth KS, Rao A, Aroor AR. Effects of *Celastrus paniculatus* on passive avoidance performance and biogenic amine turnover in albino rats. *J Ethnopharmacol* 47:101-108 (1995).

62. Gattu M, Boss KL, Terry AV, Buccafusco JJ. Reversal of scopolamine-induced deficits in navigational memory performance by the seed oil of *Celastrus paniculatus. Pharmacol Biochem Behav* 57:793-799 (1997).

63. Russo A, Izzo AA, Cardile V, Borrelli F, Vanella A. Indian medicinal plants as antiradicals and DNA cleavage protestors. *Phytomedicine* 8:125-132 (2001).

64. Kumar MH, Gupta YK. Antioxidant property of *Celastrus paniculatus* Willd: A possible mechanism in enhancing cognition. *Phytomedicine* 9:302-311 (2002).

65. Godkar P, Gordon RK, Ravindran A, Doctor BP. *Celastrus paniculatus* seed water soluble extracts protect cultured rat forebrain neuronal cells from hydrogen peroxide-induced oxidative injury. *Fitoterapia* 74:658-669 (2003).

66. Kumar MHV, Gupta YK. Cognitive enhancing and antioxidant property of *Celastrus paniculatus* in model of Alzheimer's disease in rats. *Indian J Pharmacol* 35:133 (2003).

67. Hakim RA. A trial report on *malkanguni* oil with other indigenous drugs in the treatment of psychiatric cases. *IMA Med Bull, Gujarat State Branch* 8:77-78 (1964).

68. Baranwal S, Gupta S, Singh RH. Controlled clinical trial of *jyotismati (Celastrus paniculatus)* in the cases of depressive illness. *J Res Ayur Siddha* XII(1-2):35-47 (2001).

69. Morris JV, MacGillivray RC, Mathieson CM. The experimental administration of *Celastrus paniculatus* in mental deficiency. *Am J Mental Defic* 59:235-244 (1954).

70. Nalini K, Aroor AR, Kumar KB, Rao A. Studies on biogenic amines and their metabolites in mentally retarded children on *Celastrus* oil therapy. *Alternative Med* 1:355-360 (1986).

71. *Selected medicinal plants of India. A monograph on identity, safety and clinical usage* (pp. 81-82). Mumbai: Chemexcil. Basic Chemicals, Pharmaceuticals and Cosmetics Export Promotion Council, 1992.

72. *Clinical and experimental studies on* rasayana *drugs and* pancakarma *theory* (pp. 16, 19). New Delhi: Central Council for Research in Ayurveda and Siddha, Ministry of Health and Family Welfare, Government of India, 1993.

73. *Caraka samhita,* ed. and trans. Sharma PV. (1st edn., vol. 2, p. 23, "Chikitsasthanam," chapter1, part 3, verse 30-31). Varanasi: Chaukhamba Orientalia, 1983.

74. *The wealth of India, raw materials* (first suppl. series, vol. 2, p.170). New Delhi: National Institute of Science Communication, CSIR, 2001.

75. Singh RH, Mehta AK, Sarkar FH, Udupa KN. Studies on psychotropic effect of the *medhya rasayana* drug, *shankhapushpi* (*Convolvulus pluricaulis* Chois). Part II *J Res Indian Med Yoga Homeo* 12(3):42-47 (1977).

76. Singh RH, Agrawal VK, Mehta AK. Studies on psychotropic effect of *medhya rasayana* drug, *sankapushpi* (*Convolvulus pluricaulis* Chois). Part III. Pharmacological studies. *J Res Ind Med Yoga Homeo* 12(3):48-52 (1977).

77. Shukla SP. Chemical and pharmacological studies on the indigenous drug, *sankhapuspi* (*C. pluricaulis* Chois). Part I. Barbiturate hypnosis potentiation effect of various fractions of total alcoholic extract of the whole plant. *J Res Indian Med Yoga Homeo* 14(3-4):132-135 (1979).

78. Shukla SP. Chemical and pharmacological studies on the indigenous drug, *shankhapuspi* (*C. pluricaulis* Chois). Part II. Barbiturate hypnosis potentiation effect of different successive extractives of the whole plant. *J Res Indian Med Yoga Homeo* 14(3-4):136-139 (1979).

79. Mudgal V, Srivastava DN, Singh RH, Udupa KN. Comparative studies on the hypotensive action and potentiation of barbiturate hypnosis with different parts of the plant *Convolvulus pluricaulis. J Res Indian Med* 7:74-77 (1972).

80. *Clinical and experimental studies on* rasayana *drugs and* panchakarma *therapy* (pp.15-20). New Delhi: Central Council for Research in Ayurveda and Siddha, Ministry of Health and Family Welfare, Government of India, 1993.

81. Shukla SP. A comparative study on the barbiturate hypnosis potentiation effect of *medhya rasayana* drugs *sankhapuspi (Convolvulus pluricaulis)* and *mandukaparni (Hydrocotyle asiatica). Bull Med Ethnobot Res* 1(4):554-560 (1980).

82. Singh RH, Sinha BN, Sarkar FH, Udupa KN. Comparative biochemical studies on the effect of four *medhya rasayana* drugs described by Caraka on some central neurotransmitters in normal and stressed rats. *J Res Indian Med Yoga Homeo* 14(3-4):7-14 (1979).

83. Sinha SN, Dixit VP, Madnawat AVS, Sharma OP. The possible potentiation of cognitive processing on administration of *Convolvulus microphyllus* in rats. *Indian Med* 1(3):1-6 (1989).

84. Mudgal, V. Personal communication, 1975 quoted in *Clinical and experimental studies on* rasayana *drugs and* panchakarma *therapy* (p. 17). New Delhi: Central

Council for Research in Ayurveda and Siddha, Ministry of Health and Family Welfare, Government of India, 1993.

85. Parihar MS, Hemnani T. Phenolic antioxidants attenuate hippocampal and neuronal cell damage against kainic acid induced excitotoxicity. *J Biosci* 28(1):121-128 (2003).

86. Singh RH, Mehta AK. Studies on psychotropic effect of *medhya rasayana* drug, *Shankapuspi Convolvulus pluricaulis*. Part I: Clinical studies. *J Res Ind Med Yoga Homeo* 12:18-25 (1977).

87. Bhattacharya SK, Bhattacharya A, Sairam K, Ghosal S. Anxiolytic-antidepressant activity of *Withania somnifera* glycowithanolides: An experimental study. *Phytomedicine* 7:463-469 (2000).

88. Singh RH, Malviya PC, Sarkar FH, Udupa KN. Studies on the psychotropic effect of Indian indigenous drug, *asvagandha* (*Withania somnifera* Dunol.). Part II: Experimental studies. *J Res Ind Med Yoga Homeo* 14:49-54 (1979).

89. Mehta AK, Binkley P, Gandhi SS, Ticku MK. Pharmacological effects of *Withania somnifera* root extract on GABA$_A$ receptor complex. *Indian J Med Res* 94 (B): 312-315 (1991).

90. Schliebs R, Liebmann A, Bhattacharya SK, Kumar A, Ghosal S, Bigl V. Systematic administration of defined extracts from *Withania somnifera* (Indian ginseng) and *shilajit* differentially affects cholinergic but not glutamatergic and GABAergic markers in rat brain. *Neurochem Int* 30:181-190 (1997).

91. Bhattacharya SK, Kumar A, Ghosal S. Effects of glycowithanolides from *Withania somnifera* on an animal model of Alzheimer's disease and perturbed central cholinergic markers of cognition in rats. *Phytother Res* 9:110-113 (1995).

92. Bhattacharya A, Ghosal S, Bhattacharya SK. Anti-oxidant effect of *Withania somnifera* glycowithanolides in chronic footshock stress-induced perturbations of oxidative free radical scavenging enzymes and lipid peroxidation in rat frontal cortex and striatum. *J Ethnopharmacol* 74:1-6 (2001).

93. Dhuley JN. Nootropic-like effect of *ashwagandha* (*Withania somnifera* L.) in mice. *Phytother Res* 15:524-528 (2001).

94. Ghosal S, Lal J, Srivastava RS, Bhattacharya SK, Upadhay SN, Jaiswal AK, Chattopadhyay U. Immunostimulatory and CNS effects of sitoindosides IX and X, two new glycowithanolides from *Withania somnifera*. *Phytother Res* 3:201-206 (1989).

95. Tohda C, Kuboyama T, Komatsu K. Dendrite extension by methanol extract of *ashwagandha* (roots of *Withania somnifera*) in SK-N-H cells. *Neuroreport* 11:1981-1985 (2000).

96. Kuboyama T, Tohda C, Zhao J, Nakamura N, Hattori M, Komatsu K. Axon- or dendrite-predominant outgrowth induced by constituents from *ashwagandha*. *Neuroreport* 13:1715-1720 (2002).

97. Zhao J, Nakamura N, Hattori M, Kuboyama T, Tohda C, Komatsu K. Withanolide derivatives from the roots of *Withania somnifera* and their neurite outgrowth activities. *Chem Pharm Bull* 50:760-765 (2002).

98. Jain S, Shukla SD, Sharma K, Bhatnagar M. Neuroprotective effects of *Withania somnifera* Dunn. in hippocampal sub-regions of female albino rat. *Phytother Res* 15:544-548 (2001).

99. Singh RH, Malaviya PC. Studies on the psychotropic effect of an indigenous rasayana drug, *asvagandha* (*Withania somnifera* Dunol.) Part I: Clinical studies. *J Res Indian Med Yoga Homeo* 13:15-24 (1978).

100. Karnick CR. A double blind placebo-controlled study on the effects of *Withania somnifera* and *Panax ginseng* extracts on psychomotor performance in healthy Indian volunteers. *Indian Med* 3(2-3):1-5 (1991).

PARKINSON'S DISEASE

Parkinson's disease (paralysis agitans) is a degenerative neurological disorder causing muscle tremor, stiffness, weakness, and difficulty with balance and in walking. Paralysis agitans has been described in Ayurveda as *kampavata* (*kampa,* shaking or tremor; *vata* is the principle or humor responsible for all movements). Multiplant preparations containing *Mucuna pruriens* as the source of levodopa are used in Ayurveda for the treatment of *kampavata.*[1]

Mucuna pruriens *Baker (Fl. Br. Ind.) non DC (Family: Fabaceae)*

Latin: *Mucuna prurita* Hook	Hindi: Kavach
Sanskrit: Atmagupta, Kapikachu	Tamil: Punaikali
English: Common Cowitch, Cowhage	

Mucuna pruriens (see Plate 12 in color gallery) is an herbaceous climber found growing all over India. The pods are covered with highly irritant hairs causing intense itching—the plant is named after this. Inside the pod are 4-6 black seeds, which are used medicinally. The seeds are well known in Ayurveda as an aphrodisiac agent and are also used as an anthelmintic agent, as a nerve tonic, for urinary disorders, and for fertility problems. In times of scarcity, the seeds are also used as food after repeatedly boiling and discarding the resultant liquid.[2,3]

The seeds contain up to 4-6 percent of L-DOPA – 1-3,4-dihydroxyphenylalanine,[4,5] about 0.09 percent in the pericarp and 5.28

percent in the endocarp,[5] glutathione, gallic acid, 0.53 percent alkaloids—nicotine, mucunine, mucunadine, prurienine, prurieninine, and the 5-indoles—tryptamine and 5-hydroxytryptamine, and about 6 percent of a fatty oil.[2,3]

The clinical study of *Mucuna pruriens* seeds for the treatment of Parkinson's disease[6] preceded pharmacological studies. Subsequent pharmacological studies in small animals showed that the efficacy of the seed powder against Parkinson's disease was devoid of any cholinergic effect.[7] The anti-Parkinsonian activity of the seed powder was due not only to the content of L-DOPA but also due to other components,[8-10] as seen in the activity exhibited in other fractions free from L-DOPA.[8] Comparison of the CNS profiles of 100 mg·kg^{-1} of L-DOPA and 3 g of seed powder of *Mucuna pruriens* containing 100 mg of L-DOPA showed similar activity as regards the dopaminergic pathway in showing an equivalent hypothermic and anti-Parkinsonian activity in rats and mice; however, in other aspects seed powder of *Mucuna pruriens* showed a better tolerability and improved anti-Parkinsonian activity due to the presence of other components[5,10] or adjuvants, which improve the activity of L-DOPA.[5] In addition, the alcoholic extract of the seeds has potent antioxidant activity.[11] The pharmacokinetic profile of a formulation from *Mucuna pruriens* seed known as HP-200 has been studied and found to be similar to formulations of synthetic L-DOPA.[12]

In a trial to assess the efficacy, tolerability, and acceptability of *Mucuna pruriens* in Parkinson's disease patients,[6] there was a washout period of 6 weeks, after which the seed powder was given in a dose of 15-40 g to 23 patients in divided doses, which was gradually increased until patients were receiving about 40-50 g of powder per day for an average treatment period of 20 weeks up to a maximum of 15 g four times a day. Baseline values of the patients compared with the final values showed an overall reduction in the morbidity index. Physical signs and handwriting records showed improvement. The seed powder was well tolerated; however, some patients sought a reduction in bulk. However, this bulk was useful in reducing constipation in patients. Side effects were few—dose dependent and mild— and improved on dose adjustment. These included giddiness, sweating, flatulence, diarrhea of mild nature, and dry mouth and blue-black urine in one patient of moderate intensity. Bioavailability studies with *Mucuna pruriens* showed significant absorption of L-DOPA from the seed powder.[6]

In another open multicentric study, 60 patients with Parkinson's disease were treated for 12 weeks with HP-200 derived from endocarp of *Mucuna pruriens* to assess its efficacy and tolerability. Twenty-six of the patients had earlier been on synthetic levodopa/ carbidopa combination, whereas the remaining 36 were on levodopa alone, which was discontinued before inclusion in the study. The drug prepared from the endocarp of *Mucuna pruriens* was supplied in sachets containing 33.33 mg of levodopa per sachet. Patients were assessed on the United Parkinson's Disease Rating Scale taken before the start of the trial and at the end of 12 weeks. Each patient got an average of 6±3 sachets daily. There was statistically significant improvement in symptoms seen in patients. Side effects were mild, seen infrequently, and were gastrointestinal in nature.[13]

Safety studies carried out on rats and mice have established the product as safe with no abnormalities in blood chemistry, liver and kidney observed, and no gross or histological abnormalities of brain and vital organs.[14] A long-term study, 52 weeks, of the effect of administration of the endocarp of *Mucuna pruriens* to rats found it not to exert any significant alteration on the levels of the monoaminergic neurotransmitters or cause stereotypic behavior.[9]

NOTES

1. Manyam BV. Paralysis agitans and levodopa in "Ayurveda" ancient Indian medical treatise. *Movement Disorders* 5(1):47-48 (199).

2. *The Wealth of India, raw materials* (vol. VI, pp. 442-443). New Delhi: Publications and Information Directorate, CSIR, 1962.

3. Chatterjee A, Pakrashi SC (eds.). *The treatise on Indian medicinal plants* (vol. 2, pp. 102-103). New Delhi: Publications and Information Directorate, CSIR, 1992.

4. Bell EA, Janzen DH. Medical and ecological considerations of L-DOPA and 5-HTP in seeds. *Nature* 229:136-137 (1971).

5. Hussain G, Manyam BV. *Mucuna pruriens* proves more effective than L-DOPA in Parkinson's disease animal model. *Phytother Res* 11:419-423 (1997).

6. Vaidya AB, Rajagopalan TG, Mankodi NA, Antarkar DS, Tathed PS, Purohit AV, Wadia NH. Treatment of Parkinson's disease with the cowhage plant—*Mucuna pruriens* Bak. *Neurology India* 26(4):171-176 (1978).

7. Ramaswamy S, Nazimudeen SK, Viswanathan S, Kulanthaivel P, Rajasekharan V, Kameshwaran L. Some pharmacological effects of *Mucuna pruriens*. *Procs of Madras Medical College Res Soc* 2:39 (1979).

8. Nath C, Gupta GP, Bhargava KP, Lakshmi V, Singh S, Popli SP. Study of the antiparkinsonian activity of seeds of *Mucuna prurita* Hook. *Indian J Pharmacol* 13:94-95 (1981).

9. Manyam BV, Dhanasekaran M, Hare TA. Effect of antiparkinson drug HP-200 *(Mucuna pruriens)* on the central monoaminergic neurotransmitters. *Phytother Res* 18:97-101 (2004).

10. Rajendran V, Joseph T, David J. Reappraisal of dopaminergic aspects of *Mucuna pruriens* and comparative profile with L-DOPA on cardiovascular and central nervous system in animals. *Indian Drugs* 33:465-472 (1996).

11. Tripathi YB, Upadhyay AK. Effect of the alcohol extract of the seeds of *Mucuna pruriens* on free radicals and oxidative stress in albino rats. *Phytother Res* 16:534-538 (2002).

12. Mahajani SS, Doshi VJ, Parikh KM, Manyam BV. Bioavailability of L-DOPA from HP-200 a formulation of seed powder of *Mucuna pruriens* (Bak.): A pharmacokinetic and pharmacodynamic study. *Phytother Res* 10:254-256 (1996).

13. Manyam BV. (Principal investigator). An alternative medicine treatment for treatment of Parkinson's disease: results of a multicenter clinical trial. HP-200 in Parkinson's disease study group. *J Altern Complement Med* 1:249-255 (1995).

14. Manyam BV, Parikh KM. Anti-parkinson activity of *Mucuna pruriens* seeds. *Ann Neurosci* 9:40-46 (2002).

SEDATIVE PLANTS

Sedative plants are used to calm the mind. "*Svapnajannan*" is the corresponding Ayurvedic category.[1]

Nardostachys jatamansi *DC (Family: Valerianaceae)*

Latin: *Nardostachys grandiflora* DC	Hindi: Jatamansi, Bal-chir
Sanskrit: Jatamansi	Tamil: Jatamanshi
English: Indian Spikenard, Muskroot, Spikenard	

Nardostachys jatamansi is an erect herb found growing in the Alpine Himalayas at an elevation of 3,000-5,000 m. The rhizome, covered with fine reddish brown fibrous tufts stemming from the leftover petioles of radical leaves, is used medicinally. The drug is known since the time of Caraka and has been recommended very often by Caraka, Sushruta, and Vāgbhata for nervous disorders, as a sedative, and as a tranquilizer;[2] however, it has not been much investigated. The rhizome is an official drug in the *Indian Herbal Pharmacopoeia, 2002,* as a sedative.[3]

The rhizome contains approximately 2 percent of a bitter aromatic essential oil, from which jatamansone has been isolated in 0.02-0.1 percent yields and found identical to valeranone from *Valeriana officinalis.*[3,40] Other components include a number of sesquiterpenoids such as jatamansic acid, terpenic coumarins, lignans, and neolignans.[3]

Extracts of the rhizome have shown a sedative effect in small animals.[5,6] Jatamansone has been shown to have a tranquilizing effect in experimental animals.[7] Alcoholic extract of the rhizomes cause an overall increase in central monoamines and inhibitory monoamines.[8] *Nardostachys jatamansi* shows a protective effect in focal ischemia, probably due to its antioxidant activity,[9] the petroleum ether extract of *Nardostachys jatamansi* having been shown to exhibit a dose-dependent antioxidant property.[10]

In an open exploratory study, 24 medical students were given a dose of 60 g of the root powder of *Nardostachys jatamansi* to study its sedative action. There was a prolongation of visual reaction time, the action being observed within an hour of intake, reaching a peak after 3 hours and lasting for 5 hours.[11]

In a trial on pregnant women, 6 g of *Nardostachys jatamansi* powder was given in two divided doses, and the women were observed in the 25-26th week, 33-34th week, and just before the onset of labor. The trial group women showed reduced anxiety levels and duration of labor, increased baby weight, and an increased crown and rump length in comparison to the control group, who did not receive the medication. The authors conclude that the better growth of the fetus may be due to the anxiolytic effect leading to better uterine circulation.[12]

The LD_{50} of jatamansone (valeranone) in rats and mice orally was found to be greater than 3,160 mg·kg^{-1}.[13]

Valeriana wallichii *DC (Family: Valerianaceae)*

Latin: *Valeriana jatamansi* Jones	Hindi: Tagar
Sanskrit: Tagara	Tamil: Jatamashi
English: Indian Valerian	

Valeriana wallichi is a short, hairy herb found growing in the temperate Himalayas. Caraka describes the use of the rhizome in Ayurveda; however, its use in CNS disorders is mentioned in later books such as the *Dhanvantari Nighantu* and *Bhavaprakash*.[14] In Ayurveda, it is used in delirium, insomnia, epilepsy, and in behavioral disorders.[14] Most of the scientific information with regard to Indian Valerian is in comparison with *Valeriana officinalis.* The rhizomes of *V. wallichii* have a higher percentage of valepotriates: 3-6 percent, as compared to *Valeriana officinalis:* 0.5-2 percent,[15] and therefore classified as a daytime sedative.[16] A review of scientific studies of three *Valeriana* species—*V. officinalis* from Europe, *V. edulis* from Mexico, and *V.wallichii* from India is available.[15]

NOTES

1. Vaidya ADB. The status and scope of Indian medicinal plants acting on central nervous system. *Indian J Pharmacol* 29:S340-S343 (1997).

2. *Selected medicinal plants of India. A monograph on identity, safety and clinical usage* (pp. 219-220). Bombay: Chemexcil. Basic Chemicals, Pharmaceuticals and Cosmetics Export Promotion Council, 1992.

3. *Indian herbal pharmacopoeia* (rev. new edn., pp. 265-271). Bombay: Indian Drug Manufacturers' Association, 2002.

4. Satyavati GV, Gupta AK, Tandon N (eds.). *Medicinal plants of India* (vol. 2, pp. 312-323). New Delhi: Indian Council of Medical Research, 1987.

5. Hamied KA, Bakshi VM, Aghara LP. Pharmacological investigation of *Nardostachys jatamansi. J Sci Ind Res* 21C:100-103 (1962).

6. Gupta SS, Seth CB, Mathur VS, Ghooi C, Verma RK. Central nervous system effects of some indigenous antiasthmatic drugs. *Indian J Physiol Pharmacol* 10:5-14 (1966).

7. Arora RB, Singh M, Kanta C. Tranquillizing activity of jatamansone, a sesquiterpene from *Nardostachys jatamansi. Life Sci* (6): 225-228 (1962).

8. Prabhu V, Karanth KS, Rao A. Effects of *Nardostachys jatamansi* on biogenic amines and inhibitory amino acids in the rat brain. *Planta Med* 60:114-117 (1994).

9. Salim S, Ahmad M, Zafar KS, Ahmad AS, Islam F. Protective effect of *Nardostachys jatamansi* in rat cerebral ischemia. *Pharmacol Biochem Behav* 74:481-486 (2003).

10. Tripathi E, Tripathi YB. *Effect of* B.monniera *and* N. jatamansi *in rat brain homogenate. A comparative study* (abstract A-36). Varanasi: Faculty of Ayurveda, Institute of Medical Studies, Banaras Hindu University, Procs of Internl Sem Free Radicals Mediated Diseases and Ayurveda, September 2-4, 1996.

11. Amin MG, Dixit YB, Pathak JD. Reaction time studies in relation to an indigenous drug—*Nardostachys jatamansi. Antiseptic* 58:565 (1961).

12. Ranjana, Dwivedi M. A clinical study of *jatamansi* in optimal antenatal care. *J Res Ayur Siddha* 20:120-129 (1999).

13. Rucker G, Tautges J, Sieck A, Wenzl H, Graf E. [Isolation and pharmacodynamic activity of the sesquiterpene valeranone from *Nardostachys jatamansi*]. *Arzneimittelforsch* 28:7-13 (1978).

14. *Selected medicinal plants of India. A monograph on identity, safety and clinical usage* (pp. 337-339). Bombay: Chemexcil, Basic Chemicals, Pharmaceuticals and Cosmetics Export Promotion Council, 1992.

15. Hölzl J. Baldrian. Ein Mittel gegen Schlafstörungen and Nervosität. *Deutsche Apoth Ztg* 136:751-759 (1996).

16. Schlicher H. Pflanzliche Psychopharmaka. Eine neue Klassifizierung nach Indikationsgruppen. *Deutsche Apoth Ztg* 135:1811-1822 (1995).

Chapter 13

Rasayana Drugs:
Antiaging Agents, Adaptogens,
and Immunostimulants

The term *rasayana* in Ayurveda is mentioned way back in the *Caraka Samhita* as an agent that confers long life, youthfulness, freedom from disease, a strong body, maintenance of faculties leading to a gleaming complexion, powerful voice, good eyesight, acuity of mental faculties, and acute hearing—in effect retaining one's faculties throughout one's life.[1] With such an enticing prospect, it is little wonder that this concept has aroused great interest in interpreting these outcomes in modern scientific terms.

Studies have shown that some of these effects can be explained in terms of antioxidant activity[2] protecting the body against free radical damage, stimulation of the immune system, thus protecting the body against infections by increasing host defense,[3,4] and adaptogenic activity protecting the body against the ill effects of stress, such as environmental conditions.[3,5] It has also been shown that these *rasayana* plants exhibit organ specificity, as mentioned in Ayurveda.[3] For example, there is the whole series of drugs known as *medhya* that are considered to help in enhancing memory, intellect, and retention, covered in Chapter 12. Other herbs such as *Tinospora cordifolia* are recommended for the liver, *Emblica officinalis* for the pancreas, *Asparagus racemosus* for the stomach, and *Piper longum* for the lungs.[3]

doi:10.1300/5683_13

NOTES

1. *Caraka samhita* ed. and trans. Sharma PV (vol. II, pp. 3-4 "Chikitsasthanam," chapter 1, verse 7-8). Varanasi: Chaukhambha Orientalia, 1983.

2. Scartezzini P, Speroni E. Review on some plants of Indian traditional medicine with antioxidant activity. *J Ethnopharmacol* 71:23-43 (2000).

3. Dahanukar SA, Thatte UM. Current status of Ayurveda in phytomedicine. *Phytomedicine* 4:359-368 (1997).

4. Kumar VP, Kuttan R, Kuttan G. Effect of "*rasayanas*," a herbal drug preparation on immune responses and its significance in cancer treatment. *Indian J Exp Biol* 37:27-31 (1999).

5. Rege NN, Thatte UM, Dahanukar SA. Adaptogenic properties of six *rasayana* herbs used in Ayurvedic medicine. *Phytother Res* 13:275-291 (1999).

TONIC/ANTIAGING EFFECTS

Among free radical–mediated conditions, aging is also considered to result from free radical damage. According to Caraka, *rasayanas* are drugs that vitalize cells, thereby opening up partially or fully blocked channels *(srotas)*. Many of the *rasayanas* have been shown to act as free radical scavengers exhibiting antioxidant activity with the potential to mitigate the effects of aging. Thus, just as antioxidants are taken as dietary supplements, *rasayanas* can be used both for prophylactic and therapeutic use to prevent free radical damage.[1] However, in earlier trials, modern markers of antioxidant activity were not available for evaluation.

Emblica officinalis *Gaertn. (Family: Euphorbiaceae)*

Latin: *Phyllanthus emblica* Linn.	Tamil: Nelli
Sanskrit: Amalaki	
Hindi: Amla	English: Indian gooseberry, Emblic myrobalan

The fruits of *Emblica officinalis* (see Plate 1 in color gallery) are one of the best-known *rasayana* drugs in Ayurveda, promoting health and youthfulness, protecting the heart and the body, and bestowing, on oral intake, freedom from disease. However, the antiaging, or *rasayana,* aspect has not been much investigated in the clinic, with only a few of reports of its usefulness. The fruits are very widely consumed in the form of a confection made out of the fruits and several other herbs and taken as a multiherbal preparation known as *Chyavanprash* named after the sage Chyavan, who used it for rejuvenation. In order to make it available at home throughout the year the fruit is made into jam, pickles, the whole fruit preserved in honey, or its pieces sun-dried to add, when required, into food items.

Aging has been considered to result from free radical damage, and agents displaying the antioxidant effect protect the body and mind from aging. Fruits of *Emblica officinalis* exhibit a potent antioxidant effect,[2,3] which was first attributed to the high content of Vitamin C (600-900 mg per 10 g of fresh fruit).[4] Later experiments have suggested that the fruits are devoid of Vitamin C.[5] The antioxidant activity has been postulated to arise from the tannins emblicanin A and B, punigluconin, and pedunculagin,[6] which have been shown to protect the heart[7] and the brain[8] from oxidative stress, rather than Vitamin C. The aqueous extract of *Emblica officinalis* exhibits an adaptogenic effect and protects experimental animals from a variety of stresses—physical, chemical, and biological,[9] whereas the fresh fruit homogenate on chronic administration protected the heart against oxidative stress.[10] Flavonoids from *Emblica officinalis,* apart from their potent hypolipidemic and hypoglycemic effects, also improve the blood picture by raising hemoglobin levels.[11]

Thus, there is evidence from experimental studies that the fruits are potent antioxidants, with favorable effects on several organ systems; however, evidence from clinical trials is scanty. In an early experimental study in rabbits, there was improvement in body weight and total serum protein content.[12]

In studies carried out at Varanasi, the preparation obtained from fruits of *Emblica officinalis* triturated 21 times with the fresh juice of the fruit and then dried and powdered, which is known as *Amalaki rasayan.* There was increase in body weight in clinical cases, positive nitrogen balance, increased serum mucopolysaccharides, and a decreased excretion of hydroxyproline indicating greater turnover, repair, and regeneration of connective tissues.[13]

In another study, patients undergoing surgery for inguinal hernia and senile enlargement of prostate in the age group of 55-60 years were given 10 g of *Amalaki rasayan* in three divided doses for 10 days prior to surgery. Treatment was evaluated on the basis of time taken for ambulation, early return of physiological functions such as passage of flatus, and changes in serum mucopolysaccharides, hydroxyproline, urinary nitrogen, blood picture, and blood sugar levels against the time taken by patients maintained as control. Patients treated with *Amalaki rasayan* did not show any loss of body weight, had improved hematological picture, were ambulatory earlier, and had early return of physiological functions. In addition, biochemical parameters also indicated a favorable return of connective tissue turnover.[14] The safety of *Emblica officinalis* is covered in Chapter 3, "Gastrointestinal agents."

This promising fruit needs to be further studied.

Withania somnifera *Dunal. (Family: Solanaceae)*

Withania somnifera has been covered in Chapter 8, "Antirheumatic agents" and in Chapter 12 "Central nervous system agents." The roots are considered to have a health-promoting effect, improving stamina, warding off disease, and toning up the body and mind. In a double-blind placebo-controlled trial, *Withania somnifera* has been shown to improve the health of adult volunteers over a period of 1 year. It has also been used in children to improve health.

Studies in small animals have shown that *Withania somnifera* exerts an adaptogenic effect against a variety of physical[15-17] biological,[16] and chemical stressors,[16] and in a chronic stress model.[18] There was significant increase in the physical working capacity and an increase in the heart weight and glycogen content of the myocardium and liver.[17] Adaptogenic activity has also been shown in a withanolide-free fraction from *Withania somnifera*.[19,20] The aqueous suspension[21] and the methanolic extract[22] of *Withania somnifera* and the glycowithanolides[23,24] consisting of equimolar concentrations of sitoindosides VII-X and withaferin A have been shown to exhibit antioxidant activity. *Withania somnifera* has also been shown to exhibit immunostimulatory activity with significant increase in hemoglobin concentration, red blood cell count, white blood cell count, platelet count, and body weight as compared to untreated control in different animal models of myelosupression.[25] Increased synthesis of nitric oxide by macrophages has been postulated to partly explain the immuno-stimulatory activity of *Withania somnifera*.[26]

In a double-blind placebo-controlled clinical trial to study the effect of *Withania somnifera* on normal healthy male volunteers in the age group 50-59 years, powdered root of *Withania somnifera* made into 500 mg tablets or a similar tablets made of starch, which was matched as far as possible for color, strength, and appearance, was given. A total of 331 volunteers were screened and 141 subjects, who did not have diseases such as diabetes, asthma, CHD, hypertension etc. were included in the trial and randomly allocated to receive the drug or placebo, two tablets thrice daily with milk for 1 year; 101 volunteers completed the treatment. There was significant increase in hemoglobin and red blood corpuscles in the treated group. Other significant changes included an increase in seated stature, increase in hair melanin content, reduced decrease in nail calcium, greater decrease in serum cholesterol, and erythrocyte sedimentation rate in the treated group as compared to placebo. Approximately 71 percent of volunteers reported subjective improvement in sexual performance. No side effects were seen.[27]

In another double-blind study conducted on normal male and female children, ages 8-12 years, the effect of *Withania somnifera* was compared with *Withania somnifera* and *Boerhaavia diffusa,* ferrous fumarate at two different concentrations and placebo in different groups along with milk for 60 days. Thus, group 1 received 2 g·day^{-1} of *Withania somnifera,* group 2 received 2 g of a 1:1 mixture of *Withania somnifera* and *Boerhaavia diffusa,* group 3 received 2 g lactose mixed with 5 mg of ferrous fumarate, group 4 received 2 g lactose mixed with 30 mg of ferrous fumarate, whereas group 5 received 2 g lactose powder, all medications with 100 ml of milk. All the children received similar diet and had similar environmental conditions since they were inmates of a local orphanage. Baseline values were estimated before the start of the trial. It was found that there was increase in body weight and a significant increase in mean corpuscular hemoglobin and total protein over the initial level in group 1 on *ashwagandha,* in comparison to placebo. In group 2, receiving a 1:1

mixture of *ashwagandha* and *punarnava,* although there was increase over initial values in several parameters such as hemoglobin, mean corpuscular volume, mean corpuscular hemoglobin, serum iron, and hand grip, only hemoglobin and hand grip differed significantly from placebo. In children in group 4 receiving 5 mg ferrous fumarate and those in group 5 receiving placebo, there was no significant change in any of the parameters studied, whereas in group 3 receiving 30 mg ferrous fumarate, there was significant increase in hemoglobin, corpuscular hemoglobin, serum iron, and in hand grip compared to the placebo group. The results in group 1 and 2 led the authors to recommend fortifying milk with the *Withania somnifera* and *Boerhaavia diffusa* to improve growth and strength in growing children and increasing the quantity of *Withania somnifera* in the combination in order to take advantage of the hematinic properties of *Withania somnifera,* pointing out that the quantity of iron in *ashwagandha* is equal to that in 5 mg of ferrous fumarate.[28]

In another study, *Withania somnifera* and *Tinospora cordifolia* were administered to separate groups of patients for 3 months to study potential antiaging effects, better results were achieved with *Tinospora cordifolia.* However, this study has been published in the form of an abstract and hence further details are not available.[29]

Considering the importance of the results obtained and the advances in analytical methodology it is worthwhile laying down the specifications for the material to be used, which are then followed by further trials with larger numbers of volunteers to confirm the results obtained in these studies. Aspects of the safety of *Withania somnifera* have been dealt with in Chapter 8, "Antirheumatic agents."

NOTES

1. Tripathi YB. Free radicals in Ayurveda. *Ancient Sci Life* 17(3):158-168 (1998).

2. Kumar KCS, Müller K. Medicinal plants from Nepal II. Evaluation as inhibitors of lipid peroxidation in biological membranes. *J Ethnopharmacol* 64:135-139 (1999).

3. Khanom F, Kayahara H, Tadasa K. Superoxide-scavenging and prolyl endopeptidase inhibitory activities of Bangladeshi indigenous medicinal plants. *Biosci Biotech Biochem* 64:837-840 (2000).

4. *Selected medicinal plants of India. A monograph on identity, safety and clinical usage* (pp. 231-234). Bombay: Chemexcil, Basic Chemicals, Pharmaceuticals and Cosmetics Export Promotion Council, 1992.

5. Ghosal S, Tripathi VK, Chauhan S. Active constituents of *Emblica officinalis* Part I: The chemistry and antioxidative effects of two new hydrolysable tannins emblicannin A and B. *Indian J Chem* 35B:941-948 (1996).

6. Bhattacharya A, Chatterjee A, Ghosal S, Bhattacharya SK. Antioxidant activity of active tannoid principles of *Emblica officinalis (amla)*. *Indian J Exp Biol* 37:676-680 (1999).

7. Bhattacharya SK, Bhattacharya A, Sairam K, Ghosal S. Effect of bioactive tannoid principles of *Emblica officinalis* on ischemia-reperfusion-induced oxidative stress in rat heart. *Phytomedicine* 9:171-174 (2002).

8. Bhattacharya A, Ghosal S, Bhattacharya SK. Antioxidant activity of tannoid principles of *Emblica officinalis (amla)* in chronic stress induced changes in rat brain. *Indian J Exp Biol* 38:877-880 (2000).

9. Rege NN, Thatte UM, Dahanukar SA. Adaptogenic properties of six *rasayana* herbs used in Ayurvedic medicine. *Phytother Res* 13:275-291 (1999).

10. Rajak S, Banerjee SK, Sood S, Dinda AK, Gupta YK, Gupta SK, Maulik SK. *Emblica officinalis* causes myocardial adaptation and protects against oxidative stress in ischemic reperfusion injury in rats. *Phytother Res* 18:54-60 (2004).

11. Anila L, Vijayalakshmi NR. Beneficial effects of flavonoids from *Sesamum indicum, Emblica officinalis* and *Momordica charantia*. *Phytother Res* 14:592-595 (2000).

12. Tewari A, Sen SP, Guru LV. The effect of *amalaki (Phyllanthus emblica) rasayana* on biologic system. *J Res Indian Med* 2:189-194 (1968).

13. Udupa KN. *Promotion of "health for all" by Ayurveda and yoga* (pp. 70-71, 80-81). Varanasi: The Tara Printing Works, 1985.

14. *Clinical and experimental studies on* rasayana *drugs and panchakarma therapy* (pp. 37- 40). New Delhi: Central Council for Research in Ayurveda and Siddha, Ministry of Health & Family Welfare, Government of India, 1993.

15. Singh N, Nath R, Lata A, Singh SP, Kohli RP, Bhargava KP. *Withania somnifera (ashwagandha)*, a rejuvenating herb drug enhances survival during stress (an adaptogen). *Int J Crude Drug Res* 20:29-35 (1982).

16. Rege NN, Thatte UM, Dahanukar SA. Adaptogenic properties of six *rasayana* herbs used in *Ayurvedic medicine*. *Phytother Res* 13:275- 291 (1999).

17. Dhuley JN. Adaptogenic and cardioprotective action of *ashwagandha* in rats and frogs. *J Ethnopharmacol* 70:57-63 (2000).

18. Bhattacharya SK, Muruganandam AV. Adaptogenic activity of *Withania somnifera:* An experimental study using a rat model of chronic stress. *Pharmacol Biochem Behav* 75:547-555 (2003).

19. Singh B, Saxena AK, Chandan BK, Gupta DK, Bhutani KK, Anand KK. Adaptogenic activity of a novel withanolide-free aqueous fraction from the roots of *Withania somnifera* Dun. *Phytother Res* 15:311-318 (2001).

20. Singh B, Chandan BK, Gupta DK. Adaptogenic activity of a novel withanolide-free aqueous fraction from the roots of *Withania somnifera* Dun. (Part II). *Phytother Res* 17:531-536 (2003).

21. Dhuley JN. Effect of *ashwagandha* on lipid peroxidation in stress-induced animals. *J Ethnopharmacol* 60:173-178 (1998).

22. Russo A, Izzo AA, Cardile V, Borrelli F, Vanella A. Indian medicinal plants as antiradicals and DNA cleavage protectors. *Phytomedicine* 8:125-132 (2001).

23. Bhattacharya SK, Satyan KS, Ghosal S. Antioxidant activity of glycowithanolides from *Withania somnifera*. *Indian J Exp Biol* 35:236-239 (1997).

24. Bhattacharya A, Ghosal S, Bhattacharya SK. Anti-oxidant effect of *Withania somnifera* glycowithanolides in chronic footshock stress-induced perturbations of oxidative free radical scavenging enzymes in rat frontal cortex and striatum. *J Ethnopharmacol* 74:1-6 (2001).

25. Ziauddin M, Phansalkar N, Patki P, Diwanay S, Patwardhan B. Studies on the immunomodulatory effects of *aswagandha*. *J Ethnopharmacol* 50:69-76 (1996).

26. Iuvone T, Esposito G, Capasso F, Izzo AA. Induction of nitric oxide synthase expression by *Withania somnifera* in macrophages. *Life Sci* 72:1617-1625 (2003).

26. Kuppurajan K, Rajagopalan SS, Sitaraman R, Rajagopalan V, Janaki K, Revathi R, Venkataraghavan S. Effect of *aswagandha* (*Withania somnifera* Dunal) on the process of ageing in human volunteers. *J Res Ayur Siddha* 1:247-258 (1980).

27. Venkataraghavan S, Seshadri C, Sundaresan TP, Revathi R, Rajagopalan V, Janaki K. The comparative effect of milk fortified with *aswagandha, aswagandha* and *punarnava* in children—A double blind study. *J Res Ayur Siddha* 1:370-385 (1980).

28. De RK, Tripathi PC. Role of certain indigenous drugs antioxidants in ageing (Abstract A-32). Varanasi: Internl Sem Free Radicals Mediated Diseases & Ayurveda, Faculty of Ayurveda, IMS, BHU, September 2-4 1996.

OTHER TONIC/ANTIAGING PLANTS

Centella asiatica *(Linn.) Urban. (Family: Apiaceae)*

Latin: *Hydrocotyle asiatica* Linn.	Tamil: Vallarai
Sanskrit: Mandukaparni	English: Indian Pennywort
Hindi: Brahma Manduki	

In a double-blind clinical trial carried out on 43 normal adults divided into two groups using either *Centella asiatica* (see Plate 8 in the color gallery) or *Boerhaavia diffusa* for 1 year, patients were evaluated at 6 months and 1 year. In the *Centella asiatica* group, there was a significant improvement in the number of red blood corpuscles, vital capacity, and total protein. There was also a significant improvement in hemoglobin levels with a decrease in blood urea and serum acid phosphatase.[1,2]

NOTES

1. Appa Rao MVR, Usha SP, Rajagopalan SS, Sarangan R. Six months' result of double blind trial to study the effect of *mandookaparni* and *punarnava* on normal healthy adults. *J Res Ind Med* 2:79-85 (1967).
2. Appa Rao MVR, Rajagopalan,SS, Srinivasan VR, Sarangan R. Study of *mandookaparni* and *punarnava* for their *rasayana* effect on normal healthy adults. *Nagarjun* 12:33-41 (1969).

IMMUNOSTIMULANT EFFECTS AGAINST INFECTION

Plants used as *rasayanas* have the potential to promote health by strengthening host defense against different diseases rather than specific action on the disease. This can be seen in the examples that follow and also in Chapter 4 where *Tinospora cordifolia* was used as an adjuvant to antibiotics following surgery for obstructive jaundice.[1]

Tinospora cordifolia *Miers. (Family: Menispermaceae)*

Latin: *Tinospora glabra* (N.Brum.) Merr	Hindi: Giloe
Sanskrit: Guduchi, Amrita	Tamil: Sindal

The use of *Tinospora cordifolia* (see Plate 4 in color gallery) in obstructive jaundice has been covered in section, "Hepatoprotective agents" in Chapter 4 and also as an anti-inflammatory agent in Chapter 8, "Antirheumatic agents." There has been a considerable amount of work on the immunomodulatory activity of the plant, several immunostimulating compounds having been isolated. Syringin and cordiol show anticomplementary activity, increase IgG antibodies, and increase humoral and cell-mediated immunity in a dose-dependent manner. Cordioside, cordifolioside A, and cordiol show macrophage activation.[2] An immunologically active arabinogalactan was isolated from *Tinospora cordifolia*[3] and shown to possess antioxidant activity[4] and an inhibitory effect on experimental metastasis.[5]

Tuberculosis

Tinospora cordifolia is considered a *rasayana,* which protects against infection. It has been shown in a series of experiments upon small animals to be a powerful immunostimulant, which increases host defense both in normal and in immunocompromised states[1] through activation of the immune cells such as the macrophages, and especially the peritoneal and alveolar macrophages.[6] The modulation of the alveolar macrophage function in rats by *Tinospora cordifolia* has been studied both by itself and in combination with modern anti-tubercular (anti-TB) drugs and then compared with that produced by standard anti-tubercular drugs.[7] The studies have shown that the phagocytic and intracellular killing capacity of the alveolar macrophages has been increased through stimulation of nitric oxide (NO) synthesis in alveolar macrophages by *Tinospora cordifolia,* whereas it is significantly reduced by anti-TB drugs. When *Tinospora cordifolia* was coadministered with anti-TB drugs the decrease of NO production was prevented.[8]

In a double-blind placebo-controlled trial the effect of coadministration of either 500 mg thrice daily of *Tinospora cordifolia* or placebo along with standard anti-TB drugs was evaluated in 31 patients, and these patients were assessed early on in the first 2 months of treatment. At the end of 2 months, the data available for 20 patients shows that addition of *Tinospora cordifolia* produced a number of useful effects and lowered composite clinical score faster than placebo. The patients gained weight, had reduced sputum conversion time, had improved radiological picture, and had an improved quality of life with fewer side effects and dropouts.[8] The effect of coadministration of *Tinospora cordifolia* (500 mg thrice a day) against placebo was also evaluated in TB patients on a short-term anti-TB regime for 6 months, and in a larger number of patients (24 on *Tinospora cordifolia* and 22 on placebo) confirmed results obtained earlier. At 6 months there was no significant difference between placebo and *Tinospora cordifolia.* There were fewer adverse effects reported and fewer dropouts in the *Tinospora cordifolia* group.[9]

Thus, adding *Tinospora cordifolia* (TC) to anti-TB drugs seems to hasten recovery and improve quality of life at the end of 2 months;

however, at the end of 6 months the differences seem to have evened out.[8,9] Thus in a double-blind placebo-controlled study with 50 patients—23 on TC and 27 on placebo—47 percent of the placebo group showed improvement, whereas 75 percent of the TC group showed progress including radiological improvement. In addition, there were fewer side effects in the TC-treated group (15 percent) as compared to placebo (40 percent) at the end of 2 months.[6]

Asthma

In ten chronic asthmatics treated with one 500 mg tablet of *Tinospora cordifolia* aqueous extract thrice daily for 8 weeks there was considerable improvement in the quality of life, reduced frequency of asthmatic attacks, and decrease in severity of symptoms, such as coughing and wheezing.[10]

The safety of *Tinospora cordifolia* is covered in Chapter 4, "Hepatoprotective agents."

NOTES

1. Thatte UM, Dahanukar SA. Immunotherapeutic modification of experimental infections by Indian medicinal plants. *Phytother Res* 3(2):43-49 (1989).

2. Kapil A, Sharma S. Immunopotentiating compounds from *Tinospora cordifolia*. *J Ethnopharmacol* 58:89-95 (1997).

3. Chintalwar G, Jain A, Sipahimalani A, Banerjee A, Sumariwalla P, Ramakrishnan R, Sainis K. An immunologically active arabinogalactan from *Tinospora cordifolia*. *Phytochem* 52:1089-1093 (1999).

4. Subramanian M, Chintalwar GJ, Chattopadhyay S. Antioxidant properties of a *Tinospora cordifolia* polysaccharide against iron-mediated lipid damage and γ-ray induced protein damage. *Redox Rep* 7:137-143 (2002).

5. Leyon PV, Kuttan G. Inhibitory effect of a polysaccharide from *Tinospora cordifolia* on experimental metastasis. *J Ethnopharmacol* 90:233-237 (2004).

6. Dahanukar SA, Thatte UM. Current status of Ayurveda in phytomedicine. *Phytomedicine* 4:359-368 (1997).

7. Pokharankar SL, Nagarkatti DS. Modulation of alveolar macrophage function by antituberculous agents and *Tinospora cordifolia* (p. 83). Bombay: Procs "Update Ayurveda—94," February 24-26,1994.

8. Dash A, Rege NR, Vaingankar J, Mahashur A, Thatte U, Dahanukar S. Stimulation of nitric oxide (NO) synthesis by *Tinospora cordifolia* in alveolar

macrophages and its implications in patients of tuberculosis. *Indian J Pharmacol* 33:51(2001).

9. Rege N, Vaingankar J, Dash A, Garkal P, Mahashur A, Thatte U, Dahanukar S. Stimulation of nitric oxide (NO) synthesis by *Tinospora cordifolia* in alveolar macrophages and its implications in patients with tuberculosis. *Phytomedicine* 7 (suppl. II):56-57 (2000).

10. Kulkarni K. Maintaining quality of life in chronic asthmatics with *Tinospora cordifolia. Indian J Clin Pract* 9(3):30-33 (1998).

OTHER IMMUNOSTIMULANT PLANTS

See also Chapter 5, "Respiratory tract drugs" section "Upper-respiratory tract infections."

Centella asiatica *Urban (Linn.) (Family: Apiaceae)*

Centella asiatica (see Plate 8 in color gallery) is a small creeping herb found growing throughout India near water bodies. It is traditionally used in Ayurveda for a number of conditions including cough, bronchitis, and asthma,[1] and is considered an antiaging herb that fortifies the immune system.[2] See also Chapters 6, 9, and 12.

The alcoholic extract of *Centella asiatica* has been shown to have a stimulatory effect on the reticuloendothelial system in mice.[3] In addition, the aqueous extract has been shown to have a positive effect on the complement system.[4] Rats fed orally with 100 mg$\cdot$kg^{-1} body weight per day of aqueous suspension of *Centella asiatica* for 7 days showed an immunostimulant activity, which was assessed to be comparable to 60 percent that of interferon alpha2b.[5]

Treatment for 1 month of aged persons with *Centella asiatica* was found to give significant relief in common ailments, such as cold, cough, and bronchitis. There was significant increase in serum IgM ($p < 0.01$) and IgG ($p < 0.05$) levels indicating a general increase in immunity.[6]

The safety of *Centella asiatica* is covered in Chapter 6, "Cardiovascular drugs" and in Chapter 12, "Central nervous system agents."

NOTES

1. Gogte VM. *Ayurvedic pharmacology and therapeutic uses of medicinal plants* (pp. 466-468). Mumbai: SPARC, Trans. Bharatiya Vidya Bhavan, 2000.

2. Lad V, Frawley D. *The yoga of herbs* (pp. 170-172). Santa Fe, New Mexico: Lotus Press, 1986.

3. DiCarlo FJ, Haynes LJ, Sliver NJ, Phillips GE. Reticuloendothelial system stimulants of botanical origin. *J Reticuloendothelial Soc* 1:224-232 (1964).

4. Labadie RP, van der Nat JM, Simons JM, Kroes BH, Kosai S, van den Berg AJJ, t'Hart LA, van der Sluis WG, Abeysekera A, Bamunuarachchi K, de Silva KT. An ethnopharmacognostic approach to the search for immunomodulators of plant origin. *Planta Med* 55:339-348 (1989).

5. Patil JS, Nagavi BG, Ramesh M, Vijaykumar GS. A study on the immunostimulant activity of *Centella asiatica* Linn. in rats. *Indian Drugs* 35:711-714 (1998).

6. Singh G. Immunity promoting effect of *mandukaparni (Hydrocotyle asiatica)*. (Abstract C-56 and A-43). Madras: Procs Internl Conf Traditional Medicine, 1986.

CANCER THERAPY

Cancer is a malignant growth, or tumor, formed by abnormal, rapid reproduction of cells. In Ayurveda, a number of predisposing factors have been enunciated as a result of which a tumor can develop—imbalance in the humors *(doshas)*, poor digestion, and absorption leading to formation of undigested food particles, deposition in the tissues, and enzyme malfunction that result in a tumor development.[1] From a list of 100 plants used traditionally for the treatment of cancer, 44 have been postulated as having anticancer activity. Other authors have arrived at similar figures of active plants.[2,3] Although there has been substantial pharmacological work, the clinical work is miniscule and mostly as adjuvants to modern therapy.

Boswellia serrata *Roxb. ex Coleb* (Family: Burseraceae)

Boswellia serrata (see Plate 2 in color gallery) resin has been covered in Chapter 3, "Gastrointestinal agents," in Chapter 5, "Respiratory tract drugs," and in Chapter 8, "Antirheumatic agents," where its use as an anti-inflammatory agent has been covered in a variety of conditions where leukotrienes play a key role in causation and in the persistence of the disease. Traditionally, the gum is reported to be useful in ulcers, tumors, goiter, cystic breast, diarrhea, dysentery, piles, and skin diseases.[4] The nonphenolic portion of the gum resin has been reported to possess antitumor, analgesic, and sedative activity.[4]

The 50-percent alcoholic extract of the root, fruit, and stem showed anticancer activity against several cancer screens—human epidermal carcinoma of the nasopharynx in tissue culture, lymphoid leukemia, sarcoma 180, and hepatoma 129 in mice.[5] In mice transplanted with Ehrlich ascites carcinoma and S-180 transplantable tumors, it increased longevity of mice with ascites by 24 percent and reduced tumor size of S-180 tumors by 24 percent.[6] Recent in vitro studies using human cell culture lines have also shown that the resin and the boswellic acids derived from it show anticancer activity against various cancers, notably against leukemia and brain tumors,[7] also in colon cancer cells[8] and in liver cancer HepG2 cells,[9] due to induction of cell death and modulation of enzyme activity.[7-10] In addition, the boswellic acids showed anticancer activity when applied topically against skin cancer in mice.[11]

Boswellic acids[10,12] such as 3-O-acetyl-11-keto-β-boswellic acid and 3-O-acetyl-β-boswellic acid, and β-boswellic acid have been shown to be cytotoxic to human glioma cell lines, at inhibitory concentrations (IC_{50}) ranging from 20 to 40 μM.[12] In rats with induced tumors receiving different dosages of the gum resin extract, those receiving the highest dosage (3×240 mg·kg^{-1} body weight) had twice the survival time of untreated controls ($p < 0.05$) with significantly larger number of apoptotic tumor cells.[13] Acetyl boswellic acids have been shown to be catalytic inhibitors of both topoisomerase I and II simultaneously, which could result in enhanced antitumor efficacy.[14] *Boswellia serrata* extract has been shown to be more potent than pure 3-O-acetyl-11-keto-β-boswellic acid in three hematological cell lines.[15] Acetyl-11-keto-β-boswellic acid showed a potent cytotoxic activity against meningioma cells (IC_{50} 2-8 μM), mediated partly by inhibition of the Erk signal transduction pathway that plays an essential role in signal transduction and tumorogenesis[16] by interfering/interrupting with the signals that play an important role in cell proliferation and cell death of different tumors.

Clinical studies carried out on peritumoral edema in brain tumors, such as astrocytoma and glioblastoma using much larger doses than earlier used for the treatment of arthritis, bronchial asthma, and inflammatory bowel diseases, have shown a reduction in the edema, but not of the tumor itself, perhaps due to the short treatment periods employed. It was earlier thought that there was increased formation of leukotrienes when such tumors are present.

In an open study in patients with malignant astrocytomas, there was an increased excretion of leukotrienes E_4 (LTE_4), which decreased after surgical intervention but returned to higher values when there was a relapse. Treatment with three 400 mg *Boswellia serrata* extract tablets administered thrice a day to patients for 7 days showed again a decrease in the levels of LTE_4 in the urine.[17]

In an exploratory controlled study with 29 patients with malignant glioblastoma, 14 patients received 1,200 mg of *Boswellia serrata* extract (H15) thrice daily, 9 patients received 800 mg thrice daily, and 5 patients 400 mg thrice daily 7 days before operation. Only patients receiving the highest dose had significant reduction of the perifocal edema volume, not in tumor size after 7 days intake.[18]

In another study on 12 patients with brain tumor and progressive edema, treated with 1,200 mg of *Boswellia serrata* extract (H15) for several months, two out of seven patients with glioblastoma and progressive tumors and three out of five patients with treatment-related leukoencephalopathy showed reduction in the perifocal edema volume. All patients of leukoencephalopathy showed improvement in clinical symptoms for many months.[19]

In another study, 19 children and adolescents with intracranial tumors received palliative therapy with H15 for a median period of 9 months with a maximum dose of 126 mg·kg^{-1} body weight. All the patients had earlier been treated by conventional therapy. A total of 5 out of 19 patients improved in general health, 3 out of 17 patients with malignant tumors showed a transient improvement in neurological symptoms, 3 patients showed improved muscle strength, whereas 1 cachectic patient gained weight, possibly due to the antiedematous effect of *Boswellia serrata* extract.[20]

In the glioblastoma trial[18] with increased dosages up to 1,200 mg thrice daily some patients complained of nausea and vomiting and two patients of skin irritation, which was reversible of stoppage. However, side effects were also not seen at 1,200 mg.[19] In the trial with children no side effects were seen when they received a maximum dose of 126 mg·kg⁻¹ bodyweight.[20] See also Chapter 3, "Gastrointestinal agents" and Chapter 5, "Respiratory tract drugs."

Cucuma longa *Linn. (Family: Zingiberaceae)*

Curcuma longa and the pigment curcumin derived from it have been extensively investigated and they display a range of useful effects. *Curcuma longa* has been covered in Chapter 3, "Gastrointestinal agents" for use in dyspepsia, in Chapter 5, "Respiratory tract drugs" for use in asthma, and in Chapter 8, "Antirheumatic agents" for use in rheumatoid arthritis. Both the crude drug extract and curcumin are powerful antioxidants[21,22] and exhibit anti-inflammatory effects.[23]

Curcuma longa is not classified as a *rasayana*. Turmeric and curcumin display considerable potential both for the treatment and prevention of cancer in a variety of cancers and they have been extensively investigated for their anticancer effects in vitro and in experimental animals, which have been reviewed.[24-27] Curcumin acts on a variety of tumors by suppressing proliferation,[28] through down-regulation of transcription factors,[29] down-regulation of the expression of a number of chemokines such as COX-2, lipoxygenase, NO synthase, Tumor Necrosis Factor etc., cell-surface adhesion molecules, and certain growth factors, apart from inhibition of certain kinases, which have been reviewed.[27]

In an open study carried out on 111 patients, of whom the data from 62 patients with external cancerous lesions could be evaluated, both an ethanol extract of *Curcuma longa* containing 0.5 percent curcumin and an ointment containing 0.5 percent curcumin in white Vaseline applied thrice daily gave patients considerable symptomatic relief, which was considered remarkable by the authors. A reduction in smell was noted in 90 percent cases and a reduction in itching in nearly all cases. Although 10 percent patients experienced a reduction in lesion size and pain, 70 percent of patients had dry lesions. The effects of the drug continued for several months in many of the patients. An adverse reaction was noticed only in 1 patient who complained of itching from the 62 patients treated in the study.[30]

In another study carried out on 16 chronic smokers whose urine showed positive for mutagens with Ames's test, treatment with 1.5 g of *Curcuma longa* for 4 weeks showed significant reduction in the mutagenic response in comparison to controls consisting of 6 non-smokers.[31]

Oral submucous fibrosis is commonly observed in India as a result of chewing betel nut containing masticants and their exfoliated oral mucosal cells contain significantly larger number of micro-nucleated cells when compared to healthy subjects not indulging in chewing or smoking.[32] In a trial on patients with submucous fibrosis, three treatment modalities were tried out after initial in vitro tests, on the effect of alcoholic extract of turmeric, turmeric oil, and turmeric oleoresin, were shown to protect against benzo[a]pyrene-induced increase in micronuclei in circulating lymphocytes, where-as they did not cause any increase in the number of micronuclei in lymphocytes taken from normal healthy subjects when compared to untreated controls. Patients with submucous fibrosis were treated with a total oral dose per day of 600 mg turmeric oil mixed with 3 g of alcoholic turmeric extract. Turmeric oleoresin 600 mg plus 3 g turmeric extract and 3 g turmeric extract per day served as controls. All the three treatment arms reduced the number of micronucleated cells both in the exfoliated oral mucosal cells and in circulating lymphocytes. Turmeric oleoresin was found to be more effective than the others in reducing the number of micronuclei in oral mucosal cells, although in circulating lymphocytes the decrease in micronuclei were comparable in all three groups.[33]

Curcumin

A phase I clinical trial has been carried out on 25 patients having high risk or precancerous lesions in order to check dose response and safety profile. Patients who received up to 8 g·day^{-1} of curcumin for 3 months showed no signs of toxicity. Although the study was designed to assess safety of the drug, there were preliminary therapeutic results with one out of two patients with recently resected bladder cancer, two out of seven patients of oral leukoplakia, one out of six patients of intestinal metaplasia of stomach, one out of four patients with cervical intraepithelial neoplasm (CIN), and two out of six patients with

Bowen's disease of the skin showed histological improvement of pre-cancerous lesions.[34]

In another phase I clinical trial on patients with advanced colorectal cancer refractory to standard treatment received an alcoholic extract of *Curcuma longa* in doses from 440 to 2,200 mg per day of extract for 4 months corresponding to 36-180 mg of curcumin, which was well tolerated. These dosages were considered safe and serve as reference dosages for further studies.[35]

Other aspects of the safety of *Curcuma longa* and curcumin are covered in Chapter 3.

Tinospora cordifolia *Miers.*
(Family: Menispermaceae)

Tinospora cordifolia (see Plate 4 in color gallery) has been mentioned earlier in this chapter for the treatment of tuberculosis and improving the quality of life in chronic asthmatics. Several compounds have been shown to have immunostimulating properties as discussed earlier in this chapter, the polysaccharide fraction has been shown to be effective in reducing experimental metastasis in mice.[36] The immunostimulating activity of *Tinospora cordifolia* is comparable to lithium carbonate and glucan.[37] Activation of macrophages by *Tinospora cordifolia* leads to an increase of colony-forming units of granulocyte macrophages, which again leads to leukocytosis and improved neutrophil function.[38] When the carcinogen ochratoxin A was administered to mice, *Tinospora cordifolia* was able to inhibit suppression of chemotactic activity and the production of interleukin-1 and Tumor Necrosis Factor-alpha, which is a sign of increased cancer activity.[39] In Dalton's lymphoma *Tinospora cordifolia* alcoholic extract showed antitumor activity by activating tumor-associated macrophages. The extract given intraperitoneally slowed down tumor growth and increased life span of the host.[40] Administration of the methanol extract of the *Tinospora cordifolia* stem in experimental animals increased total white blood cell count, increased bone marrow cellularity, increased the humoral immune response, and reduced tumor volume by 58.8 percent, and acted synergistically with cyclophosphamide in reducing animal tumors by 83 percent.[41] Flow cytometric measurements in mice showed that *Tinospora cordifolia* induces a dose-dependent increase in bone marrow proliferation.[42] In vitro the methanol, water, and methylene chloride extracts of *Tinospora cordifolia* caused a significant, dose-dependent increase in cell death,[43] and also enhanced the effect of radiation in cultured HeLa cells.[44] A dose-searching study on humans showed that *Tinospora cordifolia* has great potential in reducing neutropenia caused by cytotoxic drugs in patients with cancer.[45] In small animals it is also able to reduce toxicity of cyclophosphamide.[46]

In a double-blind placebo-controlled randomized study, 40 patients with breast cancer were treated with tablets of 500 mg *Tinospora cordifolia* aqueous extract thrice daily as an adjuvant in cancer chemotherapy using the combination of methotrexate, 5-fluorouracil, and cyclophosphamide. In the group receiving *Tinospora,* the number of patients whose peripheral blood counts fell below 3,000/cu.mm was 55 percent compared to 70 percent in the placebo group. In the placebo-treated group the level fell below 2,000/cu.mm 24 times as compared to 14 times in the *Tinospora* group, and below 500/cu.mm 5 times in the placebo group as compared to only once in the *Tinospora* group.[47]

In another study in 26 patients with breast cancer, use of 500 mg *Tinospora cordifolia* standardized aqueous extract thrice daily in addition to chemotherapy resulted in fewer adverse reactions in the *Tinospora* group. *Tinospora cordifolia* also increased the apoptotic index in a dose-dependent manner in 4,937 cells, apart from synergistically increasing apoptosis induced by methotrexate, cytarabine, and cisplatin.[48] These findings led the authors to conclude that *Tinospora cordifolia* shows promise as an adjuvant in cancer chemotherapy.[48]

NOTES

1. Smit HF, Woerdenberg HJ, Singh RH, Meulenbad GJ, Labadie RP, Zwaving JH. Ayurvedic herbs with possible cytostatic activity. *J Ethnopharmacol* 47:75-84 (1995).

2. Sastry JLN. *Introduction to oncology (cancer) in Ayurveda* (2nd edn., pp. 14-24). Varanasi: Chaukhambha Orientalia, 2001.

3. Pandey G. *Anticancer herbal drugs of India with special reference to Ayurveda* (1st edn., pp. 12-16, 27-121). New Delhi: Sri Satguru Publiations, 2002.

4. *The wealth of India, raw materials* (vol. 2, pp. 203-209). New Delhi: Publications and Information Directorate, CSIR, 1988.

5. Dhar ML, Dhar MM, Dhawan BN, Mehrotra BN, Ray C. Screening of Indian plants for biological activity. Part 1. *Indian J Exp Biol* 6:232-247 (1968).

6. Mukerji S, Banerjee AK, Mitra BN. Studies on plant antitumor agents. I (bark) *Indian J Pharm* 32(2):48 (1970).

7. Ammon HPT. Boswelliasäuren (Inhaltstoffe des Weihrauchs) zur Behandlung chronisch entzündlicher Erkrankungen. *Med Monatsschr Pharm* 26:309-315 (2003).

8. Liu JJ, Nilsson A, Oredsson S, Badmaev V, Zhao WZ, Duan RD. Boswellic acids trigger apoptosis via a pathway dependent on caspase-8 activation but independent of Fas/Fas ligand interaction in colon cancer HT-29 cells. *Carcinogenesis* 23:2087-2093 (2002).

9. Liu JJ, Nilsson A, Oredsson S, Badmaev V, Duan RD. Keto- and acetyl-keto-boswellic acids inhibit proliferation and induce apoptosis in Hep G2 cells via a caspase-8 dependent pathway. *Int J Mol Med* 10:501-505 (2002).

10. Heldt MR, Syrovets T, Winking M, Sailer ER, Safayhi H, Ammon HPT, Simmet T. Boswellic acids exhibit cytotoxic effects on brain tumor cells independent from 5-lipoxygenase inhibition. *Naunyn- Schmiedberg's Arch Pharmacol* 355(suppl.):R 15, Abstract 30 (1997).

11. Huang MT, Badmaev V, Ding Y, Liu Y, Xie JG, Ho CT. Anti-tumor and anti-carcinogenic activities of the triterpenoid β-boswellic acid. *Biofactors* 13:225-230 (2000).

12. Glaser T, Winter S, Groscurth P, Safayhi H, Sailer ER, Ammon HPT, Schabet M, Weller M. Boswellic acids and malignant glioma: Induction of apoptosis but no modulation of drug sensitivity. *Br J Cancer* 80:756-765 (1999).

13. Winking M, Sarikaya S, Rahmanian A, Jödicke A, Böker DK. Boswellic acids inhibit glioma growth: a new treatment option? J *Neurooncol* 46:97-103 (2000).

14. Syrovets T, Büchele B, Gedig E, Slupsky JR, Simmet T. Acetyl-boswellic acids are novel catalytic inhibitors of human topoisomerases I and II α. *Mol Pharmacol* 58:71-81 (2000).

15. Hostanska K, Daum G, Saller R. Cytostatic and apoptosis-inducing activity of boswellic acids toward malignant cell lines *in vitro. Anticancer Res* 22:2853-2862 (2002).

16. Park YS, Lee JH, Bondar J, Harwalkar JA, Safayhi H, Golubic M. Cytotoxic action of acetyl-11-keto-beta-boswellic acid (AKBA) on meningioma cells. *Planta Med* 68:397-401 (2002).

17. Heldt RM, Winking M, Simmet T. Cysteinyl leukotrienes as potential mediators of the peritumoral brain oedema in astrocytoma patients. *Naunyn-Schmiedberg's Arch Pharmacol.* 353(suppl. 4):R142, Abstract 538 (1996).

18. Böker C, Winking M. Die Rolle von Boswelliasäuren in der Therapie maligner Gliome. *Deutsche Ärtzteblatt* 94:A1197-A1199 (1997).

19. Streffer JR, Bitzer M, Schabet M, Dichgans J, Weller M. Response of radiochemotherapy-associated cerebral edema to a phytotherapeutic agent H15. *Neurology* 56:1219-1221 (2001).

20. Janssen G, Bode U, Breu H, Dohrn B, Engelbrecht V, Göbel U. Boswellic acids in the palliative therapy of children with progressive or relapsed brain tumors. *Klin Pädiatr* 212:189-195 (2000).

21. Khanna NM. Turmeric—Nature's precious gift. *Curr Sci* 76:1351-1356 (1999).

22. Scartezzini P, Speroni E. Review on some plants of Indian traditional medicine with antioxidant activity. *J Ethnopharmacol* 71:23-43 (2000).

23. Chainani-Wu N. Safety and anti-inflammatory activity of Curcumin: A component of turmeric *(Curcuma longa)*. *J Alt Comp Med* 9(1):161-168 (2003).

24. Srimal RC. Turmeric: a brief review of medicinal properties. *Fitoterapia* LXVIII:483-493 (1997).

25. Mehta Luthra P, Singh R, Chandra R. Therapeutic uses of *Curcuma longa* (turmeric). *Indian J Clin Biochem* 16:153-160 (2001).

26. Cronin JR. Curcumin: old spice is a new medicine. *Alt Comp Therap* (February):34-38 (2003).

27. Aggarwal BB, Kumar A, Bharti AC. Anticancer potential of curcumin: Preclinical and clinical studies. *Anticancer Res* 23:363-398 (2003).

28. Sikora E, Bielak-Zmijewska A, Piwocka K, Sklerski J, Radziszewska E. Inhibition of proliferation and apoptosis of human and rat T lymphocytes by curcumin, a curry pigment. *Biochem Pharm* 54:899-907 (1997).

29. Singh S, Aggarwal BB. Activation of transcription factor NF-kappa B is suppressed by curcumin (diferuloylmethane). *J Biol Chem* 270:24995-25000 (1995).

30. Kuttan R, Sudheeran PC, Joseph CD. Turmeric and curcumin as topical agents in cancer therapy. *Tumori* 73:29-31 (1987).

31. Polasa K, Raghuram TC, Prasanna Krishna T, Krishnaswamy K. Effect of turmeric on urinary mutagens in smokers. *Mutagenesis* 7:107-109 (1992).

32. Desai SS, Ghaisas SD, Jakhi SD, Bhide SV. Cytogenetic damage in exfoliated oral mucosal cells and circulating lymphocytes of patients suffering from precancerous oral lesions. *Cancer Lett* 109:9-14 (1996).

33. Hastak K, Lubri N, Jakhi SD, More C, John A, Ghaisas SD, Bhide SV. Effect of turmeric oil and turmeric oleoresin on cytogenetic damage in patients suffering from oral submucous fibrosis. *Cancer Lett* 116:265-269 (1997).

34. Cheng AL, Hsu CH, Lin JK, Hsu MM, Ho YF, Shen TS, Ko JY, Lin JT, Lin BR, Wu MS, Yu HS, Jee SH, Chen GS, Chen TM, Chen CA, Lai MK, Pu YS, Pan MH, Wang YJ, Tsai CC, Hsieh CY. Phase I clinical trial of curcumin, a chemoprotective agent, in patients with high-risk or pre-malignant lesions. *Anticancer Res* 21:2895-2900 (2001).

35. Sharma RA, McLelland HR, Hill KA, Ireson CR, Euden SA, Manson MM, Pirmohamed M, Marnett LJ, Gescher AJ, Steward WP. Pharmacodynamic and pharmacokinetic study of oral *Curcuma* extract in patients with colorectal cancer. *Clin Cancer Res* 7:1894-1900 (2001).

36. Leyon PV, Kuttan G. Inhibitory effect of a polysaccharide from *Tinospora cordifolia* on experimental metastasis. *J Ethnopharmacol* 90:233-237 (2004).

37. Thatte UM, Dahanukar SA. Comparative study of immunomodulating activity of Indian medicinal plants, lithium carbonate and glucan. *Methods Find Exp Clin Pharmacol* 10:639-644 (1988).

38. Thatte UM, Rao SGA, Dahanukar SA. *Tinospora cordifolia* induces colony stimulating activity in serum. *J Postgrad Med* 40:202-203 (1994).

39. Dhuley JN. Effect of some Indian herbs on macrophage function in ochratoxin A treated mice. *J Ethnopharmacol* 58:15-20 (1997).

40. Singh N, Singh SM, Shrivastava P. Immunomodulatory and antitumor actions of the medicinal plant *Tinospora cordifolia* are mediated through activation of tumor-associated macrophages. *Immunopharmacol Immunotoxicol* 26:145-162 (2004).

41. Mathew S, Kuttan G. Immunomodulatory and antitumor activities of *Tinospora cordifolia. Fitoterapia* 70:35-43 (1999).

42. Usha D, Thatte UM, Joshi DS, Dahanukar SA. Flow cytometric evaluation of bone marrow proliferation induced by *Tinospora cordifolia* (p. 38). Procs of "Update Ayurveda-94," February 24-26, 1994.

43. Jagetia GC, Nayak V, Vidyasagar MS. Evaluation of the antineoplastic activity of *guduchi (Tinospora cordifolia)* in cultured HeLa cells. *Cancer Lett* 127:71-82 (1998).

44. Jagetia GC, Nayak V, Vidyasagar MS. Enhancement of radiation effect by *guduchi (Tinospora cordifolia)* in HeLa cells. *Pharm Biol* 40:179-188 (2002).

45. Thatte U, Joshi D, Usha D, Kambli N, Gude R, Rao SGA, Joshi K, Rege N, Dahanukar S. The potential role of *Tinospora cordifolia* in cancer therapeutics. *Phytomedicine* 3(suppl. 1):15 (1996).

46. Mathew S, Kuttan G. Antioxidant activity of *Tinospora cordifolia* and its usefulness in the amelioration of cyclophosphamide induced toxicity. *J Exp Clin Cancer Res* 16:407-411 (1997).

47. Dhanukar SA, Thatte UM. Current status of Ayurveda in phytomedicine. *Phytomedicine* 4:359-368 (1997).

48. Oak MA, Deshmukh AS, Bagde SY, Thatte UM, Badwe R, Mitra I, Desai UM, Hardikar JV, Rege NN, Dahanukar SA. *Tinospora cordifolia* and cytotoxic chemotherapy. *Phytomedicine* 7(suppl. II):26, 2000.

OTHER PLANTS USED IN CANCER THERAPY

Withania somnifera *Dunal.* (Family: Solanaceae)

Withania somnifera has been extensively screened for possible use in cancer chemotherapy and for radio-sensitization, which have been reviewed.[1] Pilot studies in patients with advanced oral cancer indicates that it may be of use when administered alongside conventional radiotherapy. No side effects were observed and blood GSH levels showed a reduction.[1] Six patients were given 400 mg of alcoholic extract of *Withania somnifera* daily along with radiotherapy. The tumors disappeared in three patients and the response of the remaining three patients was considered good.[2]

NOTES

1. Uma Devi P. *Withania somnifera* Dunal *(ashwagandha)*: Potential plant source of a promising drug for cancer chemotherapy and radiosensitization. *Indian J Exp Biol* 34:927-932 (1996).

2. *The Hindu Business Line* dated 8/11/1994.

Chapter 14

Dental and Ophthalmological Agents

DENTAL HEALTH

Plaque formation and subsequent chronic inflammation are the major cause of problems connected with teeth and gums. Plaque is the sticky coating formed on the surface of the teeth with saliva and food debris by several bacteria, including the bacterium *Streptococcus mutans* after consumption of food. If plaque is not removed, it gets converted to tartar by deposition of the calcium salts of the saliva. Further progression by attack of the acids produced by the bacteria in the plaque can lead not only to tooth decay or caries but also to inflammation of the gums or gingiva (gingivitis). Prolonged inflammation leads to loosening of the teeth and the condition known as periodontitis.[1] In addition, the importance of maintaining the health of the oral cavity has been brought out by establishing the connection between chronic low grade inflammation and heart disease.[2]

Thus preventive care of teeth by preventing plaque formation is very important for maintaining the health of the oral cavity, and in Ayurveda dental care was carried out at three levels—prophylaxis in the form of daily care as part of the daily routine or *dinacharya,* treatment of minor conditions by drugs, and surgical interventions for serious conditions.[3]

In Ayurveda, plants play an important role in the maintenance of healthy teeth and gums and these are generally used in combination. Some 84 plants have been used for this purpose—as chewing sticks, as tooth powder for cleaning teeth and gums, for pyorrhea, for sensitive teeth, gum inflammation, toothache, and caries, which have been

doi:10.1300/5683_14

329

reviewed.[4] The herbs that were most commonly used were also the ones that were readily available such as *Azadirachta indica, Mangifera indica, Ocimum sanctum, Camellia sinensis,* and curry leaf *Murraya koenigi.*[5] However, only a few of them have been scientifically investigated.

Azadirachta indica *Linn. (Family: Meliaceae)*

Azadirachta indica has been covered in Chapter 9, "Dermatological agents" and in Chapter 11, "Antidiabetic agents." The use of *neem* twigs as chewing sticks for brushing the teeth has been known in India for a very long time. People brushing their teeth with twigs of *neem* is even today a common sight on Indian roadsides, where a twig of *neem* is selected with great care, one end chewed and softened with a stone in order to obtain a soft surface, which is used to clean the teeth and gums. Toothpastes incorporated with *neem* extracts are available in the market in India. Various parts of the *neem* tree have shown antibacterial properties, which have been summarized.[6] Aqueous extract derived from sticks of *neem* was tested against *Streptococcus mutans* and *Streptococcus faecalis* and found active at 50 percent concentration.[7] Aqueous extract from bark-containing sticks of *Azadirachta indica* have also been shown to reduce the ability of some oral *Streptococci* to colonize tooth surfaces.[8]

In an exploratory study, extracts derived from plants such as *neem, tulasi (Ocimum sanctum)*, walnut, and acacia have been used to treat plaque, periodontitis, and gingivitis in order to assess their efficacy. In the plaque-control study, the plant extracts were used for 3 days and then the plaque that was still left was scored using Quigley and Hein scoring method. A 1 percent *neem* extract was found to inhibit plaque formation by 80 percent. In the gingivitis study, a 1 percent solution of nimbidin-T reduced gingivitis by 12 percent after two applications, but maximal reduction of 70 percent reduction was seen only after 45 days. In a microbiological study, a 6 percent *neem* leaf extract eliminated aerobic organisms by the 4th day and anaerobic microorganisms on the 5th day.[9]

In another exploratory study, the antibacterial effect of *neem* mouthwash on the levels of *Streptococcus mutans* and *Lactobacillus* was assessed in the saliva for a period of 2 months. In addition, the effect on incipient carious lesions was evaluated. A total of 150 schoolchildren between the ages of 9 and 12 were selected and divided into five groups out of which three groups were test groups, one group was positive control, and one group received placebo. Out of the three treatment groups, two groups received 3 percent *neem* mouthwash with base, one with alcohol and the other without alcohol, group 3 received chlorhexidine, group 4 received base alone, whereas group 5 was on oral prophylaxis. Thus *Streptococcus mutans* was inhibited in both groups 1 and 2 using *neem* mouthwash, but not *Lactobacillus,* which was inhibited only by chlorhexidine. In addition, there is evidence from initial data that there is a reversal of incipient carious lesions, therefore, there is a need to conduct longer duration trials to confirm the initial results.[10]

In a study involving 36 subjects divided into three groups, the efficacy of a dental gel prepared from 70 percent alcoholic extract of *neem* leaf was evaluated against 0.2 percent chlorhexidine gluconate solution and against placebo gel. Subjects used the preparations twice a day for 6 weeks. Microbial evaluation of *Streptococcus mutans* and *Lactobacillus* species was carried out to determine the change in bacterial count over the treatment period. There was significant reduction in the plaque index and bacterial count in the group using *neem* extract gel over the control group using chlorhexidine gluconate mouthwash.[11]

The use of *neem* chewing sticks and neem toothpastes is widespread and no side effects or toxicity have been reported.

NOTES

1. Tyler VE. *Herbs of choice. The therapeutic use of phytomedicinals* (p.166). New York: Pharmaceutical Products Press, 1994.

2. Beck J, Garcia R, Heiss G, Vokonas PS, Offenbacher S. Periodontal disease and cardiovascular disease. *J Periodontology* 67:1123-1137 (1996).

3. Maurya DK, Mittal N, Sharma KR, Nath G. Role of *triphala* in the management of periodontal disease. *Ancient Sci Life* 17:120-127 (1997).

4. Farooqui AHA, Jain SP, Shukla YN, Ansari SR, Kumar S. Medicinal plants in oral health care in India. *J Med Aro Plant Sci* 20:441-450 (1998).

5. Patel VK, Venkatakrishna-Bhatt H. Folklore therapeutic indigenous plants in periodontal disorders in India (review, experimental and clinical approach). *Int J Clin Pharmacol Ther Toxicol* 26:176-184 (1988).

6. Gupta AK, Tandon N. (eds.). *Reviews on Indian medicinal plants* (vol. 3, pp. 356-358). New Delhi: Indian Council of Medical Research, 2004.

7. Almas K. The antimicrobial effects of extracts of *Azadirachta indica (neem)* and *Salvadora persica (arak)* chewing sticks. *Indian J Dent Res* 10:23-26 (1999).

8. Wolinsky LE, Mania S, Nachnani S, Ling S. The inhibiting effect of aqueous *Azadirachta indica (neem)* extract upon bacterial properties influencing *in vitro* plaque formation. *J Dent Res* 75:816-822 (1996).

9. Saimbi CS. Investigation of medicinal plants for dental disease (p. 22). Lucknow: Natl Sem use of Traditional Medicinal Plants in Skin Care, CIMAP, November 25-26, 1994.

10. Vanka A, Tandon S, Rao SR, Udupa N. The effect of indigenous Neem (*Azadirachta indica*) mouthwash on *Streptococcus mutans* and *Lactobacilli* growth. *Indian J Dent Res* 12:133-144 (2001).

11. Pai MR, Acharya LD, Udupa N. Evaluation of antiplaque activity of *Azadirachta indica* leaf extract gel—A 6-week clinical study. *J Ethnopharmacol* 90:99-103 (2004).

OTHER DENTAL CONDITIONS

Pyorrhea

Pyorrhea is the chronic destructive inflammation of the tissues surrounding the teeth (periodontium) characterized by bleeding, pus, and bad breath. If pyorrhea is not controlled it can lead to loss of teeth.

Adhatoda vasica *Nees (Family: Acanthaceae)*

Latin: *Adhatoda zeylanica* Medicus, *Justicia adhatoda* Linn.	Hindi: Arusa
Sanskrit: Vasa	Tamil: Adhatodai
English: Malabar Nut Tree	

Adhatoda vasica has been covered in Chapter 3, "Gastrointestinal agents" and in Chapter 5, "Respiratory tract drugs." The leaves have been used to lessen gingival inflammation. In an open trial, 25 patients with pyorrhea, bleeding gums, and pus discharge were asked to apply *Adhatoda vasica* leaf extract on the gums for 3 weeks. The herb extract was prepared by mixing two parts of crushed leaves of the plant with one part of honey and applied twice a day on the gums. The gingival inflammation (GI) index was examined once a week for 3 weeks. Most of the patients had a gingival score of 2-2.5 indicating an advanced state of inflammation, with the mean score being 1.9. The scores came down to 1.7, 1.5, and 1.3 every week showing significant reduction in all the 3 weeks offering great relief to the patients, with reduction in bleeding, pus, and halitosis.[1] Further studies are warranted in larger patient numbers in view of the promising results.

Local Anaesthetic

Anacyclus pyrethrum *DC (Family: Asteraceae)*

Latin: *Anacyclus officinarum* Hayne	Hindi: Akarkara
Sanskrit: Akaraakarabha	Tamil: Akkirakaram
English: Spanish Pellitory	

Anacyclus pyrethrum is a perennial, procumbent herb native to North Africa and cultivated on an experimental scale in Jammu and Kashmir. The roots have since long been imported into India for use in medicine. The root is used to provide relief from toothache.[2] The roots contain anacyclin—an acetylenic compound—pellitorine—the intensely pungent active principle that is a mixture of isobutylamides, although it is uncertain if it contributes to the analgesic activity— enetriyne alcohol, hydrocarolin, about 50 percent inulin, volatile oil, sesamin, and some tyramine amides.[2] In experimental animals the root extract has been shown to have local anesthetic activity.[3]

In a double-blind study on 200 patients undergoing oral surgery the anesthetic effect of a 2 percent alcoholic extract of *Anacyclus pyrethrum* root freshly dissolved in sterile water was compared with xylocaine. The effect on surgery, postoperative recovery, and rate of wound healing were also evaluated. The extract had a longer period of anesthesia when compared to xylocaine and therefore found to be useful in prolonged oral reconstructive surgery.[4] The drug was evaluated as safe.[4] The LD_{50} of the aqueous extract of the root was 750 mg·kg^{-1} in mice given intraperitoneally.[5]

Periodontitis

Chronic inflammation of the tissues surrounding the teeth (peridontium) leads to loosening of teeth and eventually to tooth loss. In Ayurveda, the periodontium is described as *dantamula* and periodontal diseases as *dantamulagataroga.*

Triphala

Triphala (*tri:* three; *phala:* fruits) is the well-known three-fruit combination of equal parts of *Terminalia chebula, Terminalia belerica,* and *Emblica offiicinalis,* which is commonly used in Ayurveda as a bowel tonic, in oral health care, and for the care of the eyes. *Triphala* has shown significant analgesic, antiarthritic, and anti-inflammatory activity.[6] When tested for putative use in pyorrhea against 22 species of bacteria, *triphala* decoction was active inhibiting growth of 16 bacteria.[7]

In a controlled study, 60 patients in different stages of inflammatory periodontal disease were selected on the basis of clinical symptoms and diagnostic criteria and divided into three groups of 20 patients each. Group I patients were treated with *triphala* decoction as mouthwash and given 3 g *triphala* powder twice daily for 1 month. Group II was the control group patients who were treated with 400 mg metronidazole thrice daily for 7 days together with *triphala* decoction as mouthwash twice daily for 1 month. Group III of 20 patients again served as control and were treated with 400 mg metronidazole thrice daily for 7 days with 0.2 percent chlorhexidine as mouthwash twice daily for 1 month. All patients had the calculus cleared before start of the trial. Patients were treated for 4 weeks, assessed every 7 days, and followed up for a further 1 month. The efficacy of the drug *triphala* was considered comparable to the modern drug, which however had faster onset of action, but also the modern drug had more rapid recurrence of symptoms.[8] Further studies are indicated.

NOTES

1. Doshi JJ, Patel VK, Bhatt HV. Effect of *Adhatoda vasica* massage in pyorrhoea. *Int J Crude Drug Res* 21:173-176 (1983).
2. *The Wealth of India, raw materials* (vol. 1, p. 248). New Delhi: Publications and Information Directorate, CSIR, 1985.
3. Gopalakrishna G, Devasankariah G, Patel VK, Bhatt HV. Local anaesthetic activity of *Anacyclus pyrethrum* root extract in laboratory animals (Abstract 36, p 29). Bangalore: Procs 74th Session Indian Science Cong (Medical and Veterinary Science), 1987.
4. Patel VK, Patel RV, Bhatt HV, Gopalakrishna G, Devasankariah G. A clinical appraisal of *Anacyclus pyrethrum* root extract in dental patients. *Phytother Res* 6:158-159 (1992).
5. Bhatt VH, Panchal GM, Patel VK. Toxicity of *Anacyclus pyrethrum* in mice. *Curr Sci* 57:912-913 (1988).
6. Ghosh D, Thejamoorthy P, Veluchamy G. Antiinflammatory, antiarthritic and analgesic activities of *Triphala*. *J Res Ayur Siddha* 10:168-174 (1989).
7. Maurya DK, Sharma KR, Mittal N, Nath G. Role of *triphala* in the management of pyorrhoea. *Sachitra Ayurved* 48:390-391 (1995).
8. Maurya DK, Mittal N, Sharma KR, Nath G. Role of *triphala* in the management of periodontal disease. *Ancient Sci Life* 17:120-127 (1997).

OPHTHALMOLOGICAL AGENTS

Plants have been used in Ayurveda to treat different eye conditions, including refractive disorders, cataract in the initial stages, and glaucoma. Although eye conditions have not been accorded a separate branch in Ayurveda, such as surgery, a large number of plants have been used.[1] In a survey[1] of seven major texts of Ayurveda, 41 single drugs are found to have been mentioned for 29 eye conditions. The various factors, which are considered to contribute to the development of eye diseases, have also been discussed.[1] Plant combinations have been mainly used for conditions such as cataract and refractive errors. The traditional formulation known as *Mahatriphaladi Ghrita* (MTG), a preparation made of various herbs cooked in *ghee* or clarified butter, which is in itself considered good for the eyes, is popularly used by Ayurvedic physicians to improve eyesight when taken internally and also applied to the eyes.[2] In a trial on 150 patients with primary open-angle glaucoma, patients were divided into three groups, group 1 served as control and patients were treated locally with standard antiglaucoma drug four times a day, group 2 received two tablespoons of MTG twice a day with warm milk, whereas group 3 received 2 percent pilocarpine with MTG, all medications for 90 days. Group 3 receiving MTG together with pilocarpine showed optimum improvement, with pilocarpine contributing to quick relief and MTG to prolonged maintenance of intraocular pressure. No side effects were seen in the MTG group, although in the pilocarpine group side effects (not specified) were reported, which were reduced in the combination group.[3] The effect of MTG on lipid parameters needs to be investigated in view of the use of clarified butter or *ghee* as base.

Conjunctivitis

Conjunctivitis is a common infectious condition of the eyes associated with redness, sticky discharge, burning and irritation, grittiness, swelling, and visual disturbances caused by pathogens of bacterial, fungal, or viral origin, and due to allergens. A review of different plant species that have been used to treat conjunctivitis has been published.[4] The modest amount of scientific work has been mostly in this area; exploratory trials with some plants having been carried out. *Curcuma longa,* with its anti-inflammatory, antioxidant, and antibacterial property, has been used to treat not only conjunctivitis, but also curcumin, the active principle has been used and tried out in chronic anterior uveitis and in orbital pseudo tumors. Other plants for which preliminary exploratory trials have been carried out are *Berberis aristata, Cyperus rotundus, and Glycyrrhiza glabra* for conjunctivitis and *Rubia cordifolia* for painful eye conditions.

Albizzia lebbeck *Benth. (Family: Mimosaceae)*

Sanskrit: Sirisha	Tamil: Vagei
Hindi: Siris	English: East Indian Walnut Tree, Siris Tree

In a comparative study on allergic conjunctivitis, 60 patients were enrolled for the study and divided into three groups of 20 each. The trial preparation was made from the aqueous extract of the bark concentrated to dryness *(ghanasatwa).* Each capsule had 500 mg of the extract and the drops were made from 2 g percent of the extract. Group 1 that served as control received standard dexamethasone two drops thrice daily for 60 days. Group 2 received *Albizzia lebbeck* eye drops two drops thrice daily for 60 days, whereas the third group received, in addition to the *Albizzia lebbeck* eye drops, one capsule containing 500 mg of *Albizzia lebbeck* extract thrice daily again for 60 days. There was a relapse rate of 100 and 60 percent in the first two groups and the third group had only a 25 percent rate of recurrence.[5]

Berberis aristata *DC (Family: Berberidaceae)*

Sanskrit: Daruharidra	Tamil: Maramanjal
Hindi: Darhald	English: Barberry

In an open trial, eyedrops made from semisolid extracts of *Berberis aristata,* honey, and distilled water were tried on 100 patients with conjunctivitis including cases not responding to antibiotics. Two to four drops of *"Madhudarvyadi"* eyedrops were instilled in each eye thrice a day. A total of 98 patients with different kinds of conjunctivitis obtained relief. About 59 percent of patients obtained relief in 1-2 days, a further 29 percent in 2-4 days, and the remaining 10 percent in 4-10 days.[6]

Curcuma longa *Linn. (Family: Zingiberaceae)*

In a comparative trial, 50 patients with conjunctivitis were treated: 25 patients with turmeric eyedrops and 25 patients with 5 percent soframycin eyedrops. The eyedrops were instilled four to five times a day for 7 days. In patients on turmeric eyedrops, symptoms improved day 3 with complete improvement by day 6, except for two cases. Patients on soframycin also improved from day 4 and complete relief took 7 days except for two patients, who needed 9 days for complete relief.[7] Thus, treatment with turmeric eyedrops was comparable to soframycin; however, further trials are required with larger patient numbers. No side effects were observed.[7]

Cyperus rotundus *Linn. (Family: Cyperaceae)*

Sanskrit: Mustaka, Musta	Tamil: Korai
Hindi: Mutha, Moth	English: Nut grass

In an open study, the effect of an aqueous solution of a methanolic extract of *Cyperus rotundus* tubers was studied in patients with conjunctivitis. Most of the patients were relieved of pain and redness and considered cured after 5 days.[8]

Glycyrrhiza glabra *Linn. (Family: Fabaceae)*

Sanskrit: Yashtimadhu	Tamil: Atimadhuram
Hindi: Mulethi	English: Liquorice, Licorice

In a comparative study, 50 patients with acute conjunctivitis were divided into two groups of 25 patients each. The first group was treated with a 5 percent aqueous solution of *Glycyrrhiza glabra* eye drops, whereas the second group was treated with chloramphenicol eyedrops, both medications being instilled six times a day by the patients while observing hygiene. Patients receiving *Glycyrrhiza glabra* eyedrops showed decrease in symptoms from day 4 onwards with complete disappearance of the symptoms in 5-7 days. There were four patients who did not respond to the treatment. In the chloramphenicol group, all 25 patients responded in 4-7 days. Symptoms such as itching, congestion, and swelling of lids subsided faster in the *Glycyrrhiza glabra* group compared to the chloramphenicol group, probably because of glycyrrhizin present, that has corticosteroid-like action.[9]

Chronic Anterior Uveitis

Curcumin

A study was carried out involving 53 patients of chronic anterior uveitis, which is characterized by pain and redness in the eye, sensitivity to light, watering of eyes, and diminution of vision, with black spots in some patients. Thirty-two patients, who were available for the trial, were divided into two groups. All 32 patients were treated orally with 375 mg of 95 percent curcumin thrice daily for 12 weeks, in addition to topical mydriatics and local hot fomentation, although one group of 14 patients, who tested positive for PPD-induced delayed sensitivity, received antitubercular drugs for 1 year, since it has been postulated that uveitis arises due to tuberculosis. The remaining 18 patients received curcumin alone. A marked clinical improvement was observed in both groups with improvement in vision, decrease in aqueous flare, and keratic precipitates, and break of anterior and posterior synechiae. Improvement was slow initially but became satisfactory after 2 weeks. No side effects due to curcumin were observed.[10] The results warrant further clinical studies.

Idiopathic Inflammatory Orbital Pseudotumors

Curcumin

In a small exploratory trial on eight patients with idiopathic inflammatory orbital pseudotumors, 375 mg curcumin was administered orally thrice daily for 6-22 months. Patients were followed up every 3 months for a total of 2 years. Of the five patients who completed the study, four patients recovered completely, whereas in the remaining one patient, swelling came down completely; however, there was restriction in movement. No side effects were observed.[11] Further studies are warranted.

Painful Ophthalmic Conditions

Rubia cordifolia *Linn. sensu Hook f. (Family: Rubiaceae)*

Sanskrit: Manjistha	Tamil: *Manjitti*
Hindi: Manji, Majit	English: The Indian Madder

Various preparations such as decoction, powder, and *ghrita* (preparation with clarified butter or *ghee* as base) of *Rubia cordifolia* were tried in painful ophthalmic conditions both internally and topically and found to relieve pain without any side effects. Further details are not available in the abstract and this study is mentioned for record.[12]

Glaucoma

Glaucoma is characterized by increasing intraocular pressure causing compression of the blood vessels to the retina resulting, over time, in loss of vision.

Coleus forskohlii *Briq. (Family: Lamiaceae)*

Forskolin, the active principle from *Coleus forskohlii,* has been evaluated for use in glaucoma only in healthy volunteers, which has been reviewed.[13]

NOTES

1. Gayathri MB, Kareem MA, Kar S, Unnikrishnan PM. Single drug therapy in *netraroga. Ancient Sci Life* XVI:122-135 (1996).

2. Ramalingayya M. *Vaidya yoga ratnavalli* (Formulary of Ayurvedic medicines) Trans. Shastri MV (pp.122-123). Madras: IMPCOPS, Indian Medical Practitioners' Cooperative Pharmacy and Stores, 1987.

3. Anand B. *Mahatriphaladya Gritha:* A remedy for glaucoma. *Sachitra Ayurved* 50:677-680 (1998).

4. Sharma P, Singh G. A review of plant species used to treat conjunctivitis. *Phytother Res* 16:1-22 (2002).

5. Mukhopadhyay B, Nagaraju K, Sharma KR. *Albizzia lebbeck:* A remedy for allergic conjunctivitis. *J Res Edu Indian Med* 11(4):17-23 (1992).

6. Padamawar RR. Clinical Trial of *"Madhudarvyadi* eye drops" in cases of *"netrabishyand"* (conjunctivitis). *Nagarjun* 23(7):138-140 (1980).

7. Srinivas C, Prabhakaran KVS. *Haridra (Curcuma longa)* and its effect on *abhisayanda* (conjunctivitis). *Ancient Sci Life* VII:279-283 (1989).

8. Saxena RC. *Cyperus rotundus* in conjunctivitis. *J Res Ayur Siddha* 1(1):21-24 (1980).

9. Srinivas C. *Glycyrrhiza glabra* in acute conjunctivitis. *Ancient Sci Life* V:151-153 (1986).

10. Lal B, Kapoor AK, Asthana OP, Agrawal PK, Prasad R, Kumar P, Srimal RC. Efficacy of curcumin in the management of chronic anterior uveitis. *Phytother Res* 13:318-322 (1999).

11. Lal B, Kapoor AK, Agrawal PK, Asthana OP, Srimal RC. Role of curcumin in idiopathic orbital pseudotumors. *Phytother Res* 14:443-447 (2000).

12. Srikanth N, Chopra KK, Hazra J. Effects of an indigenous ophthalmic drug—*Rubia cordifolia (manjistha)* in painful ophthalmic conditions (pp.163-164). Chennai: Procs Internl Cong "Ayurveda—2000," January 28-30, 2000.

13. Head K. Natural therapies for ocular disorders. Part 2: Cataracts and glaucoma. *Alt Med Rev* 6:141-166 (2001).

Appendix

List of Single Plants, Indications, and Chapters

Chapter numbers in bold print have introductory remarks about the plant.

Plant Name	Indication (Chapter Number)
1 *Adhatoda vasica*	Antiulcer agent (3), Bronchial asthma (**5**), Pyorrhea (14)
2 *Aegle marmelos*	Diarrhea (**3**)
3 *Albizzia lebbeck*	Bronchial asthma (**5**), TPE (5), Conjunctivitis (14)
4 *Aloe barbadensis*	Psoriasis (9), Wound healing (**9**)
5 *Anacyclus pyrethrum*	Local anesthetic (**14**)
6 *Andrographis paniculata*	Hepatoprotective agent (**4**), Common cold and flu (5)
7 *Asparagus racemosus*	Antiulcer agent (**3**), Galactagogue (10), Diabetic retinopathy (11)
8 *Azadirachta indica*	Skin diseases (9), Wound healing (9), Antidiabetic agent (**11**), Dental health (14)
9 *Bacopa monnieri*	Memory enhancement (**12**)
10 *Berberis aristata*	Viral hepatitis (4), Conjunctivitis (14)
11 *Berberis vulgaris* (berberine)	Chronic cholecystitis (4)
12 *Boerhaavia diffusa*	Ascites (4), Diuretic (**7**)
13 *Boerhaavia repanda*	Leukorrhea (10)
14 *Boswellia serrata*	Inflammatory bowel disease (**3**), Bronchial asthma (5), Rheumatoid arthritis (8), Cancer therapy (13)
15 *Cardiospermum halicacabum*	Skin diseases (**9**)
16 Cassia angustifolia	Laxative (**3**)
17 *Celastrus paniculatus*	Memory and learning enhancement (**12**)

Plant Name	Indication (Chapter Number)
18 *Centella asiatica*	Venous disorders (**6**), Psoriasis (9), Wound Healing (9), Memory and learning enhancement (12), Tonic antiaging effects (13), Immunostimulant effect (13)
19 *Cinnamonum tamala*	Antidiabetic agent (**11**)
20 *Cissus quadrangularis*	Fracture healing (**9**)
21 *Clerodendron phlomidis*	Antidiabetic agent (**11**)
22 *Coccinia grandis*	Antidiabetic agent (**11**)
23 *Coleus forskohlii, forskolin*	Hypertension (6), Glaucoma (14)
24 *Commiphora wightii*	Hypolipidemic agent (**6**), Rheumatoid arthritis (8)
25 *Convolvulus pluricaulis*	Memory and learning enhancement (**12**)
26 *Crataeva nurvala*	Urinary stones (7), Urinary infection (7), Benign prostatic enlargement (**7**)
27 *Curcuma longa, curcumin*	Dyspepsia (**3**), Bronchial asthma (5), Rheumatoid arthritis (8), Cancer therapy (13), Conjunctivitis (14), Chronic anterior uveitis (14), Idiopathic orbital pseudotumors (14)
28 *Cyperus rotundus*	Diarrhea (**3**), Conjunctivitis (14)
29 *Eclipta alba*	Antiulcer plant (3), Hepatoprotective agents (**4**)
30 *Emblica officinalis*	Antiulcer plant (**3**), Hypolipidemic agent (6), Tonic antiaging agent (13)
31 *Glycyrrhiza glabra*	Antiulcer (**3**), Conjunctivitis (14)
32 *Gymnema sylvestre*	Antidiabetic agent (**11**)
33 *Holarrhena antidysentrica*	Diarrhea (**3**)
34 *Inula racemosa*	Cardioprotective plant (**6**)
35 *Mimosa pudica*	Menorrhagia (10)
36 *Momordica charantia*	Antidiabetic agent (**11**)
37 *Mucuna pruriens*	Parkinson's disease (**12**)
38 *Musa sapientum*	Antiulcer plant (**3**)
39 *Nardostachys jatamansi*	Sedative plant (**12**)
40 *Ocimum sanctum*	Bronchial asthma (**5**), TPE (5), Viral encephalitis (5)
41 *Phyllanthus amarus*	Viral hepatitis (**4**), Antidiabetic agent (11)
42 *Picrorhiza kurroa*	Laxatives (3), Hepatoprotective agent (**4**)
43 *Piper longum*	Bronchial asthma (**5**)
44 *Plantago ovata*	Laxatives (**3**)
45 *Pongamia pinnata*	Skin diseases (**9**)
46 *Psoralea corylifolia*	Leukoderma (**9**)
47 *Pterocarpus marsupium*	Antidiabetic agent (**11**)
48 *Ricinus communis*	Laxative (**3**)
49 *Rubia cordifolia*	Diabetic foot (11), Painful ophthalmic conditions (**14**)
50 *Salacia spp.*	Antidiabetic agent (**11**)

Plant Name	Indication (Chapter Number)
51 *Saraca asoca*	Metromenorrhagia (10)
52 *Semecarpus anacardium*	Rheumatoid arthritis (**8**)
53 *Sida cordifolia*	Diabetic neuropathy (11)
54 *Solanum trilobatum*	Bronchial asthma (5)
55 *Solanum xanthocarpum*	Bronchial asthma (**5**)
56 *Syzygium cuminii*	*Antidiabetic agent (***11***)*
57 *Terminalia arjuna*	Cardioprotective plant (**6**)
58 *Terminalia belerica*	Bronchial asthma (**5**), Diarrhea (3)
59 *Terminalia chebula*	Laxative (3)
60 *Tinospora cordifolia*	Hepatoprotective agent (**4**), Rheumatoid arthritis (8), Immunostimulant effects (13), Cancer therapy (13)
61 *Tribulus terrestris*	Diuretic (**7**)
62 *Trigonella foenum graecum*	Hypolipidemic agent (6), Antidiabetic agent (**11**)
63 *Tylophora indica*	Bronchial asthma (**5**), Allergic rhinitis (5)
64 *Valeriana wallichi*	Sedative plant (12)
65 *Vitex negundo*	*Antirheumatic agent (***8***)*
66 *Withania somnifera*	Rheumatoid arthritis (**8**), Memory enhancement (12), Tonic antiaging agent (13), Cancer therapy (13)
67 *Wrightia tinctoria*	Psoriasis (**9**), Nonspecific dermatitis (9)
68 *Zingiber officinale*	Malabsorption syndrome (**3**) Antiemetic agent (3), Rheumatoid arthritis (8)

Index

Abdominal sepsis, 21
Abortifacient effect, vasicine, 87
Abutilon indicum, 111, 115
Acacia, in dental care, 330
Acemannan, 212, 213
Acetyl-β-boswellic acid, 34, 318
Acetyl-11-keto-β-boswellic acid, 34, 318
Acid dyspepsia, *Asparagus racemosus,* 22
Aconitum, 4
Acoustic startle response, 285
Acute phase reactants, 180
Acute viral hepatitis, 78
Adaptogenic activity, 305, 308
Adhatoda vasica, 85
   clinical trial, 29, 87, 332-333
   collection, season for, 3
   constituents, 87
   description, 86
   other names, 86, 332
   pharmacology, 87
   safety, 87-88
   traditional use, 86-87
Adhatoda zeylanica. See Adhatoda vasica
Adhatodai. *See Adhatoda vasica*
Adrak. *See Zingiber officinale*
Adraka. *See Zingiber officinale*
Aegle marmelos, 54-55
Aging and free radical damage, 306, 307
Alantolactone, 126
Albizzia lebbeck, 88-90, 336-337
   allergic conjunctivitis, 336-337
   bronchial asthma, 89-90
   constituents, 88
   description, 88
   flowers in TPE, 90, 116
   other names, 88, 336
   pharmacology, 88-89
   safety, 90
   use, 88

Albizziasaponins, 88
Aldose reductase activity, 250, 251
Alkaloids,
   in *Aconitum,* 4
   in *Adhatoda vasica,* 3, 87
   in *Aegle marmelos,* 54
   in *Bacopa monnieri,* 281
   in *Berberis vulgaris,* 82
   in *Boerhaavia diffusa,* 152
   in *Celastrus paniculatus,* 286
   in *Coccinia indica,* 234
   in *Convolvulus pluricaulis,* 288
   in *Crataeva nurvala,* 157
   in *Emblica officinalis,* 22
   in *Holarrhena antidysentrica,* 56
   in *Mucuna pruriens,* 299
   in *Phyllanthus amarus,* 77
   in *Piper longum,* 4, 95
   in *Piper nigrum,* 4
   in *Solanum xanthocarpum,* 9, 98, 100
   in *Tinospora cordifolia,* 69
   in *Tribulus terrestris,* 154, 155
   in *Trigonella foenum graecum,* 256
   in *Tylophora indica,* 101, 102
   in *Vitex negundo,* 176
   in *Withania somnifera,* 179
Allergic reaction, *Plantago ovata,* 47
Allergic rhinitis, *Tylophora indica,* 102, 104
Aloe barbadensis, 211-214
   constituents, 212
   description, 211-212
   other names, 211
   pharmacology, 212-213
   psoriasis, 208
   safety, 214
   use, 212
   wound healing, 213-214
Aloe gel, factors in use, 213-214
Aloeride, 212, 213

doi:10.1300/5683_16